Health Divided

Health Divided

Public Health and Individual Medicine in the

Making of the Modern American State

DANIEL SLEDGE

UNIVERSITY PRESS OF KANSAS

Published by the

University Press of

Kansas (Lawrence,

Kansas 66045), which

was organized by the

Kansas Board of Regents

and is operated and

funded by Emporia State

University, Fort Hays

State University, Kansas

State University, Pittsburg

State University, the

University of Kansas, and

Wichita State University

Library of Congress Cataloging-in-Publication Data

Names: Sledge, Daniel, author.
Title: Health divided : public health and individual medicine in the making of the modern American state / Daniel Sledge.
Description: Lawrence, Kansas : University Press of Kansas, [2017] | Includes bibliographical references and index.
Identifiers: LCCN 2017007057
ISBN 9780700624300 (cloth)
ISBN 9780700624317 (paperback)
ISBN 9780700624324 (ebook)
Subjects: LCSH: Health care—United States—19th century. | Medical policy—United States—19th century. | Medical care—United States. | BISAC: POLITICAL SCIENCE / Public Policy / Social Policy. | HISTORY / United States / State & Local / South (AL, AR, FL, GA, KY, LA, MS, NC, SC, TN, VA, WV).
Classification: LCC RA395.A3 S567 2017
DDC 362.10973—dc23
LC record available at https://lccn.loc.gov/2017 007057.

British Library Cataloguing-in-Publication Data is available.

Printed in the United States of America
10 9 8 7 6 5 4 3 2 1

The paper used in this publication is recycled and contains 30 percent postconsumer waste. It is acid free and meets the minimum requirements of the American National Standard for Permanence of
Paper for Printed Library Materials Z39.48–1992.

To my family

CONTENTS

ACKNOWLEDGMENTS

Writing a book like this is impossible without the support of loved ones, friends, and family. I am profoundly grateful to those who have been supportive during the long years that it took to write this book. Carolyn Sledge, George Sledge, Matthew Sledge, and David Sledge have been loving, kind, and giving. I am confident I would be nowhere without them. I thank my friends in Texas and at Cornell, as well as Jenna Green, Russell Hanson, Richard Bensel, Elizabeth Sanders, and Theodore J. Lowi. Librarians from New York to California and from Texas to Wisconsin have been critical to the completion of this volume. I also thank the anonymous reviewers who have shaped this work. I owe them a great debt of gratitude.

LIST OF ABBREVIATIONS

AALL	American Association for Labor Legislation
ACA	2010 Patient Protection and Affordable Care Act
AFL	American Federation of Labor
AMA	American Medical Association
APD	American political development
APHA	American Public Health Association
CCMC	Committee on the Costs of Medical Care
CDC	US Centers for Disease Control and Prevention; Communicable Disease Center
CES	Committee on Economic Security
CHIP	Comprehensive Health Insurance Plan
CWA	Civil Works Administration
EIS	Epidemiological Intelligence Service
FERA	Federal Emergency Relief Administration
FSA	Farm Security Administration
GEB	General Education Board
HEW	Department of Health, Education, and Welfare
HMO	health maintenance organization
IHB	Rockefeller International Health Board
MCWA	Malaria Control in War Areas
MHS	Marine Hospital Service
MMA	Medicare Modernization Act
NIH	National Institutes of Health
NRA	National Recovery Administration
PHS	Public Health Service
RSC	Rockefeller Sanitary Commission
USDA	US Department of Agriculture
WHO	World Health Organization

Health Divided

INTRODUCTION

In fall 1897, yellow fever swept through the towns and cities of the southern United States. The disease's symptoms were terrifying. Though many victims experienced only fever, headaches, nausea, vomiting, and muscle aches, others found that their eyes and skin assumed a yellow hue. Abdominal pain was paired with bloody black vomit—*vomito negro*—and additional blood escaped through their eyes, nose, and mouth.

The disease struck first in Ocean Springs, Mississippi. This Gulf Coast town was home to a cadre of Cuban refugees engaged in transporting weapons to support the ongoing rebellion against Spanish rule on the island, where yellow fever was endemic.[1] It soon spread to New Orleans, where officials proved reluctant to admit its presence. When the announcement was finally made, communities throughout the region began to panic. "Within six hours after the official declaration that fever existed here," a report from the Crescent City asserted, "every town in Louisiana, Texas, Mississippi, and Alabama was quarantined against New Orleans. Guards were placed on every road, armed with Winchesters and shotguns, and instructed to shoot down all who failed to halt properly."[2]

Throughout the region, hastily convened boards of health used the threat of violence to force trains transporting people or goods to continue on without stopping. In Jackson, Mississippi, a crowd destroyed tracks used by the Alabama and Vicksburg Railroad after a train "went through at a speed not greater than four miles an hour" rather than the twenty miles per hour mandated by local officials. "Not only was this order disregarded, but the train stopped in the heart of the city. Indignation is at a fever heat, and the people say if necessary to compel observance of their reasonable quarantine regulations, they will burn every bridge between here and Vicksburg."[3] In New Orleans, the local board of health fashioned a temporary hospital within a school. Incensed, "a riotous crowd made an attempt to burn the building. Two of the annexes were reduced to ashes, but joint efforts of the police and fire departments prevented the destruction of the main building."[4] Outside of the city, a black man was lynched for allegedly evading quarantine.[5]

Overall, the response to the epidemic was chaotic. States and localities worked against one another. Although the disease was introduced from abroad and was clearly spreading from state to state, the federal government proved incapable of asserting any meaningful role in attempting to stop its progress or coordinate the responses of the afflicted states and localities. Indeed, it was widely understood that the Cuban refugees who introduced the disease had evaded the United States Marine Hospital Service's (MHS) quarantine station at Ship Island, Mississippi.

The disorder of 1897 was extreme, but it was far from unprecedented. In 1878, another yellow fever outbreak had ravaged the lower Mississippi Valley, killing around 20,000. In both cases, the experience of epidemic disease threw local governing institutions into an unhelpful panic. Straining local resources and illuminating a dangerous lack of coordination and communication, epidemic disease also raised major questions about the appropriate role of the federal government in ensuring the health of Americans.

Public Health and Individual Medicine

This book offers a reinterpretation of the making of modern American health policy. The primary question that I ask is why the federal government created a strong national system of public health, grounded in the Atlanta-based Centers for Disease Control and Prevention, while rejecting a comparable or even integrated approach in the field of individual medicine. By "public health," I mean efforts aimed at ensuring or improving the health of populations, such as water purification, vaccination, or mosquito eradication. I use the term "individual medicine" to refer to services aimed at the health of individuals.

From the early years of the American republic, the regulation and promotion of health has been understood as a police power, left to the states under the Tenth Amendment to the Constitution, which states that all powers not given to the national government are reserved to the states or to the people. Over the course of the nineteenth century, state and local governments in the United States became engaged in increasingly sophisticated efforts to promote health.[6] Aimed largely at acute contagious illnesses such as yellow fever, typhoid, and cholera, these efforts were spurred on first by the example of the British sanitarian movement and then by the bacteriological revolution and gradual acceptance of the germ theory of disease.

The federal government's role in American health remained both modest and peripheral. Its primary health arm was the Marine Hospital Service, created by an act of Congress in 1798 and headquartered in the Treasury Department. The MHS's central task was operating a system of hospitals and "relief stations" for sailors, paid for through dedicated taxes and general revenue. During the final decade of the nineteenth century, the service secured control over most, though not all, of the nation's quarantine activities. It also operated a small Hygienic Laboratory, offered assistance to the Revenue Cutter Service (a forerunner of the Coast Guard) and on occasion to other federal agencies, and inspected immigrants at ports of entry.[7]

In the decades after the 1897 outbreak, the federal government asserted a central role in stimulating local-level public health activities and in coordinating public health efforts across political jurisdictions. The United States Public Health Service (PHS), the institutional successor to the MHS, gave birth to both the Centers for Disease Control and Prevention and the National Institutes of Health (NIH). Created by an agency originally tasked with operating a system of compulsory health insurance for sailors, these institutions made the United States a world leader in public health work and in biomedical research. The PHS also helped transform America's health care infrastructure, overseeing and funding hospital construction on a large scale through the post–World War II Hill–Burton program.

While the federal government established an overt and central position in American public health, the provision of individual medical services fell under the auspices of a complex and disjointed system. Federal influence is pervasive but often hidden from view.[8] The vast majority of individual medical services are funded through a patchwork of insurance programs, including tax-preferred employer-sponsored health insurance, Medicare, Medicaid, the Children's Health Insurance Program, and the federally regulated but state-based health exchanges created by the Patient Protection and Affordable Care Act of 2010 (ACA, also known as Obamacare). Whereas federal intervention in public health enjoys a broad, if often shallow, popular legitimacy, whether the national government should take action to ensure access to individual health services remains highly contested.[9]

A great deal of effort has been put into excavating the roots of contemporary American health policy. The scholarly literature on the development of national policies dealing with individual medicine is formidable.[10] We know far less, however, about the political development of federal policies dealing with public health.[11] With the notable exceptions of Paul Starr and Alan Derickson, scholars interested in individual medicine have paid little attention to public health.[12] No previous work has examined the interconnected political trajectories of federal policies dealing with public health and individual medicine. As we will see, however, they cannot be fully understood in isolation. In the decades after the 1897 yellow fever outbreak and the subsequent Spanish-American War, discussions of public health and individual medicine were intertwined in fundamental ways. During the New Deal era, the United States came close to creating a federal health policy regime encompassing both public health and individual medicine. Instead, a bifurcated health policy regime emerged out of the 1930s and 1940s. This regime was locked in during the decades that followed; it continues to underpin modern American health policy. Understanding the chain of events and decisions that led to the near convergence of public health and individual medicine, along with the subsequent divergence of these policy realms, is crucial to understanding the foundations of modern American health policy.

Shaping American Health Policy

In the pages that follow, I trace the foundations and development of national policies dealing with public health and individual medicine. Beginning with America's interventions in public health in the Caribbean after the Spanish-American War, I follow these policy realms through the emergence of the Communicable Disease Center (later renamed the Centers for Disease Control and Prevention), employer-sponsored health insurance, Medicare, and Medicaid.

My analysis of the making of modern American health policy is grounded in the impressive existing literature on health policy, in archival and primary research, and in the political science subfield of American political development (APD). As an approach to understanding politics and policy, APD pays particular attention to political institutions and to the temporal contexts in which they are embedded. Where other branches of political science tend to focus on stability, predictability, and the role of institutions in fostering equilibrium situations, APD focuses on questions of political change and instability over long periods of time.[13] In the influential formulation of Karen Orren and Stephen Skowronek, it is concerned with explaining durable shifts in governing authority.[14] By placing events and outcomes within a broad temporal and political context, APD is well suited to reexamining established narratives and periodization schemes.

To a great extent, this book is about the long-term impact of efforts undertaken and decisions made by small groups of people, typically government officials, operating within particular political contexts.[15] Drawing attention to the PHS and the political networks in which its leaders were embedded, I highlight the actions and relationships of federal bureaucrats, key members of Congress, presidents, and state and local officials. My analysis centers around three primary factors: (1) the strong support of Southern political leaders for federal intervention in local public health work, emerging beginning during World War I and grounded in regional concerns about the economic impact of debilitating diseases such as malaria; (2) internal divisions among policy makers during the pivotal New Deal era, particularly over the most effective and politically workable means of expanding access to individual medical services; and (3) the actions of interest groups, most notably the American Medical Association (AMA), which was both an opponent of government-backed health insurance and a supporter of public health efforts.

Sectionalism, as scholars such as Richard Bensel and Elizabeth Sanders have shown, has shaped American political development in fundamental ways.[16] During the formative stages of American social policy, Southern political representatives often played an important role in blocking the emergence of more comprehensive social welfare policies. Concerned with retaining local autonomy and preserving the region's racial caste system, Southern Democrats also opposed legislation that would benefit organized labor.[17] Where it might impact the autonomy of states and localities, Southern Democratic leaders routinely equated federal action with the Reconstruction period, black rule, and the unsettling of social, economic, and racial relationships. At its extreme, this line of reasoning viewed federal intervention in almost any form as a potential vehicle for the political rebirth and eventual social integration of black Southerners.[18]

Importantly, Southern Democrats were also a core component of the New Deal coalition. Southern Democrats, who were highly influential in Congress as a result of the seniority system and the region's one-party political system, which helped them to control key committees and wield power as a bloc when necessary, were also eager to pursue legislation that might improve conditions in the region and foster economic development. As a result, they proved integral in the development and enactment of much of the legislation that enlarged the power of the national government during the 1930s.[19] Given their antistatist reputation and often stated reservations about the threat that federal authority represented to local autonomy, this was a paradoxical role.[20]

During the foundational period of national health policy, Southern Democrats were the most powerful and influential supporters of greater federal intervention in public health. Beginning in the 1910s, officers from the PHS argued that confronting the diseases that plagued the South would be a necessary step toward future economic growth. During the first decades of the twentieth century, the South was plagued by debilitating diseases such as malaria, hookworm (an intestinal parasite that causes iron-deficiency anemia), and pellagra (a disturbing dietary deficiency disease). Together, these diseases hindered the development of human capital, curtailed agricultural and industrial productivity, and deterred outside investment and migration.

In the aftermath of the Spanish-American War, American efforts to fight yellow fever, malaria, and hookworm in the Caribbean drew attention to broadly comparable health conditions in the nearby Southern United States. Sustained American action in the Caribbean also drew attention to the inability of Southern state and local governments to effectively confront debilitating diseases at home. In a stark demonstration of federal inaction and the lack of public health capacity at the state and local levels, John D. Rockefeller funded the Rockefeller Sanitary Commission for the Eradication of Hookworm. A philanthropic venture intended to fight hookworm disease, the Sanitary Commission operated in the South from 1910 through the end of 1914. It was succeeded by the Rockefeller International Health Board (IHB), which continued to fund health work in the South into the 1930s.[21] The creation of the Sanitary Commission helped to fuel a brief push for a national department of health, which culminated in an expansion of the PHS's research mandate.[22]

The emergency of mobilization for World War I led to an unprecedented federal government intervention in local-level public health work. Beginning in 1917, the PHS undertook a massive effort to control the spread of diseases such as malaria in areas surrounding military installations, largely in the South. Working closely with state and local officials, the PHS used techniques first developed to fight disease in the Caribbean. After the war, PHS officers worked to extend the effort. Operating on a significantly smaller scale and with a greatly reduced budget, the PHS's Leslie Lumsden built a modest but highly consequential program intended to stimulate the development of local public health infrastructure. Known as the rural sanitation program, Lumsden's initiative set the PHS down the path that ultimately culminated in the creation of the Centers for Disease Control and Prevention. An at times controversial figure, Lumsden led a small group of men that included several future PHS leaders.

Focused largely on the health problems of the South, the rural sanitation program worked to gain the support of local leaders and communities. Typically justified in terms of the economic interest of Southern elites, public health interventions were nonetheless aimed largely at improving the health status of low-income Southerners, both black and white. As one might expect, discussions about disease in the South were often infused with ideas about race. Public health officials characteristically viewed race as a biological and social fact with significant implications for successfully understanding and confronting disease.

Arguments about race and public health fell into two broad categories. The first, which emphasized the impact of black health on the health of whites, portrayed blacks as a "reservoir of disease." Because black Southerners often lived in close proximity to whites or worked in white homes, public health workers argued, they represented a direct threat to white health. Less impacted by "tropical" diseases such as malaria and hookworm, blacks could continue to function under their strain, heightening the chance that they would pass the diseases along to whites. Fighting disease in the black population, by this logic, was necessary for the physical protection of whites.[23]

The second broad category of racial arguments about public health emphasized economics. If black Southerners were subject to debilitating diseases such as malaria, hookworm, and pellagra, they would be incapable of being fully productive workers. Given the importance of black workers in the Southern economy, this argument often proved persuasive. Arguments such as this overlapped with arguments about class and the threat of blacks to white health. In the case of hookworm, for instance, poor white tenant farmers were portrayed as the economic victims of a disease imported by West African slaves and carried continuously in the intestines of blacks. Redeeming poor whites and furthering regional economic development, by this logic, was dependent on improving the health status of blacks.

Officers from the PHS's rural sanitation program, often cooperating with private philanthropies such as the Rockefeller International Health Board and the Red Cross, gradually cultivated strong relationships with state and local officials. Although the PHS worked to expand its effort to help stimulate the development of local public health infrastructure beyond the South, the region's ongoing unique health problems and major natural disasters (the 1927 flood of the lower Mississippi Valley and the 1930–1931 drought) reinforced the program's Southern orientation.

During the 1930s and 1940s, the PHS's reputation for competence and the close relationships its officers had cultivated with Southern politicians became the key to the PHS's political power and ability to impact national health policy. Beginning with the New Deal and on an even larger scale after mobilization for World War II, the PHS constructed a permanent framework for federal intervention in local-level public health work, based on the foundation of the rural sanitation program. The location of the Centers for Disease Control and Prevention in Atlanta, near the heart of the nation's former malaria belt, is a physical testament to the Southern origins of national-level public health policy.

Policy Disputes, Strategy, and Interest Groups

The processes underpinning the making of modern American health policy were, in the language of political science, path dependent. In path-dependent processes, early decisions or occurrences set in motion lines of political development that become increasingly difficult to turn back over time. Beginning with an initial state of affairs in which a variety of outcomes are possible, movement down a particular path reshapes future alternatives. As institutions or policies become entrenched, changing course becomes increasingly challenging. Options that were once plausible become both more difficult to implement and less politically acceptable.[24]

Early interventions in public health laid the ground for a strong and politically legitimate federal role. At key moments, proponents of expanded federal intervention were able to point to existing institutions and to rely on the support of politically powerful Southern Democrats. Federal officials were unable, however, to establish a comparable role in the realm of individual medicine. For some, this meant a contributory health insurance program, on the model of Social Security's old-age pensions. For others, this meant a system of direct funding for the care of the indigent and for expensive health services and diagnostic procedures, explicitly connected to and integrated with public health work. Far from preordained, this outcome was shaped in crucial ways by disputes among policy makers over what form federal action should take and by interest group alignments. These disputes, and the alignment of interest groups during the 1930s and 1940s, were shaped by events that stretched back to the Progressive Era.

During the 1910s, the American Association for Labor Legislation (AALL), a progressive group that had effectively pushed for workers' compensation laws in a number of states, embarked on a campaign for state-level compulsory health insurance. Confident that health insurance was a natural next step in American social policy, the AALL nonetheless faced major obstacles. These obstacles included opposition from the life insurance industry, the opposition of business interests, and the ambivalent positioning of organized labor, which was divided over whether to pursue health benefits through state action or through collective bargaining. Although the AMA was initially supportive of insurance proposals, rank-and-file opposition and fears that insurance might affect physician autonomy ultimately led the AMA's leadership to come out against government-backed health insurance. These factors, along with the success of attempts to tie the idea of insurance to fears about German authoritarianism and Soviet Bolshevism during and after World War I, ensured that no state adopted compulsory health insurance during the 1910s.

The long-term impact of the Progressive-Era debate over insurance was substantial. To begin with, it led to the mobilization of organized medicine against government-backed insurance and to the emergence of effective and ideologically based arguments against insurance. Although the PHS's work on the topic has attracted little scholarly attention, Progressive-Era debates over insurance prompted the service to begin investigating the relationship between public health and individual medicine. Insurance, PHS officials argued in a major report issued in 1916, should be linked to state and local public health efforts, which should also be expanded. Insurance should be used to reorganize and modernize the practice of medicine as well as to shift physicians away from traditional fee-for-service medicine, which created perverse incentives for physicians.

With the costs of individual medical services being borne by workers, business, and government via compulsory insurance, the true cost of poor health would become evident. The result would be an increased emphasis on preventive medicine and public health work. While the AALL engaged in a state-level campaign for insurance, the PHS report maintained that a federal system was constitutional. The long-standing existence of the marine hospital system, according to the report, offered a clear precedent for federal government taxation of industry for the purpose of facilitating access to individual medical services.

In the wake of the PHS's World War I intervention in local-level health work, these arguments helped to fuel an expansive vision of what role the federal government might play in ensuring the health of Americans. In proposals for a postwar health system, PHS officials argued in favor of an intergovernmental system that would seek to collapse distinctions between public health and individual medicine. While these plans did not become law, the vision of health policy that they articulated had a long and complex life within the PHS.

Two distinct but closely related conceptions of the role that the federal government should play in the provision of individual medical services grew out of the Progressive Era. Connected in their origins and far from inherently at odds, they came into conflict during the 1930s and 1940s. The first emphasized the importance of creating stable access to services through compulsory insurance for workers and viewed federally backed insurance as a path toward reorganizing the delivery of medical services in a more efficient manner. This contributory social insurance model, which became associated with policy makers from the Social Security Board, would remain the ideal for liberal policy makers for decades to come.

The second major conception of the nation's health priorities and of the role that the federal government might play emphasized the importance of integrating individual medicine with public health work. Highlighting the political challenges confronting insurance, the proponents of this approach urged a conciliatory approach to the AMA. The most ardent advocate of this approach was Thomas Parran Jr., a veteran of the PHS's World War I intervention in local public health work and of the rural sanitation initiative that followed. From 1936 to 1948, Parran served as surgeon general of the PHS. Although Parran and the PHS were often at the center of health policy making during this period, the vision of national health policy that they articulated during the New Deal era and the 1940s has received little sustained scholarly attention.[25]

Beginning during the development of what became the Social Security Act, Parran laid out an alternative approach to expanding access to individual medical services and integrating them with public health efforts. In doing so, he built on the work of men such as public health theorist C.-E. A. Winslow (who had challenged the division of health policy into population-based and individual-based realms) and on the "health center" concept articulated by Hermann Biggs during the early 1920s.[26] Under the Biggs proposal, which was developed in part as an alternative to compulsory health insurance, government-funded centers would house laboratories and expensive diagnostic equipment that could be used by local physicians. In addition, the state government would help to fund consultations with expensive (and in rural areas often scarce) specialists.[27]

Parran also built on ideas that the AMA had endorsed in principle, and sometimes in practice. He pushed for direct federal payments for the care of the indigent, a concept that the AMA viewed as far less threatening than insurance for workers. During the early New Deal, such payments were made through the Federal Emergency Relief Administration (FERA). Where the AMA had signaled that it would accept catastrophic insurance coverage for the working population, Parran proposed instead federal funding for particularly expensive medical care. Funneled through states and localities, federal money would help Americans pay for chronic illnesses such as cancer and arthritis, for childbirth, for expensive diagnostic procedures, and for the treatment of contagious diseases such as syphilis and tuberculosis.

Proponents of extensive federal funding for individual medical services, Parran and other PHS leaders were also firm believers in decentralization, experimentation, and flexibility. Under the plans proposed by the PHS, federal money would flow through state and local health departments. In addition, Parran's approach emphasized the importance of building a framework capable of integrating public health and individual medicine.

Parran's vision of American health policy, I argue, was both potentially transformative and highly pragmatic. Throughout the 1930s, the AMA signaled its willingness to support options for expanding access to health services as long as government-backed insurance for noncatastrophic care was kept off of the table. Given the financial strain that physicians faced during the Great Depression and the interest of organized medicine in heading off the threat of national health insurance, I argue, compromise with the AMA was possible. During the development of the Social Security Act, and again after the National Health Program unveiled by the PHS, Social Security Board, and Children's Bureau in 1938, Parran's approach might have formed the basis for a new health policy regime that actively sought to integrate public health and individual medicine.

This outcome, however, would have required a consensus among leading health policy makers that was not present. From the perspective of the staunchest proponents of government-backed insurance, Parran's proposals in the realm of individual medical services were half measures. If enacted, they might sap the strength of the political coalition necessary to pass insurance into law. Compromise with the AMA, it seemed clear, was a fool's errand. Presenting itself as the voice of a unified profession, the AMA leadership routinely used caustic and irresponsible rhetoric in denigrating and demonizing the proponents of insurance. Insurance, according to the AMA, would transform the United States into Nazi Germany or the Soviet Union. Organized medicine would do anything to ensure that an insurance plan did not become law, and disingenuous gestures toward compromise were simply part of an attempt to block very necessary changes in the American health care system.

Health Divided

The window of opportunity opened up by Franklin Roosevelt's ascension to the presidency in 1933 proved brief. It began to close with the emergence of the conservative coalition of Southern Democrats and northern Republicans in 1937 and the strong Republican showing in the 1938 midterm elections; it was shut decisively when the United States began mobilizing for World War II. Rooted in earlier developments and strongly accentuated by policy decisions during the New Deal era, the divergent paths of policies dealing with public health and individual medicine were further reinforced by World War II. As it had in 1917, mobilization for war once again rendered the diseases that plagued the Southern United States an issue of national security.

The PHS's successful work during World War II and ongoing support from its key Southern constituency gave it a great deal of clout as the war came to end. In 1946, the PHS renamed its Atlanta-based Malaria Control in War Areas program the Communicable Disease Center. Under legislation passed in 1944, the service's National Institute of Health also gained greater power and authority. In 1946, the PHS was given control over the Hill–Burton hospital program, through which it helped to fund the construction of the nation's postwar hospital infrastructure.

At the same time, wartime wage controls and federal tax policy helped to foster a system in which increasing numbers of Americans accessed health insurance through their employers.[28] Even as President Harry Truman came out in favor of national health insurance after the war, major regional divisions within the Democratic Party over race and the ongoing opposition of the AMA worked to make government-backed insurance increasingly unlikely. After Republicans gained control of Congress in the 1946 midterm elections, organized labor turned decisively toward collective bargaining agreements as a means of securing access to individual medical services through tax-preferred employer-sponsored health insurance plans.[29] Ultimately, the proponents of insurance turned toward the incremental approach that led to the enactment of Medicare and Medicaid in 1965.

From the perspective of the twenty-first century, the series of attempts to pass government-backed health insurance plans that began during the Progressive Era and culminated in the 1940s may too easily be seen as leading almost inexorably toward these outcomes. The integrated approach to American health policy articulated by Thomas Parran and other PHS leaders during the New Deal era and into the 1940s, meanwhile, has been largely forgotten. In the pages that follow, I hope to refocus our attention on these alternatives, which, while perhaps difficult to imagine given the path that American health policy took instead, once appeared both viable and highly plausible.

CHAPTER ONE

HEALTH AT HOME, HEALTH ABROAD

The early contours of federal health policy were shaped by two factors: federalism and international relations. For constitutional reasons and for purely practical reasons, the lion's share of health-related government action in early America was highly local. Writing in 1824, Supreme Court chief justice John Marshall declared "health laws of every description" to be among the wide array of powers "not surrendered to the general government" by the states.[1] Federal action was sparked, however, by trade and by war.[2] As early as 1798, Congress created the Marine Hospital Service, an organization charged with operating a system of compulsory hospital insurance for sailors. During the second part of the nineteenth century, the service's mandate grew to include quarantine efforts, the inspection of immigrants, and basic scientific research.

Expanding into the Caribbean after the Spanish-American War, American authorities encountered serious and debilitating diseases, including yellow fever, malaria, and hookworm. For the first time, national authorities became involved in public health operations on a large scale. American public health work abroad drew attention to conditions in the American South, where many of the same diseases were present, and also to the inability of Southern state and local governments to confront these diseases. With the promotion and regulation of health broadly understood to be an area of state authority under the Constitution, it was private philanthropy that took the first major step against these diseases at home. In 1909, John D. Rockefeller announced the creation of the Rockefeller Sanitary Commission for the Eradication of Hookworm, an endeavor that sought to rid the South of hookworm.[3]

These developments, which I explore in this chapter, would have important implications for health policy in the United States, leading to a debate over the appropriate role of the federal government in public health and ultimately paving the path toward expanded federal intervention.

States, the Federal Government, and Health

Following the Elizabethan poor law tradition, local governments in America were obliged to help the indigent sick access health services beginning during the colonial period. Localities typically hired a physician to treat the poor, usually on a part-time basis. States, townships, and counties also had responsibility for the health needs of prisoners and other public charges. Beyond this, some illnesses, such as tuberculosis and venereal disease, were considered issues of special public concern, demanding government action even where the sick individual was not indigent or a public charge. Over the course of the nineteenth century, most states built tuberculosis sanitoriums, as well as facilities to house those with mental illnesses and the blind.

Private philanthropy supplemented and in many cases preceded government action to promote health. In northeastern cities, charities founded "dispensaries," which distributed drugs to the urban poor and treated minor ailments. Dispensaries also administered vaccinations, a crucial public health function.[4] As a general rule, they remained privately funded, although some received state and local funding. Their great strength was the role they played in medical education, offering clinical experience to future physicians and serving as a stepping-stone to higher status within the profession.[5] Often private philanthropies contributed funds to combat specific diseases such as tuberculosis and to improve maternal and infant health. Private philanthropy also played a central part in the development of hospitals, which were typically geared toward care for the indigent sick.

In addition to their role in individual medicine, states and localities were the primary sites of action in public health work. During the second half of the nineteenth century, these efforts were vastly expanded. Inspired by the growing sanitarian movement in Great Britain, attempts to regulate sanitary conditions became commonplace in American cities. In the final decades of the century, the bacteriological revolution further accelerated the development of local health regulation and promotion. The germ theory of disease drew attention to the role of specific pathogens in causing illness, leading officials to further focus attention on the relationship between individual health status and the health of the community.[6]

The extent and quality of health efforts varied significantly across the nation. Health efforts were concentrated in the industrializing North, where municipal governments and states issued regulations intended to further goals such as access to clean water, a hygienic milk supply, improved infant and maternal health, a population vaccinated against smallpox, and adequate reporting of deaths from contagious disease. Health work lagged behind in much of rural America, and particularly in the South.

Although health work was primarily local, the federal government had a role in promoting the health of Americans almost from the beginning. In 1798, Congress created the United States Marine Hospital Service, which was given the task running a system of hospitals and compulsory health insurance for sailors. Connected to the nation's system of customhouses and founded with an eye toward the relationship between trade and disease, the service was a bureau of the Treasury Department. Sailors, a highly mobile group, often crossing international and interstate boundaries, were taxed, and in return they received access to medical care.

Throughout much of its early existence, the MHS was a disjointed and patronage-prone operation. Legislation passed in 1870, however, placed the service on firmer ground. Among other organization matters, the legislation created the coordinating position of supervising surgeon general. During the early 1870s, supervising surgeon general John Maynard Woodworth (a former Union Army medical officer) reorganized the service along military lines, with its physicians holding rank in a uniformed corps. This system was later enshrined in statute, with service officers receiving formal commissions from the president.[7]

These patterns of government activity were broadly accepted. Large-scale epidemics, however, called prevailing approaches into question. In 1878, with the Caribbean's ongoing yellow fever problem apparently growing in magnitude, Congress passed legislation granting the MHS a role in overseeing local quarantine efforts and allowing it to engage in its own. Already on the ground in the port cities where it operated hospitals for sailors, the MHS appeared the best candidate for policing the nation's borders against the threat of yellow fever. Before an appropriation could be made for the MHS's new quarantine powers, however, a major outbreak of yellow fever struck the lower Mississippi Valley, killing as many as 20,000.[8]

With Southern politicians briefly mobilized in support of federal action, the 1878 quarantine legislation was superseded by an even more ambitious project: the formation of a new National Board of Health. Created in 1879, the board was authorized "to advise state and local boards of health, to obtain and publish pertinent health information, to inquire into public health questions, and to plan for a permanent national health organization."[9] Asserting a connection between public health and the regulation of commerce, the board's authorization might under different circumstances have provided a framework for greater federal involvement in public health.

Southern states, however, rapidly became antagonistic toward the agency's perceived intrusions on their quarantine prerogatives. When no major yellow fever epidemic occurred between 1879 and 1883, Congress declined to continue funding the board.[10]

The passing of this experiment allowed the MHS to reclaim the limited quarantine role it had been granted in 1878.[11] Now the service began cooperating with American representatives abroad, collecting information on the threat of disease aboard ships calling at foreign ports, including Havana, Vera Cruz, London, and Liverpool. Later in the decade, it created its own series of quarantine stations to supplement the existing state-based system.[12] During the 1890s, the MHS's role was further expanded, both in response to increasing immigration and in response to growing knowledge of bacteriology and acceptance of the germ theory of disease. In 1890, its officers were given control over the medical inspection of immigrants at the port of New York; the next year, the MHS gained formal control over the medical inspection of all immigrants. Also in 1890, Congress passed legislation giving the president authority to direct the surgeon general to issue regulations intended to stop the interstate spread of four diseases: cholera, yellow fever, smallpox, and plague.[13]

This limited assertion of authority over the interstate spread of disease was complemented and expanded in 1893 by new legislation intended to pave the way for a fully national system of quarantine. The surgeon general was directed "to examine the quarantine regulations of all state and municipal boards of health, and to cooperate with and aid the local boards in the enforcement of the regulations." Where regulations did not exist or were deemed insufficient, the secretary of the treasury was "authorized to make additional regulations, which must operate uniformly." The legislation also granted the MHS authority to combat the interstate spread of all contagious diseases through the use of the quarantine.[14] In 1899, the MHS opened a tuberculosis sanatorium in Fort Stanton, New Mexico, and began investigating the need for a federal facility for caring for lepers—clear signs of its growing interest in the domestic transmission of disease.[15]

Significantly, the new legislation did not bar states from operating their own quarantine stations, providing that they could instead transfer them to the MHS as they saw fit. As a result, state and local authorities continued to control the quarantine at important ports into the twentieth century. Louisiana did not transfer its facilities, including the station in New Orleans, to the service until 1907. Boston, meanwhile, transferred its station in 1915. New York became the last state to fully cede its quarantine stations in 1921.[16]

Yellow Fever

Dramatic events often contain the seeds of potential change. They focus the attention of the media, the public, and politicians, placing interested leaders in a position to define or redefine both the nature of a problem and its appropriate remedy. Disruptive and unpredictable occurrences, it is often argued, are the central driving force behind significant policy change in the United States.[17] The yellow fever outbreak of 1897 was, at least potentially, one such event. Introduced from Cuba into Mississippi, the disease swiftly spread throughout the South. With state and local governments throughout the region at odds, the federal government largely looked on from the sidelines. The MHS's poor response during the episode was particularly glaring, as was the likelihood that the disease had been introduced by individuals who slipped past the MHS-operated quarantine at Ship Island, Mississippi.

As the epidemic subsided with the onset of colder weather, Congress began considering proposals aimed at expanding the role of the federal government in public health and addressing the failures of coordination made clear over the course of the outbreak.[18] These plans were quickly forgotten, however, after April 25, 1898, when the United States declared war against the Spanish empire. The energy that briefly sparked a debate over how the United States might better coordinate public health activities was now redirected toward Havana, Cuba, the point of origin for the 1897 outbreak.

Though the Spanish-American War was over in a matter of months, its consequences were, in the early assessment of Massachusetts senator Henry Cabot Lodge, "many, startling, and of world-wide meaning."[19] The fruits of American victory were formalized in December, when the two nations signed a treaty granting the United States possession of the Philippines, Puerto Rico, and Guam. The US Army also began an occupation of Cuba, home to both yellow fever and the insurgency against Spanish rule whose brutal suppression had played a prominent part in the American decision to go to war. For the Americans, ridding Havana of yellow fever was a central goal of the occupation.

Understandings of the disease had changed significantly during the nineteenth century. It was long thought that miasma, a noxious vapor believed to emanate from decaying organic matter, caused the disease. There were always critics of this theory, however, who pointed to yellow fever's apparently contagious nature and its connection to trade. The miasma approach faced a potent challenge with the advancement of bacteriology and was dealt a strong blow among American physicians and public health workers by the 1878 epidemic. In the wake of that outbreak, a new germ theory of the disease emerged: it was spread by "fomites—objects that had been infected with the vomit or excrement of earlier victims."[20]

Taking charge of Cuba, the US Army operated on the assumption that yellow fever could be controlled through intense cleaning and fumigation. Whether it emanated from decaying matter or was transferred by fomites, the key to ridding Havana of yellow fever, it appeared, was to thoroughly clean the city. Where the Spanish had allowed it to become filthy and disease ridden, American authorities would ensure that it was cleaned up and remained so. Despite the imposition of stringent sanitary measures, however, the American occupation's efforts proved a failure, and the disease continued to thrive. Their assumptions shaken, the Americans created a Yellow Fever Commission, headed by US Army medical officer Walter Reed and charged with rethinking the causes of the disease.

Reed and his men were influenced in part by Cuban physician Carlos Finlay, who had collaborated with a group sent to Cuba by the short-lived National Board of Health in 1879.[21] Since then, Finlay had argued that mosquitoes spread yellow fever. They were also inspired by the work of the MHS's Henry Rose Carter, whose research suggested that the disease required a period of incubation in an intermediary host such as the mosquito. Setting aside the idea that yellow fever could be eliminated through an attack on Havana's filth, the Yellow Fever Commission soon determined that Havana's large mosquito population was spreading the disease.

This was an important development, and one that would prove the beginning of a major American effort to combat mosquito-borne illness in the Caribbean. Under the command of the US Army Medical Corps's William Gorgas, American authorities developed techniques for destroying the breeding sites of Havana's mosquitoes and limiting the transmission of yellow fever. A system was devised for inspecting homes within the city to ensure that standing water was not left in artificial containers.[22] At Gorgas's insistence, physicians were required to report cases of yellow fever to the American authorities.[23] Successful and increasingly confident, the Americans broadened their efforts, developing methods for interrupting the breeding of the *Anopheles* mosquitoes that spread malaria on the island. As in the case of yellow fever, they were breaking new ground. Working in India, British physician Ronald Ross had only recently demonstrated the role of mosquitoes in the disease's transmission. Before the Cuba campaign, no antimalaria work had been undertaken based on this knowledge.[24]

Though neither disease was fully banished from Cuba, the efforts of

Gorgas and his men were impressive: both yellow fever and malaria now represented far less significant health threats than they had before. In the United States, yellow fever soon became a minor threat, both because of the work in Cuba and because of increased action against mosquito breeding in Southern cities. A final outbreak occurred in New Orleans in 1905, but the occupation of Cuba and its aftermath marked the end of yellow fever as a recurrent terror for Americans. In 1904, the United States began work on the Panama Canal, an enterprise that—as the failed earlier French attempt to build a canal across the Panamanian isthmus demonstrated—would have been impossible without the knowledge of how to control mosquito-borne illnesses developed in Cuba. The army's William Gorgas again supervised the work.

The canal opened in 1914, evidence of what could be accomplished through the marriage of epidemiology, rigid public health regulation, and engineering. A source of pride for many Americans, Gorgas's successes abroad also laid bare the inadequacies of public health work at home. Yellow fever was a serious but essentially episodic threat: at times introduced from abroad (typically from Cuba), it pulsed through the cities and towns of the South before disappearing with the onset of cold weather. Malaria, however, was a disease of massive domestic importance and impact.

As the twentieth century dawned, the malaria-causing parasites *Plasmodium vivax* and *Plasmodium falciparum* were both endemic throughout large swaths of the Southern United States. The disease's impact on Southern life had been widely known since the colonial period, when it served to deter migration into the region. As in the Caribbean, malaria was used to justify the importation of West African slaves, who were recognized as being less affected by the disease than Americans of European descent. Often present at the frontiers of white settlement throughout the United States, malaria had—outside of lingering pockets in California, some marshy regions of New Jersey, and heavily irrigated portions of New Mexico—receded from most of the North and West by the beginning of the twentieth century (Figure 1.1).

The men engaged in the enormous antimalaria effort taking place in Panama, as well as those who witnessed its fruits, were well aware of its potential applications at home.[25] It was in the states where the disease thrived, however, that local public health infrastructure was the least effective. Indeed, no former Confederate state had the ability to adequately collect vital statistics during the first decade of the twentieth century. As a result, it was impossible to document the full extent of malaria's devastating impact

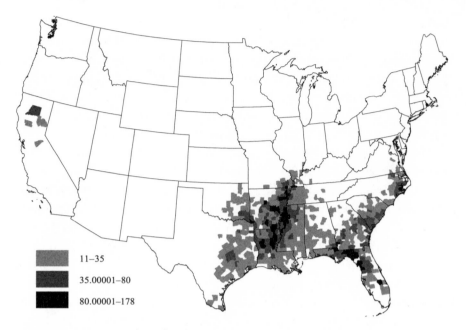

Figure I.I. Average number of malaria deaths per 100,000 people, 1919–1921. *Source:*
Maxcy, "Distribution of Malaria in the United States." Maxcy's data exclude counties
with a mortality rate of less than 10 per 100,000.

on the region's economy and people, or to plan effective efforts against it.
From the perspective of the federal government, meanwhile, the South's
malaria problem was an issue of local, rather than national, concern. While
American officials confronted malaria on a large scale in Cuba and in the
Panama Canal Zone, no serious steps toward applying the techniques developed
in the Caribbean were taken within the United States itself.[26]

Hookworm in Puerto Rico

The American fight against mosquito-borne illness in the Caribbean
highlighted the failures of public health efforts at home. American expansion
into the region also drew attention to the domestic impact of another
debilitating disease: hookworm. The intestinal parasite, which causes
iron-deficiency anemia, had been widespread in the South for centuries.
Its presence, however, was only recognized in the aftermath of the Spanish-American War.

While American officials in Cuba worked to understand yellow fever,
an army medical officer in Puerto Rico identified hookworm among the

newly acquired territory's rural *jibaros*. Dr. Bailey K. Ashford was stationed in Ponce (on Puerto Rico's southern shore) when a major hurricane hit on August 8, 1899, destroying the coffee crop as well as most of the banana and plantain crops. As part of the army's response to mounting disease and starvation, Ashford was ordered to "establish a field provisional hospital for the purpose of accommodating at least some of the thousands of sick jibaros who were thronging the streets of the city."[27]

Many of those who entered into his care were, he found, severely anemic, even to the point of death. Attempting to "feed up" the *jibaros*, Ashford found that they disliked the American-style food they were issued, which apparently gave them diarrhea. "With a Spanish cook," he reported, "the food was made more palatable and the diarrhea subsided, as did the complaints of the barbarous food of the 'Americanos,' but not one whit more color came into their faces, and the daily death toll was about the same as it had been at first."[28]

After "two months' examination of many patients and much speculation, it became evident that these chronic sick, the anemics of many years, not of a few months, were all suffering from a common malady." After excluding malaria as a cause through the use of blood tests, Ashford examined the feces of a number of anemic patients. Consulting British physician Patrick Manson's text on tropical diseases, he determined that the fecal samples indicated hookworm infection. "With the recovery of the worms," he later wrote, "the cause of the anemia of Porto Rico was demonstrated."[29]

In 1904, at Ashford's behest, the Puerto Rican legislative assembly agreed to fund an "anemia commission" comprising Ashford, quarantine officer W. W. King of the recently renamed Public Health and Marine Hospital Service, and Pedro Gutierrez Igaravidez, a health officer from Bayamon, Puerto Rico.[30] From the beginning, the Anemia Commission focused on the operation of dispensaries, temporary clinics where "the physician . . . fixed a definite place and hour when he might see the anemics." If found to be infected, dispensary patients were treated for free. From 1904 to the end of June 1910, the Anemia Commission and related government organizations recorded the treatment of 287,568 hookworm cases in Puerto Rico. During the same years, its leaders estimated that "at least 30,000 more have been treated apart from Government work and of which we have no record." Writing in 1911, Ashford and Gutierrez Igaravidez reported that they felt "entirely safe in saying that over 300,000, or nearly one-third of the population of Porto Rico, have received specific treatment for uncinariasis [hookworm]."[31]

Dirt Eaters

In the United States, Bailey K. Ashford's discovery struck a chord with Dr. Charles Wardell Stiles, a European-trained scientist and expert in medical zoology employed by the US Department of Agriculture (USDA). Since the early 1890s, Stiles had given lectures at Georgetown, the Army Medical School, and Johns Hopkins urging students to consider hookworm infection as a potential cause when they encountered iron-deficiency anemia in tropical or subtropical climates.[32] Ashford had heard Stiles lecture at the Army Medical School and had almost certainly learned of the disease from him. Proud of his discovery, he provided a sample of the Puerto Rican hookworm to Stiles.[33]

Stiles soon became convinced that Ashford's findings in Puerto Rico were only the tip of the iceberg. In 1901, Dr. Allen J. Smith of Galveston, Texas, reported finding hookworm in a patient who had spent time as an overseer on a plantation in Mexico.[34] The same year, Smith found hookworm eggs in the stool of eight students at the University of Texas Medical School in Galveston and sent a specimen to Stiles at the USDA.[35]

Inspired by the findings of Ashford and Smith, Stiles began an exhaustive inquiry into presence of hookworm in the United States. His initial finding, using samples from Puerto Rico and Texas, was that the hookworms in question were a different species from those known to exist in Europe. Though it would later be found that the parasite had originated in Africa, Stiles designated the new species *Necator americanus*.[36]

Despite his growing interest in the question of hookworm in the United States, Stiles was employed as a zoologist with the USDA. Human diseases were outside of his purview. His prominence in the field of medical zoology and his mounting fascination with hookworm, however, serendipitously intersected with organizational changes in the United States MHS. As the service acquired an increased authority in international and interstate quarantine efforts, MHS leaders worked to build up the service's research and laboratory capabilities.

Beginning in 1899–1900, the threat of plague on the West Coast offered the MHS a compelling argument for further expanding and formalizing its research activities.[37] Near the end of 1899, plague appeared in Honolulu, Hawaii. In January 1900, the Honolulu Board of Health began setting sanitary fires in areas where the disease appeared. One fire, set on January 20, burned horribly out of control, displacing as many as 6,000 residents of

Honolulu's Chinatown.[38] In March, the disease appeared in San Francisco, where the MHS's Joseph Kinyoun identified it.

The recognition of plague set in motion a series of events in which the MHS found itself at odds with local officials, many of whom were at pains to deny that plague existed in San Francisco. When the state directed the city to quarantine its Chinatown, a lawsuit brought in federal court found that the quarantine represented "an unwarranted act of racial discrimination."[39] Authorities could not quarantine individuals simply because they were born in China or were of Chinese descent. In an attempt to smooth things over with local authorities, Surgeon General Walter Wyman reassigned Kinyoun, who soon resigned from the service in protest. Rupert Blue, a South Carolinian who would later become surgeon general, took over the service's antiplague efforts in the critical Bay area. Blue proved successful at courting local support, building an effort that, among other features, included a program that employed local hunters to reduce the Bay area's plague-carrying ground squirrel population.[40]

The appearance of plague on the West Coast, and its connection to trade with the East and emigration from China, placed the MHS in a strong position to ask Congress for an enlargement of its activities. Meanwhile, a series of deaths among St. Louis children who had been exposed to tetanus when given the diphtheria antitoxin provided further cause for Congress to look to the service as a source of high-quality laboratory work.[41] In 1902, Congress passed legislation that provided a clear framework for further growth, with a particular emphasis on research. Under the 1902 legislation, the service was renamed the Public Health and Marine Hospital Service. Its small Hygienic Laboratory, which would ultimately become the National Institutes of Health, was expanded and formally organized.

Under the new legislation, the surgeon general was authorized "to appoint heads of the [laboratory's] Divisions of Chemistry, Zoology, and Pharmacology from outside the service."[42] The Hygienic Laboratory was tasked with regulating the production of biological products, such as the diphtheria antitoxin.[43] Research and laboratory work would be key functions of the Public Health and Marine Hospital Service going forward, and the service would have increased discretion in recruiting noncommissioned personnel for its efforts. Each of these developments would play an important role in the growth of the service's functions, conception of its own mission, and reputation.

The reorganization of the MHS into the Public Health and Marine Hospital Service also had immediate implications for hookworm disease in the United States. Charles Wardell Stiles, the USDA scientist now leading the way on research into the disease, was not a medical doctor and as a result could not be a member of the service's commissioned corps. Under the service's new charter, however, Surgeon General Wyman asked Stiles to serve as the head of the Hygienic Laboratory's new zoology division. Stiles, who hoped to concentrate his energies on research into hookworm, eagerly accepted.

Almost immediately, he warned Surgeon General Wyman that, although hookworm likely already existed in the United States, "the return of our troops from the West Indies and the Philippines might result in the importation of additional infection."[44] In September 1902, Stiles set out from Washington, DC, to conduct some initial fieldwork, making his way through Virginia, the Carolinas, Georgia, and into Florida. His conclusions were stark. Hookworm, he came to believe, was "one of the most important factors in the inferior mental, physical, and financial condition of the poorer classes of the white population of the rural sand and piney woods districts which I visited."[45]

The disease, Stiles reported, represented an ongoing threat to the South's economic livelihood, "resulting in loss in wages, loss in productive-ness of the farms, loss in the school attendance of the children, extra expenses for drugs and for physicians' services, etc." Its causes, moreover, were evident: "The heavy and frequent infections found are amply explained by the almost total absence of privies and closets on the farms visited. Defecation occurs at almost any place within a radius of 50 meters from the house or hut, and as a result the premises become heavily infested with the [hookworm] embryos."[46]

In time, it would be established that the disease ranged throughout the Southern United States, though it was particularly severe in sandy coastal areas. The discovery of hookworm offered a clear explanation for the South's derided "dirt eaters" and "clay eaters," economically marginalized whites who lived on the region's poorest land. In a typical description of Georgia's clay eaters during the 1840s, New England schoolteacher Emily Burke wrote, "when a person has once seen a clay-eater, he can, ever after, instantly recognize any one of their number by their sickly, sallow, and most unnatural complexions. . . . Children, by the time they are ten or twelve years of age, begin to look old, their countenances are stupid and heavy and they often become dropsical and loathsome to the sight. Those who survive this practice [clay-eating] thirty or forty years, look very wrinkled and withered, their flesh shrunken to their bones like that of very aged people."[47]

Many Southern physicians found that Stiles's discovery offered a welcome means of making sense of an all too recognizable condition. "For a long time," Alabama's Dr. C. A. Mohr noted at the 1903 meeting of the AMA, "we were unacquainted with the disease and were treating for this, that, and the other thing, and especially for malarial anemia. . . . Only when our attention was drawn to the true nature of the trouble did we get any good results."[48] After a presentation by Stiles in Texas the same year, physicians were generally in agreement with his contention that the disease stretched as far west as the Lone Star State. "I have been familiar with these cases all my life," reported Dr. Bethel Nowlin, "but never knew what was the matter with them. I had always heard them called dirt eaters; a name that was always an insult to the patient."[49]

Outside of the South, the discovery of the region's hookworm problem was taken to be something of a joke. After Stiles announced his findings, a journalist published an account reporting that he had discovered "the germ of laziness," a turn of phrase that quickly caught on.[50] In a typical comment, one newspaper mockingly reported that there was there was "no doubt" that "the lazy man's respect for himself will go up amazingly, and self pity will also be in evidence when he realizes that he is in reality suffering from a disease."[51]

In time, Stiles's efforts to publicize his discovery and convince Southerners to adopt sanitary practices that would help them to avoid hookworm infection gained the attention of the John D. Rockefeller philanthropy, laying the ground for a substantial external intervention in Southern public health. Dispensaries like those held in Puerto Rico, at which hookworm sufferers were publically diagnosed and then given hookworm purgatives to ingest at home, were the core feature of the initial Rockefeller intervention, which lasted from 1910 through the end of 1914. After the conclusion of this campaign, the Rockefeller International Health Board (IHB) would become actively involved in attempting to stimulate the development of county-level public health capabilities in the South, cooperating with federal authorities into the 1930s.

For the time being, however, Stiles was on his own. Whenever possible, he traveled the South, attempting to persuade physicians and anyone else who would listen of the ongoing threat that hookworm posed to the region. In doing so, he defined the disease's impact in economic terms and its victims in racial terms.

Tapping into long-standing stereotypes of Southern "poor white trash," Stiles portrayed impoverished whites as the primary victims of hookworm disease.[52] The discovery of hookworm disease, he argued, offered an avenue for their rehabilitation into productive contributors to a new and more dynamic South. Invoking the ideology of the New South, which imagined an industrializing South released from the indignity of second-class status within the national Union, Stiles developed a powerful argument in favor of organized action against hookworm.

Drawing attention to the role of hookworm disease in their economic plight, Stiles hoped to use the sympathetic image of the diseased but redeemable poor white to rouse political backing for a more extensive campaign against the parasite. In meetings with groups of physicians, in lectures, and in journal articles, Stiles linked the presence of hookworm with the poor white stereotype and aspirations for Southern economic development.

"I believe that there are millions of people in our Southern States who are affected by the hookworm who can be saved," Stiles told the *Washington Post* in 1908. "Not saved from disease alone, but saved from that laziness which has given them the title of 'shiftless' and 'poor white trash.'" Hookworm, he continued, "causes much of the economical poverty of the States which are infested most with the germ which produces it."[53] As a 1909 article in *McClure's Magazine* summarized Stiles's argument, "Two million dollars will pay the whole bill for the cure of the South . . . and when the cure is complete, the South will take her place with the North and West in agricultural and industrial prosperity, for her two million sick whites will be two million able workers."[54]

The flip side of defining the victims of hookworm as poor whites was a portrayal of the disease, soon determined to be of West African origin, as fundamentally African and of black sufferers of hookworm as a "reservoir of disease."[55] Like malaria, Stiles noted, hookworm appeared to have a greater physical effect on whites than blacks: "This fact . . . is one of great importance, for it points us to a conclusion from which there is no escape, namely, that the negro race forms a great reservoir of supply for these infections."[56] Because the disease was less severe in blacks, Stiles maintained, they were able to continue working and were less likely to seek treatment. As a result, the disease would continue to be transferred to whites.[57] Speaking to the American Society for the Advancement of Science, Stiles stated plainly that the South's hookworm problem resulted from "the fact that in the United States we are violating a law of nature; namely, in attempting to lodge different races of man side by side in the same area."[58]

Offering a clear portrait of the victims and perpetrators of hookworm, Stiles elaborated on the implications of his understanding of the disease for any meaningful attempt to confront it. Racial discrimination in the battle against hookworm, he maintained, could only serve to harm the health and well-being of white Southerners. As long as disease was allowed to endure among blacks, whites would remain in danger and the region's economic resurgence would be hampered. "It is absolutely necessary," Stiles argued, "to avoid any distinction between the white and the negroes in this campaign of sanitary education."[59] The responsibility of white landowners, to black tenants as well as their own families, was unambiguous: "The white man who fails to recognize the important necessity of improving the sanitary conditions under which the negro is living fails to go to the root of the evil, and he unconsciously invites disease and death, especially to the women and children of his own race."[60]

Public Health and Private Philanthropy

Though obsessed with hookworm, Stiles had a variety of other responsibilities, including overseeing the service's research into Rocky Mountain spotted fever, a deadly and poorly understood disease first identified in the 1890s. The Public Health and Marine Hospital Service, meanwhile, had neither the means—nor, it was believed, the authority—to become any more involved. When the secretary of the North Carolina State Board of Health wrote to request that the Public Health and Marine Hospital Service detail "an officer to cooperate and assist his board in efforts to eradicate the disease from the State," service officials were inclined to respond by sending an officer. Nonetheless, "it was found impossible to make the detail requested," as there was no legal means available to them for paying for an officer to engage in "such field investigations and cooperation with state and local health authorities."[61]

Unable to take on the direct role he would have liked in combating the disease, Stiles began to pursue private support for an antihookworm campaign. Ultimately, he secured the backing of the John D. Rockefeller philanthropy. On October 27, 1909, Rockefeller announced that he would donate $1 million to bring hookworm disease to an end in the American South. In order to fight the disease, Rockefeller's men assembled a commission comprising "prominent educators and scientists, selected in large part from institutions in the South, where the disease is prevalent." The new organization was named, with a degree of optimism that would prove highly misplaced, the Rockefeller Sanitary Commission for the Eradication of Hookworm.[62]

The turn to private philanthropy for support was, in many ways, a natural one. Both individual medical services for the poor and public health had long received substantial private support. American hospitals had their origins as charitable institutions, often funded by religious organizations or through contributions from wealthy individuals.[63] Northeastern dispensaries represented another prominent model of privately backed medical care. There were numerous other precedents. In New York City, for instance, prominent businessman Nathan Straus funded milk stations "to provide free or low-cost cure milk to tenement families" beginning in the 1890s, an act of philanthropic support for adequate nutrition that wealthy donors in other cities soon mirrored.[64]

Maternal and child health was a particular area of interest for private philanthropy, but individual diseases such as tuberculosis and cancer also received significant attention, as did venereal disease and mental health. In a 1904 move that presaged the Rockefeller hookworm donation, Henry Phipps, a wealthy associate of Andrew Carnegie, endowed an institute for the study and treatment of tuberculosis at the University of Pennsylvania. In 1908, Phipps paid for a new psychiatric clinic at Johns Hopkins. In the years to come, private foundations would play a significant role in American health care, particularly in medical education.[65] Often, interventions by nongovernmental actors were intended to provide a framework that governments might ultimately model their own public health work on. In some cases, such as the New York milk station program, governments even assumed direct responsibility for initiatives originally funded privately.

The John D. Rockefeller philanthropy, notably, was already collaborating with federal officials as part of the USDA's farm demonstration program. Beginning in 1903, the USDA's Seaman Knapp developed a system of farm demonstration projects intended to introduce Southern farmers to techniques for improving the overall quality of their crops and to ward off the quickly spreading cotton boll weevil. Following his apparent successes, Congress appropriated funds to the USDA that could be used for extending Knapp's farm demonstrations.[66]

The congressional appropriation, however, was limited to areas that were infested with the boll weevil. Knapp and the USDA believed that the effort would benefit farmers outside of the areas subject to the pest. In 1906, hoping to expand its reach, the USDA made an agreement with the Rockefeller-funded General Education Board (GEB), which was focused on fostering a better educational environment in the South. Using money from the board, the USDA would extend the farm demonstration program into areas beyond those envisioned by the existing congressional authorization.[67] USDA agents working in areas that had not yet been hit by the boll weevil were paid by the GEB; the USDA, meanwhile, retained total control over the program.[68] The leaders of the GEB believed that supporting farm demonstration projects would create increased prosperity and economic stability in the South, laying the groundwork for educational improvements.

Although the collaboration played an important role in the growth of the farm demonstration program, it was not highly publicized. Indeed, after the 1914 Ludlow massacre—in which five coal miners, two women, and eleven children were killed in a standoff at a Rockefeller-owned mine in Colorado—the role of the GEB in paying the salaries of farm demonstration agents became something of a scandal, with members of Congress accusing Rockefeller of perniciously extending his influence into seemingly neutral government activities.[69]

Stiles hoped that the Public Health and Marine Hospital Service would work closely with the newly formed Rockefeller Sanitary Commission (RSC), but the Treasury Department proved unwilling to become involved in the effort. Although scientists at the service's Hygienic Laboratory continued to engage in hookworm-related research, Stiles was the only federal public health official involved in the new Rockefeller effort. Long the face of the antihookworm crusade, he was given a largely ceremonial role as the RSC's "scientific secretary." Nonetheless, he was elated.[70]

Public reaction to the Rockefeller gift was decidedly skeptical. John D. Rockefeller was a wildly unpopular individual, embroiled in the antitrust suit that would lead to the dissolution of his Standard Oil empire in 1911. For some, the gift appeared to be an attempt to distract public attention from his questionable business dealings. In the South, widespread apprehension was further fueled by the unwelcome symbolism of a wealthy Northerner offering, through the grant of a shockingly large sum of money, to cure the region of its intestinal parasites.

A few prominent Southerners openly denounced the gift. Southern Methodist bishop Warren Candler, brother of the inventor of Coca-Cola and soon to become the first chancellor of Emory University, was among the most vocal of the Rockefeller opponents. "It is to be hoped," Candler announced indignantly, "that our people will not be taken in by Mr. Rockefeller's vermifuge fund and hookworm commission. The habit of singling out the South for all sorts of reforms, remedies, and enlightenment is not for our benefit, and the too ready acceptance of these things on the part of some of our people is not to our credit."

For Candler, the sectional insult represented by the donation was unmistakable: "The South is represented to be filled with a wretched brood of dirt eaters. Who that knows the South can for a moment believe this?"[71] Other Southern leaders voiced similar reservations. Former Mississippi governor James Vardaman and prominent North Carolina progressive journalist Josephus Daniels both expressed disdain at the idea that the region was blighted by intestinal parasites and concern about Rockefeller's motives in donating money to be spent on such a large scale in the region. In time, however, both would become supporters.[72]

The Rockefeller Sanitary Commission

The RSC operated dispensaries—which diagnosed hookworm victims and then gave them purgatives that they could take at home to rid themselves of their worms—in eleven Southern states from 1911 through the end of 1914.[73] Operating for approximately one month in individual counties within participating states, the hookworm dispensaries generated a great deal of publicity for the disease. They did not, however, bring an end to the South's hookworm problem.

There were significant limitations to the dispensary approach. Rather than targeting a limited area such as Puerto Rico, the Rockefeller effort was aimed at a vast region. Because the campaigns were brief, unforeseen events could easily affect the effectiveness of a campaign in a given area. Poor weather or the overlap of the campaign with a particularly busy time in local agriculture might easily mean failure. In a number of cases, rumors spread that taking the thymol treatment would have potentially disastrous health effects.[74]

Beyond this, the lack of access to sanitary privies in much of the region meant that the threat of reinfection was significant. Of the 250,680 homes surveyed by the RSC between 1911 and the end of 1914, fully 125,584 had no privy at all.[75] In 1910, working with the Public Health and Marine Hospital Service's Leslie Lumsden and Norman Roberts, Charles Wardell Stiles developed a blueprint for the "LRS" sanitary privy, a relatively inexpensive model that could ensure that feces containing hookworm, typhoid, or dysentery did not make its way into the soil.[76] Blueprints for the LRS privy were widely distributed, and the men who ran dispensary campaigns attempted to convince rural Southerners that building one would contribute to both their personal health and economic prospects. Nonetheless, the RSC faced consistent indifference in its attempts to persuade rural Southerners to construct privies. Dispensary campaigns could draw large crowds, gin up a great deal of local excitement, and distribute thymol to substantial numbers of hookworm sufferers, but building privies took time and money that many simply did not have.[77]

By 1914, the men in charge of the RSC had decided that the dispensary approach could not accomplish the goal of ridding the South of hookworm. In August, John D. Rockefeller announced that the commission would cease to exist at the end of the year. Significantly, he did not claim that the disease had been eradicated. Although the commission did not have a clear sense of the extent of hookworm infection in the region, its leaders knew that the problem remained a substantial one.

Extrapolating from county-level data on hookworm incidence in school-children collected by the RSC, it is possible to calculate a rough estimate of the extent of hookworm disease in the states where the RSC operated.[78] An estimate based on these surveys and county-level population data from the US Census suggests that, of the 23,929,700 individuals living in the states in which the RSC operated, approximately 6,749,216 (28.2 percent) were infected.

From 1911 through the end of 1914, only 440,376 (6.5 percent of those estimated to be infected) were given the purgative thymol through the RSC's dispensary campaigns (Table 1.1). Because the treatments were administered at home, rather than under the supervision of field agents or physicians, it is impossible to know how many actually took the drug. Of those who did, we do not know how many succeeded in purging themselves of their hookworms. Among those who were successfully treated, the general lack of access to sanitary privies in the region likely ensured that a significant number became reinfected.

The decision to discontinue the RSC was part of a larger shift within the Rockefeller philanthropy. As it wound down the commission, the Rockefeller Foundation created a new International Health Board intended to combat diseases such as hookworm on a more global scale. Also continuing work within the Southern United States, the IHB explicitly attempted to confront the weaknesses that had hampered the dispensary campaigns.

The dispensary campaigns had relied on individuals, often encouraged by publicity efforts and community leaders, to seek out treatment. The IHB's new approach, however, required the creation of more permanent institutions, capable of actively seeking out individuals and households.

Table 1.1. Estimated Extent of Hookworm Infection as Indicated by Rockefeller Sanitary Commission Surveys and Total Number of Cases Recorded Treated through Dispensary Campaigns, 1911–1914

State	1910 Population	Hookworm Infections		Hookworm Cases Treated	
		n	%	n	%
Alabama	2,138,093	868,076	40.6	43,520	5.0
Arkansas	1,574,449	268,496	17.1	6,970	2.6
Georgia	2,609,121	1,349,350	51.7	45,494	3.4
Kentucky	2,289,905	373,720	16.3	37,916	10.1
Louisiana	1,656,388	346,358	20.9	37,225	10.7
Mississippi	1,797,114	600,059	33.4	73,919	12.3
North Carolina	2,206,287	873,335	39.6	98,990	11.3
South Carolina	1,515,400	716,218	47.3	38,411	5.4
Tennessee	2,184,789	444,121	20.3	23,332	5.3
Texas	3,896,542	548,487	14.1	17,490	3.2
Virginia	2,061,612	360,995	17.5	17,109	4.7
Total	23,929,700	6,749,216	28.2	440,376	6.5

Source: Calculated from the Annual Reports of the Rockefeller Sanitary Commission, 1910–1914, State Economic Areas (after IPUMS), and the 1910 Census of Population and Housing, accessed through the National Historical Geographic Information System (https://www.nhgis.org/). Numbers are rounded.

Rather than just targeting hookworm, officials would map out and address other major diseases, such as typhoid and malaria. Seeking to build permanent institutions and fully document local conditions, the new approach would ultimately prove far more effective than the ephemeral dispensary campaigns.[79]

Health at Home, Health Abroad

Throughout early American history, the regulation and promotion of health was a largely local endeavor. The federal government, however, played a distinct if limited role in health, first through the operation of marine hospitals and later through quarantine efforts and the inspection of immigrants. In the years after the Spanish-American War, American public health efforts in the Caribbean drew increasing attention to the debilitating diseases that plagued much of the American South. They also underlined the failures of local public health in the region, where state and local government proved incapable of dealing with threats such as malaria and hook-worm. The 1909 announcement that John D. Rockefeller would donate $1 million to fight hookworm in the South dramatized both the severity of the problem and the inability of American government at all levels to confront it. As we will see, it also helped to bring to a head a movement to create a national department of public health that had been gathering steam in the preceding years.

CHAPTER TWO

PUBLIC HEALTH AND HEALTH

INSURANCE

After the Rockefeller hookworm announcement, Oklahoma senator Robert Owen introduced legislation that would have created a national department of public health, modeled on the powerful USDA.[1] Owen's bill soon gained the support of the Committee of One Hundred on National Health, an organization created by progressive academics and committed to consolidating and expanding the public health powers of the federal government. It also gained the support of the life insurance industry and the AMA, both of which would later emerge as highly influential opponents of government-backed health insurance.

The push for a national department of public health failed, but it clarified the challenges that any effort to expand the role of the federal government in domestic health matters would face. The Public Health and Marine Hospital Service was among the staunchest opponents of the plan, which Surgeon General Walter Wyman viewed as a threat to the service's relative independence. Ultimately, the service was able to capitalize on the debate over Senator Owen's proposed department, using it to help secure an expanded research mandate and reorganization as simply the US Public Health Service.

With a broader mandate and a new set of appropriations, the PHS entered into an expansionary stage. Much of its new research was focused on the problems of rural America, and the PHS's Hygienic Laboratory began to make a name for itself through research into pellagra, a disturbing disease recently identified in the South. The PHS also initiated research into issues such as stream pollution and industrial hygiene. In addition, it began an important study of the relationship between health insurance and public health. Published in 1916, the study staked out a strong position in favor of compulsory health insurance. It was coauthored by Edgar Sydenstricker, who would head the development of the Social Security Act's health provisions nearly twenty years later. Citing the service's marine hospital system, Sydenstricker and leading PHS thinker Benjamin S. Warren argued that a clear precedent existed for a national system of compulsory health insurance. Such a system, they maintained, should be integrated with public health efforts. Indeed, health insurance would help to strengthen public health efforts: with workers, business, and government collectively footing the bill for individual medical services, each would become more interested in pursuing less expensive public health efforts.

A National Department of Public Health

On February 10, 1910, only a few short months after the announcement of the Rockefeller donation, Senator Owen introduced a bill to create a national department of public health. Owen's bill was short and to the point. It listed the organizational shifts necessary to bring a Department of Health into being, and it declared its purpose to be the consolidation of "all matters within the control of the Federal Government relating to the public health and to diseases of animal life."[2] In consolidating federal health efforts, the bill proposed changes for a number of federal agencies, including the Public Health and Marine Hospital Service, the revenue cutter service, Indian affairs, and even the Government Printing Office.[3]

After the Public Health and Marine Hospital Service, the two most prominent affected agencies were the Census Bureau and the USDA. In 1880, the US Census Bureau created a Death Registration Area, initially comprising Massachusetts, New Jersey, Washington, DC, and a number of other cities. States were admitted to the Death Registration Area as the bureau confirmed that they were capable of accurately collecting mortality statistics. Beginning in 1900, the bureau reported death rates annually. As of 1910, a number of states remained outside the Death Registration Area (Figure 2.1).

Under Owen's plan, the effort to collect nationwide vital statistics would be moved into the new health department, as would the USDA's work in regulating nonbiologic drugs and inspecting meat entering interstate commerce under the 1906 Pure Food and Drug Act.[4] Bringing together functions housed in a variety of agencies, Senator Owen's proposed Department of Public Health would collect health-related data, develop and implement quarantine measures, and enact standards for the safe production of chemical, biological, and other materials.[5] It would, Owen hoped, lay the groundwork for both the coordination of existing national-level health efforts and for a significant increase in the national government's role in ensuring the public's health.

At first, there appeared to be strong momentum in favor of Owen's proposal.[6] In 1907, the American Association for the Advancement of Science

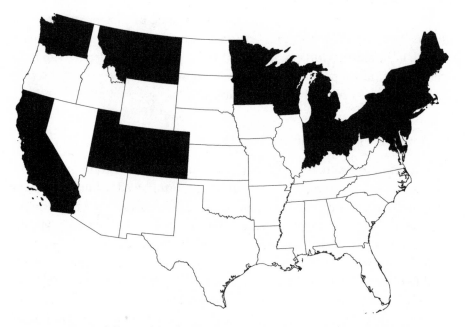

Figure 2.1. States fully capable of collecting mortality data, as indicated by inclusion in the Census Bureau's Death Registration Area, 1910. *Source:* Department of Commerce and Labor, Bureau of the Census, *Mortality Statistics: 1910,* https://www .cdc.gov/nchs/data/vsushistorical/mortstatbl_1910.pdf.

created a Committee of One Hundred on National Health.[7] Headed by progressive Yale economist Irving Fisher, the committee began working on a proposal for consolidating and expanding federal health activities. Bringing federal health activities under the auspices of one federal agency, Fisher hoped, would transform the science of public health "just as the Department of Agriculture has revolutionized the science of American agriculture."[8] President Theodore Roosevelt offered early support for the committee's efforts, though he believed federal health activities should be consolidated within a bureau, rather than—as the committee initially hoped—a Cabinet-level department.[9]

After taking office in 1909, Roosevelt's successor, William Howard Taft, offered clear support for a unified federal health agency. Like Roosevelt, he favored the more cautious approach of a sub-Cabinet-level bureau. As precedent, Taft—like Fisher, the Committee of One Hundred, and nearly all supporters of Senator Owen's bill—pointed to the work of the USDA. Along with its growing farm demonstration program, the USDA had engaged in well-publicized interventions against pleuropneumonia in cattle as well as against hog cholera.

Speaking at the Georgia–Carolina fair in Augusta, Georgia, less than two weeks after the announcement of Rockefeller's $1 million fund to eradicate hookworm, Taft maintained that such an agency would be particularly beneficial for the South, "for as you reach nearer to the tropics the danger of the spread of diseases is much greater."[10] Earlier Taft had served as governor general of the Philippines, where American authorities had developed a distinct and highly invasive approach to confronting local public health problems.[11] Now he directly contrasted the situation in the South with American efforts abroad. In the decade since the Spanish-American War, Taft explained, "we have found out through the study of our army officers and our army surgeons how the yellow fever can be suppressed, how malignant malaria can be suppressed. Without the knowledge, my dear friends, it would have been impossible to build the Panama Canal." As a result of American efforts, he continued, "we have less malaria, or certainly not more on the Isthmus of Panama than you have in your Southern States, and there has not for three years been a case of yellow fever."[12]

When introducing his legislation, Senator Owen also highlighted the benefits that a national department of public health might have for places like his home state of Oklahoma, where diseases such as hookworm, typhoid (increasingly confined to rural America as cities improved their water supplies), and malaria represented ongoing threats. Detailing the need for a national health agency on the floor of the Senate, Owen singled out hookworm as precisely the sort of preventable disease that a national department of public health might take on. "I am informed by a high authority," he told his Senate colleagues, "that more than 90 per cent of the children of one of the Southern States are afflicted with the hookworm, a preventable disease, curable at a cost of less than 50 cents apiece, with two doses of thymol and a little careful treatment."[13]

Owen's timing was exceedingly poor. In the next few months, the RSC would begin a successful program of outreach to state governments. When Owen introduced his bill, however, Southern leaders remained highly sensitive to claims about hookworm's prevalence and impact such as those being made by Owen. As he spoke on the Senate floor, Owen's invocation of the hookworm threat was met with hostility. Alabama's Joseph F. Johnson, responding to Owen's claims about the extent of hookworm infection in the region, complained that they were simply unbelievable. Mississippi's Hernando De Soto Money, meanwhile, demanded to know where Owen had gotten his information. Told it came from a "high authority," Money angrily declared that he did not "care who the expert is, I don't believe a word he says."[14]

Owen's supporters consistently pointed to the Rockefeller donation as a prime example of federal impotence in the face of a grave threat to the heath and economic livelihood of millions. That the USDA had a long and celebrated history of intervention where the health of livestock was concerned, they asserted, only made it worse. Testifying in favor of the bill, former army surgeon general George Sternberg expressed his disgust with the situation: "I do not believe in leaving all these things to philanthropists and to private enterprise. We do not depend upon private enterprise for the defense of our seacoasts from foreign foes or for the prevention of infectious diseases among our hogs and cattle." The lack of federal action in domestic public health, he maintained, was unacceptable. "Why," Sternberg asked, "should we depend upon the altruistic efforts of a few citizens of the Republic and the munificence of a Henry Phipps or a John D. Rockefeller for the extinction of tuberculosis and hookworm disease?"[15]

George Kober, dean of medicine and professor of hygiene at Georgetown, expressed similar concerns. There was, he maintained, "a certain line of work which should not be left to private philanthropy." In Puerto Rico, the army's Bailey Ashford had for years been engaged in efforts to combat hookworm. Within the United States, however, the same work "is practically left to private philanthropy." Fighting hookworm was "an example of what might be done if we had an efficient federal health department that would look into such problems and take them up with the respective States. It is clearly the duty of every State to protect the lives and health of its people. It ought not to be left to private philanthropy to undertake work in health protection any more than in fire or police protection."[16]

Supporters and Opponents of the Owen Bill

Senator Owen's primary base of support was among two interest groups: the life insurance industry and the American Medical Association. The life insurance industry had straightforward economic motives for favoring the creation of a national department of public health. Industry leaders hoped that a national department would lead to a more accurate collection of vital statistics. With information on mortality and rates of sickness in hand, they would be better able to accurately price policies, leading to increased profits.[17] Industry leaders also believed that expanded public health efforts would result in a healthier—and as a consequence more insurable—population.[18] Already in 1909, Metropolitan Life had started to dispatch visiting nurses to its industrial life insurance policyholders. Metropolitan Life's visiting nurse program had a dual function: it gave subscribers a tangible short-term benefit, and it offered a means of improving their health and longevity, meaning that they would be able to pay into insurance accounts for longer periods of time. In time, other insurance companies would follow the visiting nurse innovation.[19]

The AMA, meanwhile, had favored an expanded federal health role for years. Long engaged in a battle to professionalize and standardize the practice of medicine in the United States, the AMA had by 1910 amassed a significant and rapidly growing degree of prestige. The organization's leadership was dominated by a coterie of academics and physicians involved with large research hospitals who believed strongly in the Progressive vision of a government embodying scientific knowledge and expertise. For these men, creating a national department of public health appeared an uncontroversial means of furthering the unambiguously positive goal of improving the nation's health.

Along with the insurance industry and the AMA, Owen secured an impressive list of backers, including the Conference of State Boards of Health, the surgeons general of the army and navy, Harvey Wiley of the USDA's Bureau of Chemistry, various prominent academics, the Grange, the Tennessee Federation of Women's Clubs, and the American Federation of Labor (AFL). Although the progressive Committee of One Hundred worried at first that Owen's proposal was poorly thought out, the committee swiftly decided that it made sense to throw its full support behind the proposal.

Senator Owen worried that fears about the preservation of states' rights would be at the core of opposition to his proposed department. Such concerns, however, were quickly overshadowed by the emergence of an unexpected source of opposition. Soon after Owen introduced the bill, a group calling itself the League for Medical Freedom began to run advertisements against the legislation in major newspapers. The league's base of support was opaque, but it appeared to be well funded. Among its known supporters were some members of the "irregular" branches of medicine, such as osteopaths, eclectics, homeopaths, and chiropractors.[20] Other league supporters included Christian Scientists and those opposed to compulsory vaccination. The funding and impetus for the league, however, appeared to come from the patent medicine industry.[21]

The league's central line of argument, which appeared in a series of newspaper advertisements and in pamphlets, revolved around the AMA. The AMA, according to the league, planned to use the new public health department to create a "medical trust," which would discriminate against the practitioners of nonmainstream medicine, force individuals to be vaccinated, and grant the AMA and the federal government a controlling role in the health decisions of millions of Americans.[22]

Although the league positioned itself as a defender of individual liberty, Committee of One Hundred president Irving Fisher maintained in a June 18, 1910, letter to the *New York Times* that its real strength "evidently comes from commercial interests, such as those of the quack medicine interests and others who have reason to fear the Food and Drugs act." The purveyors of patent medicines, he asserted, were using groups such as the Christian Scientists to further their own agenda: "While Christian Scientists and other 'drugless' cults are denouncing drug doctors and denouncing a 'medical trust' which does not exist, these cults are themselves playing into the hands of a drug trust that does exist." The idea that the legislation was a vehicle for nationalizing control over American medicine and furthering the interests of the AMA, he asserted, was manifestly ridiculous: "Under our Constitution, the Federal Government could not, if it would, regulate the practice of medicine."[23]

Opposition from the Public Health and Marine Hospital Service

The League for Medical Freedom's opposition was highly publicized, but it was the behind-the-scenes hostility of the affected federal bureaucracies that ensured the defeat of Owen's bill. When the House Committee on Interstate and Foreign Commerce informally surveyed officials from the affected agencies, they offered almost unanimous opposition.[24] Walter Wyman, the surgeon general of the Public Health and Marine Hospital Service, perceived the Owen bill as a threat to the service's standing and independence. Already before Owen introduced his plan, Wyman was lobbying members of Congress in favor of his own legislation, which would expand the research capabilities of the service, grant it a broader investigative mandate, and increase the salaries of its officers. Rather than denouncing the proposal for a national department of public health, however, he continued to quietly lobby members of Congress to support his own set of proposals.[25]

It gradually became clear that Owen's position was weak. The League for Medical Freedom's arguments about the creation of a national medical monopoly were bizarre, but they appeared to be gaining traction. In addition, Senator Owen had failed to secure the support of political representatives from the rural parts of the nation that were most likely to benefit from his bill. Members of Congress from more industrialized areas, meanwhile, viewed his proposal with skepticism because it was being framed in large part as a program that would benefit poorer states with less developed public health capabilities.

When Surgeon General Wyman died of cancer in 1911, the Treasury Department and the Public Health and Marine Hospital Service moved to capitalize on the surge of interest in federal public health activities that surrounded the Owen bill. The need for a greater federal health role, officials from the Treasury Department and the service maintained, was real. It was just that Owen's proposed national department of public health was a half-baked plan. Testifying before Congress, Treasury Secretary Franklin MacVeagh explained that the progress of the Public Health and Marine Hospital Service had been held back by "an effort to erect a health department with a new member of the Cabinet at its head." Rather than continuing to pointlessly consider the merits of consolidation under the Owen bill, it was time to "sufficiently concentrate attention upon the public health work already in hand to develop it to the utmost." Surgeon General Wyman's sudden death, Secretary MacVeagh continued, "brings this service into special notice; and no better recognition of this man who did so much to build the service up and who was so eager to carry it forward, could be made than to promote and expand its usefulness."[26]

Initially threatened by a proposed consolidation of federal health efforts that would have rendered the surgeon general the subordinate of a new Cabinet-level health official, the service now instead emerged triumphant. In 1912, Congress passed Wyman's proposals into law. Following his recommendations, the new legislation raised the pay of the service's commissioned officers, renamed the organization the Public Health Service, and substantially increased its research authority. Under the new legislation, the PHS was granted the vague, and as it turned out expansive, authority to "study and investigate the diseases of man and conditions influencing the propagation and spread thereof, including sanitation and sewage and the pollution either directly or indirectly of the navigable streams and lakes of the United States."[27]

"A New Epoch"

President Taft appointed Rupert Blue, the South Carolinian who had headed the service's antiplague work in the San Francisco Bay area, to fill the vacancy created by Surgeon General Wyman's death. Blue, as it turned out, had a far more expansive view of the role that the service should play in American life than his predecessor. Pleased with the changes to the service's mandate and eager to preside over its expansion, Blue interpreted the new authorization broadly. According to the surgeon general's report for 1912, it marked "a new epoch in the history of the health activities of the Federal Government, and it is believed [that the act] clearly recognizes the Public Health Service as the central health agency in the Nation."[28]

Before 1912, the service's most substantial inland endeavor had been the Blue-led attempt to kill plague-infected ground squirrels in the counties surrounding the San Francisco Bay.[29] After Blue took over as surgeon general, the PHS embarked on a broad range of new research activities. In July 1913, the service secured an appropriation of $200,000 "for field investigations" and $20,000 for the operation of its Hygienic Laboratory.[30] It soon embarked on research into malaria, typhoid, and other diseases of rural America. It also began investigations of industrial hygiene, occupational diseases, and stream pollution. In New York, the service began a study of the occupational diseases faced by garment workers, and in Cincinnati, it began a study of tuberculosis in industry. In Indiana, it initiated research into the health of female workers. The service began a study of the problem of trachoma among steelworkers, and it started working with the Bureau of Mines to investigate the health problems faced by American miners.[31]

In a few cases, the PHS became actively involved in domestic public health efforts. In 1914, it supervised a campaign, funded by local textile mill operators, in Roanoke Rapids, North Carolina. Directed by service officers, local workers dug ditches, oiled lakes, and removed blockages from streams. A similar effort, funded by a local lumber company, was undertaken in Electric Mills, Mississippi.[32] In 1916, the PHS engaged in a cooperative effort with the Rockefeller International Health Board. At two locations in Arkansas, service officers oversaw antimalaria efforts that were funded with Rockefeller money.[33]

In eastern Kentucky, and later in the mountains of Virginia, West Virginia, and Tennessee, the service began surveying and treating people for trachoma, an infectious and often-blinding eye disease that was widespread in southern Appalachia. This effort was funded through the service's epidemic fund, which could be used at the service's discretion; it was justified as necessary for preventing "the spread of the disease in interstate traffic."[34] Taking place deep in the interior of the nation, this effort was a substantial departure from earlier practices. Tiny in scope, it nonetheless suggested a new and even bold avenue of action for the PHS.

Pellagra

Pellagra, a dietary-deficiency disease that was widespread in the South, was singled out as a disease of special importance in the newly reorganized PHS's first major appropriation. Along with the general grant of funds for field investigations and new money for the service's Hygienic Laboratory, Congress earmarked an additional $47,000 for the PHS to operate a new pellagra hospital and research center, to be located in Spartanburg, South Carolina. Spartanburg was chosen both because pellagra was rampant in the area and because of the welcoming nature of local mill owners, who had earlier embraced a privately funded investigation of pellagra, the Thompson–McFadden Commission.

Pellagra caused something of a panic when it was first recognized in the United States in 1907. In an article published that year in the *Journal of the American Medical Association,* Alabama physician George Searcy documented pellagra cases among the patients at Alabama's Mount Vernon Insane Hospital.[35] The disease was known to be widespread among Spanish and Italian peasants, but it was generally not believed to exist in the United States (although some earlier cases had been reported).[36] Now physicians across the South recognized its characteristic symptoms: dermatitis, dementia, and diarrhea.

Like hookworm, pellagra made life and work difficult for its victims. In its early stages, signs of pellagra included "lassitude, weakness, loss of appetite, mild digestive disturbances and psychiatric or emotional distress (anxiety, irritability and depression)."[37] Diarrhea contributed to feelings of weakness and discomfort. In time, symmetrical patterns of dermatitis appeared on victims' skin. The afflicted found it increasingly difficult to work or concentrate. Eventually, "fatigue and insomnia" led "to encephalopathy characterized by confusion, memory loss, and psychosis." As the disease progressed, patients became "disoriented, confused and delirious, then stuporous and comatose." For some, the disease would lead to death.[38]

Pellagra's causes were unknown. As in Spain and Italy, the Americans most likely to develop pellagra were those who subsisted on a monotonous diet heavy in corn. That this diet had some relationship to the disease seemed apparent. Cesare Lombroso, a leading Italian expert on the disease, had argued that spoiled corn caused the disease. As pellagra emerged as a major public health concern, many within the United States adopted the spoiled corn theory.[39] Alternative explanations, however, quickly emerged. The most prevalent was that pellagra was the result of an unknown infectious agent, possibly transmitted by protozoa carried by flies.[40] In its Spartanburg-based study, the privately funded Thompson–McFadden Commission concluded that the spoiled corn theory did not hold up and that pellagra was almost certainly contagious.

Starting in April 1914, the PHS's pellagra research activities were placed under the direction of Joseph Goldberger. A childhood immigrant from the Austro-Hungarian empire who grew up in New York City, Goldberger was considered a rising star within the service. An astute observer of individuals and society, he had spent much of his early career in Texas and Louisiana combating yellow fever and dengue.

From the beginning, Goldberger was skeptical of the major explanations of pellagra's causes. Focusing on the question of what made poor rural Southerners distinct from other population groups, and observing that pellagra often afflicted inmates but not staff in institutional settings such as mental hospitals, Goldberger came to believe that the disease was the result of a dietary deficiency.[41] At two orphanages in Mississippi, he fed children high-protein diets and found that the disease largely disappeared.[42] At the Georgia State Sanitarium, he administered a similar diet to a group of white female inmates and a group of black female inmates. Both were soon cured of the disease.[43]

In 1915, Goldberger persuaded Mississippi governor Earl Brewer to allow him access to inmates at Mississippi's Rankin Prison Farm. Pellagra was known to be particularly prevalent among Southern women and African Americans, a fact that would later be attributed to their poor diets relative to white men's.[44] Since they were the population least prone to pellagra, Goldberger proposed inducing the disease among a group of healthy white men by feeding them a highly monotonous diet similar to that eaten by Southern tenant farmers. The remaining prisoners would serve as a control group. Governor Brewer agreed to offer pardons to twelve inmates in return for their "voluntary" participation in the study.

Beginning in April 1915, Goldberger subjected the prisoners to his highly monotonous diet.[45] Because of the long-standing belief that spoiled corn was responsible for pellagra, he ensured that they were fed "the best quality of both meal and hominy grits obtainable on the local market."[46] Perhaps atypical in its extreme lack of variety, the prisoners' diet was essentially an exaggerated form of the familiar Southern "meat, molasses, and maize" regimen.[47] In six of the prisoners, the diet produced pellagra, a diagnosis confirmed by a team of experts.[48] Although the remaining inmates had not yet developed pellagrous lesions when the experiment was concluded, they exhibited other characteristic symptoms of pellagra. "In other words,"

Goldberger wrote, "we are of the opinion that every one of the volunteers developed pellagra, six or seven with skin lesions and four or five without."[49] While Goldberger felt confident that he had demonstrated the role of diet in causing pellagra, many physicians remained skeptical.

Even if Goldberger's research had swiftly been recognized as definitive, it was far from clear how the underlying problems that fueled Southern pellagra might be addressed. In a later study of pellagra in seven South Carolina cotton mill villages that he devised and conducted with his close collaborator, PHS statistician Edgar Sydenstricker, Goldberger demonstrated that the principal difference between families with cases of pellagra and those without was the presence of animal protein in the diets of those without the disease. Both pellagrous and nonpellagrous households, they found, ate corn products from the same sources in similar quantities.

The mill village study showed that those afflicted by pellagra were not just victims of poverty but also victims of location and political economy. In some mill towns, poor residents remained entirely free of the disease, while in others the disease ran rampant. The key to understanding these differences, Goldberger and Sydenstricker found, was the nature of farming in the surrounding countryside. Where cotton was prevalent, pellagra was too. Where farmers grew vegetables and raised dairy cows, the disease was largely absent. Pellagra was a major problem in the South because a significant portion of the population lived in areas that focused heavily on growing cotton and where there was little access to a high-quality and varied diet.[50]

Goldberger's research into pellagra made him nationally known and significantly added to the stature of the PHS's Hygienic Laboratory. His findings, however, were in many ways devastating. In the decades after the Civil War, cotton came to dominate large swaths of the South. For many tenant farmers, growing a cash crop such as cotton was required by either landlords or by the furnishing merchants who gave them loans. As long as this economic system persisted, Goldberger recognized, it was likely that pellagra would continue to be a major public health problem in the South. An improved diet was, for many, simply not attainable. Deeply affected by the plight of the victims of the disease, Goldberger would spend the next decade working on an alternative solution.

Health Insurance

The reorganized PHS embarked on important new research into the diseases of both rural and urban America. Joseph Goldberger's research on pellagra was highly innovative and proved a milestone in modern epidemiology. In addition to research focused on specific health problems, the service also began exploring the administration of health services. This led the service to become involved in one of the most controversial health-related issues of the Progressive Era: health insurance.

Compulsory sickness insurance for workers was first introduced in Germany in 1883 under Otto von Bismarck. There, it was part of a broader project of shoring up support for the governing institutions of the recently consolidated German empire and mitigating the appeals of socialism.[51] Interest in health insurance among American progressives, however, mounted only after 1911, when Britain passed its National Insurance Act, a comprehensive piece of legislation that created a system of compulsory sickness, disability, and unemployment insurance aimed at British wage earners. Britain's David Lloyd George, then chancellor of the exchequer, was a strong admirer of the German system. Like Bismarck, he also viewed compulsory sickness insurance as a means of heading off a threat from the political left, this time in the form of the rapidly growing Labour Party's challenge to his own Liberal Party.[52]

In the United States, the most prominent early supporter of compulsory sickness insurance was former president Theodore Roosevelt. Hoping to regain the presidency and denied the 1912 Republican nomination, Roosevelt launched a new Progressive Party. Speaking at the party's convention, Roosevelt asserted that "the hazards of sickness, accident, invalidism, involuntary unemployment, and old age should be provided for through insurance."[53] In its platform, the new party endorsed the "protection of home life against the hazards of sickness, irregular unemployment and old age through the adoption of a system of social insurance adapted to American use."[54] The full implications of this endorsement were not fleshed out, however, and the issue did not play a role of any note in the campaign. Nonetheless, Roosevelt's vision of a New Nationalism, in which the federal government would assume social welfare functions in areas traditionally dominated by the states, suggested a future in which health insurance might well be an arena in which the national government would become involved.

In the years after Roosevelt's defeat, the AALL began pushing for health insurance laws within the United States. An archetypical progressive organization, the AALL largely comprised academics committed to the idea that scientific expertise could be applied neutrally to address major social problems.[55] Before taking on the issue of health insurance, the association had engaged in a successful campaign to persuade states to adopt workman's compensation laws.

In state after state, the AALL persuaded large corporations and state legislatures that workman's compensation would, in addition to providing a safety net for injured workers, protect corporations against ruinously large court settlements and create a more stable business environment.[56] The success of the workman's compensation campaign convinced the leaders of the AALL that a similar approach could be used in the realm of health insurance.

The AALL expressed supreme confidence about what could be achieved through health insurance, often framing its arguments in terms of a healthier and more productive workforce. Access to health services through insurance, AALL leaders argued, "would yield handsome returns for employers by creating a healthier and more productive labor force."[57] This, it was assumed, was an argument that employers would embrace. The AALL released its model health insurance bill in 1915, which it hoped would provide the basis for state-level action. The organization pursued state legislation because its leaders believed that constitutional challenges would likely derail any national-level insurance legislation.[58]

Under the model bill, workers earning up to a specified amount (which presumably would vary by state), employers, and the state would contribute to an insurance fund. Workers earning less than a specified amount would be enrolled but would not contribute. The model bill brought together what in the present day would be called health insurance and disability insurance. When a worker was incapacitated by an illness or accident not covered by workman's compensation, "the workman would be entitled to receive at the expense of the fund adequate medical, surgical and nursing care and two-thirds of wages until able to resume work." These benefits would be available for up to twenty-six weeks in a given year. A funeral benefit was also included in the bill, as was maternity care for female workers and the wives of insured men.[59]

The reasons that a funeral benefit was included are worth highlighting because the benefit resulted in major pushback from the life insurance industry. For many working-class families, funeral costs represented the threat of either severe financial hardship or a pauper's burial. The AALL hoped that compulsory health insurance would replace the industrial life insurance policies that many working-class families purchased to ward off these dangers. These policies—which paid out a lump sum on the death of the policyholder—were administratively expensive, as a company would dispatch an insurance agent on a regular basis to canvas working-class neighborhoods and collect premiums. Under the AALL's model bill, this money would instead go into more efficient health insurance funds. Intending to control costs, and convinced that profit should not be a motive in the proposed health insurance system, the leaders of the AALL explicitly excluded existing for-profit insurance companies from operating the insurance funds that would be created under the model bill.[60] The result, predictably, was that the life insurance industry viewed the AALL's proposal for state-based compulsory health insurance as a threat to its economic well-being.

Insurance and Health Promotion

In Britain, Germany, and the growing number of European nations adopting similar legislation related to the health of workers, the term "sickness insurance" was commonplace. As originally adopted under Bismarck, sickness insurance was first and foremost a system for providing workers with cash benefits during a period in which they were unable to work because of illness. Payments for physician services, however, were also an aspect of the system. Lloyd George and other British proponents, who believed that insurance could be used to improve the health of the British population, viewed such payments as an important part of sickness insurance.

In the United States, the AALL attempted to frame its model bill as "health insurance," a term intended to evoke a broader conception of its purposes. When AALL leaders listed its benefits, coverage for the costs of medical care, rather than for wages lost to sickness, came first. In promising to cover medical costs through insurance, the model bill was, for the United States, breaking new ground. For a variety of reasons, insurance companies had been uninterested in offering policies covering such costs.

To begin with, insurance companies faced a major adverse selection problem: the people most likely to enroll in a plan insuring against medical costs were those who anticipated having high medical costs. Insurance companies also believed that it would be difficult to establish whether an individual was actually ill. Given the uneven availability of mortality statistics and even worse reporting of nonfatal cases of disease, it was believed that accurately pricing policies would prove an insurmountable task.[61] Finally, there was a general lack of demand. Although medical costs were increasing and medical technology was improving, most working families remained far more concerned with the loss of wages resulting from a bout of sickness than with the costs of medical care.[62] Put plainly, insurance companies did not believe they could profit from health policies, and few Americans were interested in purchasing them.

In its campaign for workman's compensation, the AALL had argued that compulsory insurance would lead employers to create safer working environments so as to cut down on compensation costs. The AALL applied the same logic to health insurance. If workers, employers, and governments were forced to contribute to funds that would insure against wages lost from sickness and against medical bills, all three would have the incentive to avoid such costs by pursuing disease prevention.[63] The PHS wholeheartedly embraced this line of thought, which suggested that compulsory health insurance might prove an asset for the proponents of public health efforts. In 1916, as the AALL launched a campaign to persuade state legislatures to consider its model bill, the PHS issued a major report on health insurance, titled "Health Insurance: Its Relation to Public Health."

The PHS's Benjamin Warren and Edgar Sydenstricker wrote the report. Warren, a career PHS officer and native of Alabama, had a long track record as a policy innovator. He helped to draft both the 1902 and 1912 legislation that had reorganized and expanded the service, setting the stage for its growth during the 1910s. Sydenstricker, born in China to missionary parents before returning to Virginia, was not a physician but a statistician. As such, he was not a commissioned PHS officer. Detailed to assist Warren, he also worked closely with Joseph Goldberger in the service's pellagra studies. In time, Sydenstricker would emerge as a towering figure in American health policy, ultimately leading the development of the health aspects of what became the 1935 Social Security Act. Isidore Falk, a close colleague and also a major figure in the development of American health policy, described Sydenstricker as "a very thoughtful person, a gentle person, but a very strong person. . . . He had a Southern twang about him, a little bit, because he was of a Southern background. He had a very good sense of humor. He had an intense sense of integrity. He was a scientist, every inch of him." [64]

Warren and Sydenstricker's report laid out an ambitious vision of the role of government in ensuring the health of the American people. European systems of sickness insurance, they argued, were far too heavily oriented toward providing relief for lost wages. Worse, they were not integrated with preventive and population-based health efforts. As a result, they should not be taken as the model for insurance in the United States. "To obtain the highest degree of success in America," Warren and Sydenstricker wrote, "it would appear that health insurance systems should be very closely correlated with national, State, and local health agencies. If these agencies are at present inadequate, they should be enlarged and strengthened instead of attempting to create new and independent health agencies."[65] With compulsory insurance making the full costs of a sick population visible to both business and government, a strong political base could be created for increased public health efforts, which would help to keep the population healthy and which would prove less costly.[66]

In a notable departure from the state-based approach of the AALL, Warren and Sydenstricker argued that although state-level insurance was acceptable, a clear precedent for a federally backed system of health insurance existed in the form of the PHS's marine hospitals. "Taxation by the Federal Government for benefits to employees," they wrote, "has been in operation for over a century in the maintenance of marine hospitals, and the Federal Government has been a frequent contributor, in appropriations by Congress, to the Marine Hospital Service."[67] If the federal government could operate a system of compulsory insurance for sailors, then it could certainly create an insurance system for other employee groups.

The PHS report was presented as a scientifically neutral study of sickness among industrial workers, European approaches to insurance, and the question of how such approaches might by improved on in an American system. Nonetheless, it had an unmistakable undercurrent of advocacy. For Warren and Sydenstricker, it was evident that insurance should be tied to existing public health agencies, then used to improve their administrative capabilities and their ability to take on preventable disease. They also had little doubt about the constitutionality of a federally backed insurance system. "The taxation of industry by the Federal Government in a health-insurance system," they concluded without equivocation, "has been thoroughly established."[68] If contributions were collected and disbursed by the federal government, health insurance could be used as the basis for a more integrated approach to public health and individual medical services, both locally and across political jurisdictions. Perhaps the existing marine hospital system might even provide a framework for federally operated insurance.

Indicative of the PHS's quickly expanding horizons, Warren and Sydenstricker's report was widely read by those interested in government-backed health insurance. Writing in late 1916, Isaac Rubinow, a leading figure in the AALL, asserted that their analysis had already played "a historic role, the importance of which can not be overestimated." Bearing the imprimatur of the PHS, "the study of Dr. Warren and Mr. Sydenstricker has already succeeded in doing a very great amount of publicity work. It was the most quoted and perhaps the most widely read of all the propaganda publications on health insurance which appeared during the last year." Lee Frankel of the Metropolitan Life Insurance Company, meanwhile, cited "the studies in sickness insurance made by Warren and Sydenstricker" as among the factors that "indicate strongly the present trend of thought and the need for consideration of a subject which promises to loom large in the immediate future."[69]

As 1917 began, Warren and Sydenstricker pushed even further. In a paper read at the annual meeting of Maryland's state medical association in April, they repeated their argument that an effective system of health insurance would have to be administratively linked to public health efforts if it was to "not be merely a variety of commercial or mutual insurance or another type of public relief, but a practicable method of improving and extending the present facilities for the prevention of disease."[70] In order for such a system to function properly, they continued, insurance would have to be used to reorient the practice of medicine itself.

Traditional fee-for-service medicine, they suggested, would have to be dispensed with. In addition to creating perverse financial incentives for physicians, fee-for-service created conditions in which it was likely that preventive health measures would be subordinated to curative medicine. "Under present practices of the medical profession," they explained, "there is a premium placed on sickness. That is to say, the patient who is sick often, or for long periods, is worth much more to his doctor than the patient who is seldom sick." This situation, they continued, "should be reversed; the premium should, in so far as practicable, be placed on health. With a premium on health payable to the doctor, it goes without saying that it would be an added incentive to him to keep his patients well, and to cure them as quickly as possible when sick."[71] Achieving these ends, Warren and Sydenstricker acknowledged, was not a simple proposition, but compulsory insurance provided a potential means of achieving it.[72]

In 1916, Surgeon General Rupert Blue was elected president of the AMA. In his inaugural address, he echoed Warren and Sydenstricker in emphasizing the idea that compulsory health insurance could be used to draw attention to the importance of preventive health efforts. There were "unmistakable signs," Blue told the association's members "that health insurance will constitute the next great step in social legislation." He suggested that an adequately designed health insurance system would "distribute the cost of sickness among those responsible for conditions causing it and thereby lighten the burden on the individual." With business, government, and the broader community aware of the costs of care, "financial incentive may thus be given for the inauguration of comprehensive measures for the prevention of disease."[73]

By establishing itself as an important player in the debate over health insurance, the PHS had staked out an innovative position in favor of a system that would link public health and individual medical services. Federal action, Warren and Sydenstricker argued, would be constitutional, and health insurance should be used to transform the practice of medicine.

Employers and Labor

Although a number of states considered the AALL's model bill, no state adopted compulsory health insurance legislation. From the beginning, the life insurance industry was mobilized against the bill, which it viewed as a serious threat to its bottom line. This, however, was only one of a myriad of factors working against state-level proposals for health insurance. Earlier, workman's compensation bills succeeded because they contained elements that offered clear material benefits to both employers and labor.[74] From the perspective of employers, state-based compensation plans made the business environment more predictable by helping to ensure that courts would not award financially ruinous settlements to injured employees. Compensation bills appealed to workers and labor unions because of the promise that settlements would actually be awarded, and without the delays that might come from being processed through the court system.

Most employers and many workers, however, were skeptical of the idea of compulsory health insurance. Though the AALL argued that health insurance would mean healthier and more productive workers, employers saw little reason to accept this claim. More likely, they believed, an insurance program would promote laziness and shirking among workers, who might pretend to be sick in order to receive cash benefits and avoid work. In the debate over insurance, the opposition of employers was critical. Businesses, members of state legislatures worried, might relocate to states without insurance if they were forced to contribute to insurance funds that did not in the end have the effect of creating more productive workers.[75]

Organized labor was fragmented. One reason for labor's lukewarm response was the manner in which workman's compensation legislation was being implemented. Employers, it appeared, were now less likely to hire employees with physical problems. In addition, they were using the pretext of company physicals to dismiss workers found to have, in the words of one AFL leader, "the disease of unionism."[76]

For some labor leaders, government action appeared the wrong road to take: insurance should be achieved through collective bargaining. AFL president Samuel Gompers was the most prominent proponent of this view. "Compulsory sickness insurance," Gompers maintained, "is based upon the theory that [the workers] are unable to look after their own interests and the State must interpose its authority and wisdom and assume the role of parent or guardian."[77] Rather than binding workers to state governments through insurance legislation, workers should be bound together and to the union that secured their benefits through collective bargaining. Other labor leaders, importantly, took different positions. In California and New York, two states where the mood appeared at times to be turning toward compulsory insurance, the state branches of the AFL formally endorsed it.[78] The much-remarked-on opposition of Gompers, however, guaranteed that labor would not present a unified front. It also proved a boon to opponents within the business community, who eagerly highlighted his opposition.

Failure of the AALL's Proposal for Compulsory Health Insurance

The opposition of the life insurance industry, business opposition, and divisions within organized labor would likely have been enough to seal the fate of compulsory health insurance. Two additional factors, however, ensured that compulsory insurance legislation would not pass. The first was the steadily mounting opposition of organized medicine. When the AALL model bill was first introduced, AMA leaders expressed openness to the idea of compulsory insurance.[79] Designed with the hope of cultivating physician support, the bill offered only an outline of how insurance might relate to actual medical practice. After introducing it, the organization explicitly asked the AMA to suggest an approach that it would find acceptable. As AALL leader John B. Andrews wrote, the AMA "immediately accepted the invitation in good spirit," creating an investigative committee that included as its executive secretary prominent AALL member Isaac Rubinow.[80]

While the AMA's leaders were open to the idea of insurance, convinced that it was likely inevitable, and largely in agreement that the organization should try to influence the form it would take, the AMA's rank-and-file members came to view compulsory health insurance as a threat to their professional autonomy and financial well-being.[81] The AALL was circumspect on the issue of how medical financing would relate to the practice of medicine, but there were good reasons for physicians to believe that compulsory insurance would lead to changes that they were not eager to experience. Detailing the system that he hoped to see created, Isaac Rubinow wrote that he favored a "state of affairs in which all the medical work to be done for the members of a health-insurance fund would be done by physicians and surgeons. . . . who are specifically employed for the purpose."[82] As examples of how this might work in practice, he cited the salaried physicians employed by some industrial companies, the military, "Russian village medicine," and the "brilliant results achieved by thorough organization of medical service in the building of the Panama Canal."[83]

For Rubinow and other AALL leaders, as for the PHS's Warren and Sydenstricker, it was critical that compulsory insurance be used to begin shifting physicians away from the established fee-for-service system, which AALL leaders had concluded created perverse incentives toward quantity over quality in the supply of health care. A financially workable system of health insurance, from the perspective of the AALL, would have to require either flat payments to physicians per individual policyholder or the employment of salaried physicians. If compulsory insurance was blindly wedded to fee-for-service medicine, the result might easily be spiraling costs as physicians provided increasing amounts of care that they knew would be compensated by insurance funds.[84] Government-backed insurance would have to mean change.

For many physicians in private practice, these were not arguments to be taken lightly. A system based on capitation or salaries, some worried, would lead to an overuse of services because people would no longer be constrained by costs associated with additional services. Being paid by insurance funds, meanwhile, might easily mean a decline in their ability to make decisions about who they treated and how they treated them. There was also the obvious threat that insurance funds might seek to control costs by limiting payments to physicians.[85] Although the AALL viewed workman's compensation as a triumph, physicians were less sure. In instances where workman's compensation programs had included provisions for medical services for injured workers, physicians noted, payments were often stingy. Their disbursement, meanwhile, was often delayed or administered in a manner that alienated those physicians who participated.[86] Insurance, it seemed, might quickly lead to a loss of control.

Physician opposition to the AALL proposal, initially subdued, took on a strident tone as it became clear that physician concerns about individual and professional autonomy were widespread. At the state level, AMA leaders supportive of health insurance found themselves increasingly swamped by an unhappy and agitated membership. Why, physicians at the grass roots asked, was the organization working with the proponents of health insurance, nonphysicians who appeared bent on bringing government-backed insurance funds into their relationships with patients and limiting their professional freedom? Tapping into these concerns, the insurance industry began working to organize local physicians in opposition to government-backed insurance. As opposition became increasingly well organized, the AMA leadership at both the state and national levels was forced to respond. In 1920, the national AMA formally condemned compulsory health insurance, designating it a threat to both the quality of American medicine and the very fabric of American life.[87]

American participation in World War I added an additional factor to the debate. In 1916, incumbent president Woodrow Wilson had campaigned on the slogan that "He Kept Us Out of War." After a period in which it suspended the sinking of neutral ships so as to avoid antagonizing the United States, Germany announced in early 1917 that it would resume unrestricted submarine warfare. British authorities, meanwhile, intercepted the so-called Zimmerman Telegram, in which German officials proposed a military alliance with Mexico against the United States. With Germany suggesting that it would assist Mexico in reconquering the territory lost in the Mexican-American War and again sinking American ships in the Atlantic, the United States joined the war on the side of the Allied Powers in April 1917.[88]

This turn of events was decisive for the already imperiled prospects of compulsory health insurance. Almost immediately, the opponents of insurance latched on to the anti-German sentiment that became commonplace in much of the nation. In a series of pamphlets, the AALL's program was tied to German authoritarianism and portrayed as an alien encroachment on the American way of life. When the Bolsheviks took over Russia and signed a peace treaty with Germany and Austria-Hungary, health insurance opponents gained a new and potent rhetorical tool. From then on, proposals for overt government involvement in health insurance would routinely be tied to the threat of Soviet communism.

Ideological opposition to insurance, it is important to point out, did not simply emerge out of a popular sense of unease with government intervention. During debates over workman's compensation, the antistatist arguments that became commonplace in debates of health insurance were absent. Instead, ideological opposition was cultivated by groups, such as the insurance industry and organized medicine, that had a material stake in guaranteeing that insurance proposals did not become law.[89] The AALL and other proponents of insurance pointed out that America's ally, Britain, also had an insurance system, but their arguments gained little traction. Attempts to portray insurance as necessary to the war effort because it would improve the health of workers proved similarly ineffective. In California and New York, the two states where proposals for compulsory insurance had progressed the furthest, the dual threats of German authoritarianism and Russian Bolshevism came to dominate the public debate.

In November 1918, California voters considered a constitutional amendment that would have authorized the legislature to create an insurance program if it saw fit. "Made in Germany," a prominent opposition pamphlet asked. "Do you want it in California?"[90] The amendment was resoundingly defeated. The push for health insurance continued in New York, where newly elected governor Al Smith supported it, even in the aftermath of the war. In 1919, insurance legislation passed in the state senate. Subjected to a campaign in which it was portrayed as both too German and as an entering wedge to Bolshevism, the bill died in the state assembly. Smith, for his part, soon chose to direct his energy elsewhere.[91]

Public Health and Health Insurance

The announcement that a private philanthropy—the Rockefeller Sanitary Commission—would launch a campaign against hookworm in the American South led Oklahoma senator Robert Owen to introduce legislation in Congress proposing a national department of public health. Promoting the health of Americans, Owen and his supporters believed, should be a function of government rather than an initiative of private individuals. For the Public Health and Marine Hospital Service, however, the Owen bill represented a threat. Under it, the service would have been made a subordinate unit of a department covering a broad range of health activities.

When the Owen bill proved incapable of mustering significant support and came under fire as an attempt to create a "medical trust" through which the AMA and the federal government would control American health care, the service was able to turn the tide in favor of its own goals. After the sudden death of Surgeon General Walter Wyman, Congress passed legislation that significantly expanded the service's mandate and funded a new series of research initiatives. Now known simply as the Public Health Service, the agency bolstered its reputation with studies of major diseases. Most prominently, the PHS's Joseph Goldberger established that pellagra, a debilitating disease that afflicted large sections of the American South, was caused by a dietary deficiency.

The PHS also became deeply involved in the debate over compulsory health insurance. Insurance, the PHS maintained, should be administratively linked to public health efforts. By making the costs of illness apparent to the employers and governments that would have to contribute to insurance funds, compulsory insurance would draw attention to the need for preventive medicine and strengthen the case of public health work. Insurance should also be used to transform and streamline the practice of medicine. The existing marine hospital system, according the PHS's Benjamin Warren and Edgar Sydenstricker, offered a clear precedent for federal action.

The movement for compulsory health insurance, however, proved a failure. With the defeat of insurance proposals in California and New York, the issue was essentially banished from the political agenda. Organized medicine, meanwhile, was mobilized against insurance, which many physicians came to view as a significant threat. In a crucial sequencing of events, significant opposition to government involvement in health insurance emerged on both economic and ideological grounds before the American public had any real experience in using insurance to help cover the costs of medical services. World War I sealed the fate of compulsory health insurance, offering its opponents ideological ammunition that would prove extremely powerful. As we will see, the war had an opposite effect in the realm of public health, creating an immediate need for federal intervention against the debilitating diseases that threatened troops stationed in the South.

CHAPTER THREE

WAR AND ITS AFTERMATH

When the United States declared war against Germany in April 1917, the PHS was ready with plans for addressing wartime health threats. Under an executive order issued by President Woodrow Wilson, the service was made part of the US military. Within months, most of its prewar plans were being put into practice. The service's efforts focused on war industries, venereal disease control, and the management of diseases such as malaria around military encampments in the South.

Working with the army's ordnance department, PHS officers examined hygienic conditions in a number of explosives factories. In West Virginia, the PHS helped build the town of Nitro, which supplied gunpowder for the war effort. There, service officers examined job applicants, vaccinated new employees, installed a water and sewer system, and examined housing conditions. In addition to public health work, they provided individual medical services to Nitro residents.[1] The effort in Nitro was unique but indicative of the importance accorded to the health of workers in an essential industry. The PHS's effort against venereal disease, meanwhile, got off to a somewhat slow start. Viewing the problem as one of education, regulation, and criminal enforcement, the service focused on providing expert advice to state governments. As the nation mobilized, the PHS entered into agreements in which it detailed officers to state health departments, who in turn paid half of their salaries.

In terms of personnel, planning, and public prestige, the most significant component of the PHS's wartime work was its effort to confront the daunting health problems of the Southern United States. Although most essential war industries were located in the industrial North, a significant number of industrial sites were located in the South. In addition, a disproportionate number of military encampments were located in the region, where training would be less hampered by the threat of cold weather.[2]

Endemic malaria, hookworm, typhoid, and the South's underdeveloped public health infrastructure quickly became pressing issues of national concern. Although the federal government had not previously engaged in large-scale domestic public health work, the PHS, with the support of Congress

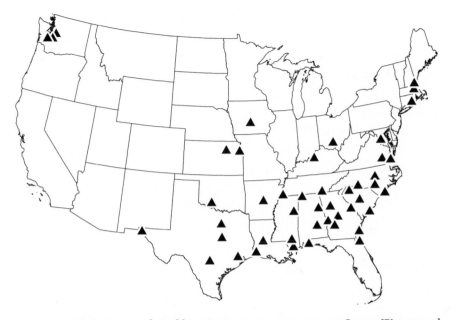

Figure 3.1. Headquarters of World War I extracantonment zones. *Source:* Warren and Bolduan, "War Activities of the United States Public Health Service."

and the president, moved quickly to establish a series of extracantonment zones, or areas of intensive public health work in the civilian areas surrounding military installations. By the end of the war, the PHS oversaw public health work in forty-eight extracantonment zones. All but nine were located in the South (Figure 3.1).[3]

Particularly for young PHS officers, the war was a transformational experience, suggesting an exciting new direction for the service. In its aftermath, the PHS proposed an ambitious postwar program, which sought to establish a role for the service in promoting health both in industry and in rural America. Benjamin Warren, author along with Edgar Sydenstricker of the service's report on health insurance, began calling for a "unified health service," capable of bringing together the nation's disparate health efforts, coordinating health work across political jurisdictions, and bridging the gap between public health and individual medicine.

Ultimately, Congress did not adopt the PHS's postwar program. Although the service imagined a powerful role for itself in promoting health among American workers, it had little political support in industrialized states, where local authorities were already creating high-quality public health institutions. As a result of its work in the wartime extracantonment zones, however, the service could now count on significant support from the Southern states where diseases such as malaria played an important role in restraining economic development. Working with the PHS, South Carolina Democrat Asbury "Frank" Lever introduced a Rural Health bill, which would have placed the PHS in charge of a program of federal assistance to states and localities for the development of local public health infrastructure. The Republican takeover of Congress in 1919 ensured that this bill, whose base of support came from Southern Democrats, would not become law. Nonetheless, the PHS was able to build on its wartime effort in important ways. Indeed, the wartime extracantonment effort provided the basis for a new initiative that would ultimately help to transform the role of the federal government in American public health.

Public Health Efforts in Extracantonment Zones

The PHS's domestic efforts during World War I were both unprecedented and wide-ranging. Sanitary work was undertaken in 170 shipyards, and inspections were conducted in a wide variety of industrial locations. The service's extracantonment effort, which was concentrated in the South, encompassed an estimated population of 3.75 million people. In many areas, health conditions were desperate. Throughout the region, what local services existed were completely overwhelmed by an influx of civilian workers, who lived in low-quality temporary housing, often unscreened against mosquitoes and without access to safe water or to sanitary privies.[4] Active public health work was rudimentary at best in most extracantonment zones, and successfully monitoring health conditions required the creation of new systems of disease surveillance.[5]

PHS officer Leslie Lumsden supervised the extracantonment effort, which was in many ways an improvised affair. A charismatic leader and native of Virginia, Lumsden had long been interested in developing a program for improving health conditions in rural America. He was particularly interested in typhoid, and in 1910 he worked with Charles Wardell Stiles to create the privy model that the RSC attempted to persuade rural Southerners to build. In 1911, after investigating a typhoid outbreak, Lumsden persuaded the government of Yakima County, Washington, to begin funding a health department, among the first effective rural public health departments in the nation.[6]

After the 1912 expansion of the service's research mandate, Lumsden pushed for increased funding for his research into the nation's rural health problems, securing a $25,000 appropriation for "studies of rural sanitation" in 1916. With the money, Lumsden began surveying health conditions in typhoid-prone rural counties in the South, Border States, and Midwest.[7] This effort proved short-lived, however. When the United States entered the war, Lumsden and his small staff were detailed to the war effort.[8]

Thomas Parran Jr., a freshly commissioned officer, was among those under Lumsden's command at the time. Later, Parran would play a key role in the development of the Social Security Act. As surgeon general under presidents Roosevelt and Truman, he was often at the center of major developments in American health policy, including the creation of the Communicable Disease Center (CDC), expansion of the NIH, passage of the 1946 Hill–Burton hospital construction act, and crucial debates over the role of the federal government in individual medical services.

First assigned to extracantonment work around Ft. Worth, Parran was placed in charge of the crucial effort around Muscle Shoals, Alabama, in 1918. As he later recalled, the extent of the PHS's authority was often far from clear. In most cases, PHS officers were deputized as agents of state boards of heath as a means of circumventing concerns about the constitutionality of the intervention. Although PHS officers possessed "some powers of enforcement," Parran later explained, they tended to use them only sparingly: "In those days in the South there still were memories of the Civil War, and the federal officer coming around to tell them what to do was not very palatable."[9]

Leslie Lumsden, Parran recalled, would pay "periodic visits to try to help us with whatever problems seemed to be most urgent, figuratively to give us aid and encouragement, hold our hands, and give us support. He was the supervisor and a very wise, old man."[10] On the ground, the American Red Cross proved a key resource, providing funding, equipment, and personnel. In particular, home visits by Red Cross nurses helped PHS officials to build community trust and support.[11]

Malaria Control

Extracantonment work included the building of privies, vaccination against smallpox, administration of diphtheria antitoxin, efforts aimed at controlling typhoid, and efforts aimed at providing clean water and safe milk. Although record-keeping was at times spotty, the service recorded 260,338 vaccinations against smallpox during the war and 435,066 inoculations against typhoid.[12] Venereal disease control was also a major concern, and the Red Cross provided funding for clinics.[13]

Extracantonment zones were concentrated in the South, however, for a straightforward reason: the threat of malaria. In the years after 1912, the service began documenting the region's malaria problem. Because most of the affected states were outside of the Census Bureau's Death Registration Area, this was a difficult task. As of 1917, only a general outline of the disease's incidence was available. Worse, Southern officials had done little to address it. "There are few diseases," Assistant Surgeon General John Trask wrote in 1916, "to which health departments have given so little attention."[14] Southerners, he believed, simply accepted malaria's presence. In contrast to newly recognized problems such as pellagra, the disease offered little drama. While "an exotic disease which threatens invasion or an occasional malady of which little is known will arouse a general clamor," Trask lamented, "ailments which are widely prevalent and are thoroughly understood receive the most meager attention."[15]

The situation was a difficult one, but the PHS possessed much of the expertise necessary to begin controlling malaria. Assistant Surgeon General Henry Rose Carter was among the nation's leading experts on mosquito-borne disease. A Virginian, Carter was considered for a Nobel Prize for his research into the role of mosquitoes in transmitting disease. He had joined the PHS in 1879, and most of his early assignments were to quarantine positions on the Gulf Coast. In Cuba, his theory of the extrinsic incubation of yellow fever influenced the work of Walter Reed, leader of the Yellow Fever Commission, that determined that the disease was spread by mosquitoes. In Panama, he served as chief quarantine officer from the beginning of the American effort until 1909.[16]

Joseph A. LePrince, who oversaw most of the service's wartime antimalaria work, had been at the center of American efforts against mosquito-borne disease since Havana. First in Cuba and then in Panama, LePrince was William Gorgas's "right hand" in fighting yellow fever and malaria. His 1915 book, *Mosquito Control in Panama*, "was to remain a bible for mosquito control workers for many years."[17] A preeminent figure in public health, he returned to the United States after the completion of the canal, joining the PHS in the newly created position of senior sanitary engineer.

In Panama, LePrince and other officials possessed a great deal of leeway. Behaviors that heightened the likelihood of infection, such as sitting out at night, could be sharply regulated. His powers were far more limited in the United States, although the approach remained broadly similar. The PHS's work focused on draining low-lying areas and oiling the ponds where *Anopheles* mosquitoes bred. A heavy emphasis was placed on ensuring that mosquitoes would not breed within flight range of military installations. Screening windows, a highly effective means of ensuring that individuals would not become infected, were an important component of the work in Cuba and Panama. In the United States, however, the cost of screening and concerns about compliance and maintenance generally meant that screening was not a major aspect of the extracantonment effort.

PHS officials working in extracantonment zones concentrated heavily on cultivating the support of local governments, political leaders, and businessmen. In addition to financial support from the Red Cross, money from local governments was typically required for an extracantonment effort to function. Seeking to build local support, PHS officers highlighted the long-term economic benefits of malaria control. Ridding the South of malaria, they argued, would increase agricultural output and allow for the development of new industries. Consistently pushed by PHS officials, such arguments would become ubiquitous.

By the end of the war, according to Joseph LePrince, the region's leaders were well aware of the full economic impact of malaria on the South. Southern business interests, he maintained, had been made "fully aware that an absence of mosquitoes has an important bearing on the availability and efficiency of skilled and unskilled labor as well as on the proper development of real-estate values."[18] In addition to being a patriotic duty, malaria control was now understood as an investment that would provide very real financial benefits: "The President of a large association of cotton-mill interests has stated that the elimination of mosquitoes near the mill properties has paid a higher return on the money expended than any other investment that the corporation has ever made."[19]

Along with many others in the PHS, Joseph LePrince viewed the service's wartime efforts as a stepping-stone to an expanded postwar effort against malaria. Not just the South, he argued, but the entire nation could be persuaded to embrace the economic virtues of large-scale malaria control. Even Northern industry could be mobilized in support of such a program. "The business interests of the North," LePrince suggested in a burst of optimism, "will be quick to see that if we reduce malaria in the South by 100,000 or 1,000,000 or more cases, that just so much more earning capacity (now dormant) will be created." Increased purchasing power in the South would have significant financial benefits: "The Northern manufacturer will have an increased market for his products and the Northern laborer will prosper."[20]

LePrince's optimism was fueled by the service's clear successes. Ultimately, the PHS concluded that its efforts eliminated *Anopheles* mosquito breeding from over 12,000 square miles.[21] Within the extracantonment zones, only 3,160 malaria cases were reported during the 1918 malaria season. Although this figure was likely less than comprehensive, and data from earlier years were sketchy at best, the small case rate appeared to indicate that antimalaria activities were having a significant impact. "From such data as are obtainable from previous years," the service concluded, "this was a tremendous reduction in the malarial rate in these communities. These results may well be compared with those in Panama, especially since they were obtained, not under military conditions but through the voluntary work of a civil population."[22]

"A Unified Health Service"

The PHS's generally successful wartime effort was punctuated by the fall 1918 wave of the Spanish flu epidemic. Striking first in Boston, the disease spread along railroad lines and other transportation routes. It hit naval bases, army installations, and training camps with particular ferocity. Cramped military quarters, filled beyond capacity with men from all over the nation, served as incubators of the disease.[23] The mounting severity of the situation was compounded by an acute shortage of physicians and nurses, many of whom were serving in the military.

Pressed for help by officials from state governments, Congress appropriated $1 million to be used by the PHS to fight influenza in October 1918.[24] Already stretched past its limit, the PHS was forced to appeal for help in staffing its effort to the AMA and the Volunteer Medical Corps, an organization created by the Council of National Defense. Although it worked to create state-level organizations for combating the disease, the PHS's response to the epidemic was generally chaotic.

Most control efforts were directed by local governments, which focused on limiting public group interactions. The Red Cross, for its part, provided vital nursing care. In many areas, schools, churches, theaters, and dance halls were closed down. In some, quarantine and isolation measures were put in place. Though such efforts at times proved effective, the disease's virulence and the need to continue supplying the war effort ensured that it would continue to spread. Typically, the incidence of influenza rose again in areas where restrictions on public meetings were relaxed. Ultimately, between 500,000 and 676,000 people died in the United States. Between 50 and 100 million died worldwide.[25]

In November, with the influenza epidemic still raging, the war came to an end. For the Public Health Service, this was a critical moment. PHS officers were engaged in an unprecedented attempt to contain public health threats at home. Congress's willingness to look to the service as a means of controlling the influenza epidemic, meanwhile, indicated a significant degree of confidence in its capabilities. Already the PHS had persuaded Congress to create a reserve officer corps, a long-standing service goal. By executive order, the Treasury Department had been placed in charge of all nonmilitary health functions of the federal government. Earlier in 1918, Congress had passed the Chamberlain–Kahn Act, authorizing new expenditures for venereal disease control and education. An Interdepartmental Social Hygiene Board, comprising the surgeons general of the army, navy, and PHS, would administer the funding, which required state matching grants. Congress also funded the creation of a new venereal disease division within the PHS.[26]

The end of the war represented both an opportunity and a threat. The service might emerge stronger, or it might find its budget trimmed and authority rolled back. On December 3, 1918, the PHS sent Congress its plan for building on the wartime effort and transforming the service into a comprehensive agency aimed at improving the health of Americans in a variety of realms. Its two central proposals were for a grant-in-aid program aimed at improving health and safety conditions in industry and for a grant-in-aid program aimed at promoting the development of county health departments in rural areas.[27]

The industrial hygiene component of the PHS plan had little chance of becoming law. Some aspects of it were mundane, such as proposals that the wartime surveys of health conditions in industry be continued and that funding be directed toward improving the collection of vital statistics. Others, such as a proposal to create federal minimum health and safety standards for industry in cooperation with the Department of Labor, challenged the limits of federal power as it stood at the end of the 1910s.

Notably, the plan pushed beyond public health and into the realm of individual medical services, suggesting a role for the PHS and cooperating state and local governments in ensuring access to medical care for workers. Under one component of the plan, the PHS would direct the development of "adequate systems of medical and surgical supervision of employees in places of employment."[28] Although the full meaning of the proposal was left somewhat vague, its precedent was apparently the PHS's intensive sanitary and medical effort in Nitro, West Virginia, during the war. There was essentially no prospect that such an effort would receive congressional backing in the absence of the war emergency.

More realistic was the service's plan for extending the extracantonment effort into the postwar period, which centered on the creation of a grant-in-aid program aimed at stimulating the development of county health departments in rural America. Under the plan, the PHS, states, and localities would jointly fund rural health departments. The PHS would detail officers to help in the development of new infrastructure and to target specific problems such unsafe milk, contaminated water supplies, and a lack of sanitary privies. Following the precedent set during the war, the officer in charge of a local health department, along with the department's sanitary inspectors and public health nurses, would be appointed a field agent in the PHS. By these means, state, local, and national health work could be coordinated.[29]

Like the PHS's industrial hygiene proposal, the service's plan for "rural hygiene" blurred the lines between public health and individual medicine. In addition to federal assistance for preventive health work aimed at populations, the plan pointed out the importance of "bedside control of cases of communicable disease." Individual medical services for those with contagious diseases, this suggested, would be conceived of as part of an enlarged public health program. This was a provocative proposal, which Benjamin Warren would soon flesh out in greater detail.[30]

Along with its proposals for confronting disease in industry and in rural America, the PHS's postwar plan contained a variety of smaller measures. Among them were proposals for cooperation with the Children's Bureau and the Red Cross on the issue of infant and child mortality, a national effort to stimulate water purification work and provide clean water supplies, a national program for controlling malaria, the extension of venereal disease control efforts, and a new program for collecting morbidity statistics.

It was an ambitious proposal, but PHS officials were confident. Benjamin Warren, author with Edgar Sydenstricker of the PHS's 1916 report on health insurance, was a prominent and articulate advocate. Recently promoted to the rank of assistant surgeon general, Warren had earlier helped draft and push for the 1902 and 1912 bills expanding the PHS's mandate. The PHS's new postwar proposal, he maintained, should provide the basis for moving the United States toward what he termed a unified health service.

Speaking in his home state of Alabama in January 1919, Warren cited fellow Alabaman William Gorgas's successes in Panama and the wartime extracantonment effort as precedents for a more integrated national approach to combating disease. The federal government, states, and localities, he asserted, all possessed similar interests in ensuring the health of their people, and diseases had no interest in respecting political boundaries. A "case of typhoid fever in a remote rural district of Alabama," he maintained, "is a matter of joint interest to the county, State, and Federal health authorities. The typhoid germ does not recognize county or State lines and may well find its way into intra- and interstate traffic and cause the loss of many human lives and the expenditure of large sums of State and Federal funds." The "rational procedure," Warren continued, would be to form an intergovernmental partnership "and prevent or control all preventable diseases at their source."[31]

Preventing infant mortality was possible, Warren asserted, and the nation's mothers would certainly be willing to pay for it. Preventing malaria was also possible, and controlling the disease would easily pay for itself through the economic energy it would unleash. Public officials should not, however, think only in terms of prevention. "In these days of progress in preventive medicine," Warren warned, "there is some tendency to separate too sharply the preventive from curative medicine." Prevention as it was generally understood was only one side of the coin, however: "It should not be forgotten that an adequate medical service to the whole people will do more to prevent disease and disability than any other single measure to be considered."[32]

Warren had previously argued that public financing of medical services through compulsory health insurance would make the costs of sickness more visible, resulting in an increased focus on public health work. Now he went a step further, expanding on the PHS's postwar program and explicitly redefining curative medical services as a critical aspect of public health work. The United States, Warren asserted, was already spending more than enough money on drugs, physicians, and hospital care. If the system were reorganized and rationalized, access could be guaranteed to everyone. "With a proper organization, distribution, and training of the medical and sanitary personnel of the country, and a proper expenditure of the funds now being spent for medical purposes, there would be available, to every person, adequate medical and hospital services and supplies." With such a system of medical services "closely coordinated with, or forming part of, the health department, it needs no argument to show that disease prevention would begin at the source—the bedside, and eliminate a large proportion of disease spread."[33] The vision of governmental responsibility for health articulated by Warren and embodied in the PHS's postwar program was a sweeping one. Ensuring access to health care for all Americans, Warren maintained, was possible. In addition, curing disease was the best means of ensuring that contagious diseases would not spread. Government should be involved in reorganizing medical services in order to ensure that these goals could be met.

Warren was well aware of the limitations of any health program, particularly one that attempted to unify prevention and cure across a variety of political jurisdictions. A "perfect health machine," he admitted, "is not to be expected." Instead, a "unified health service" should "be planned so that it will be elastic and easily adjusted, as changing conditions or experience of operation may indicate."[34] Inevitably, different levels of government and agencies within governments would possess different formal responsibilities. Where there was overlap or potential conflict, government agencies should strive to cooperate.

Private philanthropy, however, was problematic. Over the preceding decade, both the Carnegie Foundation and the Rockefeller Foundation had become deeply involved in American medicine, financing public health work, new research efforts, and pushing for a reorganization of American medical education. In 1916, the Rockefeller Foundation funded the creation of a school of public health at Johns Hopkins.[35] Warren viewed these developments as troublesome. More than just an issue in terms of coordination, Warren suggested that philanthropy and charity might at times represent a threat to democratic control of governing institutions. Such concerns were becoming commonplace as huge amounts of private money poured into America's health care system. Although there was a role for philanthropy to play, Warren maintained, the danger posed by such groups should not be ignored. Private entities were in some instances "exercising some sort of direction in Government health affairs." This was not acceptable: "In a democratic government there should be no agency directing governmental administration which is not responsible to the people. Such agencies must be controlled and made auxiliary to Government administration."[36]

The Lever Rural Health Bill

While the PHS's plan for expanding its role in industrial hygiene had no obvious political base, the service had forged fairly strong relationships with Southern state and local governments over the course of the war. In its aftermath, the economic significance of disease in the region, and particularly of malaria, proved a major theme of the service's push for an expanded mandate. Like hookworm control, service officers explained, malaria control needed to be aimed at both black and white Southerners if the region's agricultural and industrial productivity was to be improved. The PHS's arguments were often paternalistic, but in framing disease as an economic issue, PHS officers tied together the interests of elites and of the South's most marginalized residents.[37]

The service found its most influential postwar supporter in Asbury "Frank" Lever, a Democratic congressman from South Carolina and chairman of the House agriculture committee. Coordinating with the PHS and its supporters in the American Public Health Association (APHA), Lever moved to introduce legislation that would bring the "rural hygiene" aspect of the service's postwar proposal into being. His proposed Rural Health bill would authorize an initial $250,000 for cooperative health work, which would in time grow to $1 million a year.[38]

Surgeon General Rupert Blue soon began contacting state health officers, forwarding copies of the Lever bill and requesting that they ask their state legislatures for appropriations for rural health work "contingent upon the appropriation of a similar amount by the federal government."[39] APHA president and North Carolina state board of health head Watson Rankin also contacted the nation's health officers and asked for their help in ensuring that the legislation was passed. State health officers were asked to lobby their elected representatives either in person or through the mail. Prominent citizens, he suggested, should be persuaded to write their senators and representatives. Farm demonstration agents and farmers' organizations should be mobilized, as should the press.[40]

Congressman Lever, it was agreed, was an ideal sponsor for the legislation. Eager to continue the flow of federal money into South Carolina, he was a driving force behind the 1914 Smith–Lever Agricultural Extension Act, which created a cooperative program between the federal government and land grant universities intended to "carry practical scientific information about farming and home economics to farm families."[41] As APHA's Watson Rankin noted, Lever had "taken a leading, I might say initial, part in federal aid extension legislation. He is an experienced legislator, and an expert in legislation directed to the rural interests." The "prospects for this bill passing Congress during its present session," Rankin concluded, "are exceptionally bright."[42]

Rankin's mention of the "present session," however, hinted at trouble. In November 1918, with the nation still at war, the Republican Party won control of both the House of Representatives and the Senate. The party would take control of Congress in March 1919, meaning that Lever, a Democrat, would lose his position as chair of the House agriculture committee.

In February, PHS officers appeared before Lever's House committee on agriculture, where they received a generally favorable hearing. Making the case for the Rural Health bill were J. W. Schereschewsky, the assistant surgeon general in charge of scientific research, and Leslie Lumsden, the man who had overseen the extracantonment effort and who now hoped to head up the new program. As part of the war effort, Congress raised the appropriation for Lumsden's rural sanitation program, increasing it to $150,000. Now he hoped for a clear mandate to begin an expanded program based on the extracantonment intervention.

Explaining the need for federal aid in improving rural public health capabilities, Lumsden emphasized the economic impact of disease in the South. Although pervasive, the diseases that plagued the region were subtle in their cruelty. Under current conditions, he noted, the full extent of hookworm's reach was difficult to establish. "There are so many cases we do not know of. Persons are affected, a little below par, pulled down a little, anemic, incapacitated but able to keep going at a reduced rate. The economic loss from hookworm is tremendous."[43] Malaria's impact on day-to-day life was similarly subtle, and also devastating: "A man with chronic malaria, though able to keep going, only goes at half speed." He did not know of anything, Lumsden contended, "from an economical standpoint, that we can make as strong an argument for as we can for this health business."[44]

Failure of the Lever Bill

The window of opportunity for the PHS's postwar program was brief. The service's plan for an expanded role in industrial hygiene was set aside fairly quickly, given the lack of support in Congress. By March 1919, when the new Republican Congress was sworn in, the Lever Rural Health bill had still not moved forward in Congress. PHS officials nonetheless remained optimistic, and Congressman Lever reintroduced the legislation. The rural sanitation program's Leslie Lumsden, still anticipating that the bill would become law, directed his men to continue pursuing cooperative projects with local officials. Reports from what were still being called extracantonment zones, meanwhile, were generally positive.[45]

Nonetheless, the political context was unwelcoming. In response to the wartime growth of the national government, Republicans in Congress were pursuing a policy of retrenchment. The Southern Democrats who were the staunchest supporters of the Rural Health bill held little influence in the new Congress. By June, when the nation's state and territorial health officers came to Washington for their annual conference with the surgeon general, the PHS's confidence had been significantly diminished. Urging the health officers to meet with their political representatives while in Washington, APHA president Watson Rankin and the PHS's Leslie Lumsden both noted that the service had a solid backup plan. The state health officers should tell their congressional representatives to support the PHS's request to Congress that, if the Lever bill was not passed, the existing appropriation for rural sanitation be expanded from $150,000 to $500,000. "In case the Lever bill should fail to pass," Rankin told the health officers, "our only chance is in getting through this appropriation of $500,000 which is contained in the sundry civil bill."[46]

The sectional implications of the Rural Health bill were laid bare at the meeting of state and territorial health officers, with representatives from more industrialized states expressing skepticism. "To be perfectly frank between ourselves," the health officer from Massachusetts told the meeting, "there are some States that are not financially benefited by this act. My state is one of them. We stand to lose." The Rural Health bill would redistribute resources away from industrialized states and toward those where public health capabilities remained underdeveloped. Some members of the Massachusetts congressional delegation had informed him they would either support or remain neutral on the bill, but "others have come out very frankly and flatly said they were getting rather tired (to use the exact phrase that one Congressman used) of having $2 of Massachusetts money taken out of the taxpayers of Massachusetts, about 25 cents of it returned in the form of Federal aid, and the rest distributed over the South, the West, and the Middle West."[47]

Ohio's public health commissioner, Dr. Allen Freeman, acknowledged and attempted to justify the sectional nature of the Rural Health bill. Earlier in the decade, he had served as the director of the RSC's antihookworm work in Virginia.[48] "So far as Federal Aid is concerned," Freeman told his fellow state health officers, "I think we can get along in Ohio without it." Still, he realized, "having worked a large part of my time in the South, that a Federal subsidy supplemented by a State subsidy is of the greatest value in stimulating the progress of the work." "There are many counties in the South," he continued, "whose economic condition is such as to make it wholly impossible for them, without some sort of aid, to sustain an adequate health administration." The benefits for the South were clear, but the

Rural Health bill would benefit the entire nation: "It is not a question of north or south. Rhode Island and South Carolina and Ohio and Texas are all tied together in the same bag, and we are going to progress in sanitation as in every other line just so far as we progress together."[49]

The next month, the discussion over the sectional implications of the bill became moot. In July, Representative Lever accepted an appointment from President Wilson to fill a vacant position on the federal farm loan board.[50] Though PHS officials such as Benjamin Warren continued to hope that the nation might somehow begin moving toward a "unified health service," the PHS's postwar push for expansion had ended with a whimper.[51] The Rural Health bill, the aspect of the service's plan with the most realistic chance of becoming law, ran up against a new Congress uninterested in expanding the wartime effort. Ultimately, the bill even lost its sponsor, who did not wish to continue serving in Congress without the power he had possessed as chair of the House agriculture committee.

Rural Sanitation

As the PHS's plans for postwar expansion stalled, service officers nonetheless worked to build on the wartime intervention in the South as best they could. In late June 1919, with the new fiscal year swiftly approaching, Surgeon General Rupert Blue and Assistant Surgeon General J. W. Schereschewsky appeared before the Senate Appropriations Committee, requesting that $150,000 be appropriated for the service's rural sanitation program rather than the $50,000 that had been allowed by the House. The committee appeared indifferent. Warned that "we have a list of engagements and ask you to be as brief as possible," Blue and Schereschewsky made short statements. They received only one question, from Senator Reed Smoot, a well-known opponent of federal growth in the realm of health: "You want $150,000 instead of $50,000?"[52]

When the appropriations bill was finally passed, the appropriation for rural sanitation, raised to $150,000 during the war, was lowered to $50,000.[53] Leslie Lumsden, who had envisioned heading a large-scale program that would build up the nation's rural health capabilities and put them on a pace to begin catching up with developments in urban areas, was supremely disappointed. "On account of the reduction in the appropriation," an irritated Lumsden wrote, "the work in a considerable number of areas in which it was yielding excellent results had to be discontinued."[54]

The PHS's work combating disease in the extracantonment zones would be dramatically scaled back, and Congress had declined to authorize the hoped-for grant-in-aid program for the development of local public health infrastructure in rural America. Still, it was not a total defeat. A $50,000 appropriation for "studies" of rural sanitation was clearly better than nothing. Lumsden, for his part, was unwilling to take the defeat as a sign of Congress's intention to limit his work.

More and more, Lumsden and other PHS leaders simply asserted that both the Constitution and the service's existing mandate already allowed for a quite expansive federal health role. Speaking in May 1919, Lumsden argued that poor sanitary conditions in the rural areas of one state were, "through commerce and otherwise, a menace to contiguous States especially; and, on account of modern transportation facilities, a menace to the whole country." Disease was by its nature an interstate issue, uninterested in political boundaries. Moreover, it suppressed labor productivity and constrained the nation's potential military might. The implications, Lumsden argued, were obvious: "The problem of rural sanitation appears to be one with which the National Government under constitutional authority may deal, and one with which the National Government from a standpoint of general welfare should deal.[55]

Benjamin Warren, writing later in the year, explained that the service did not have to wait for its program to be adopted or for legislation such as the Lever bill to be passed to begin building a unified health service. Already, he claimed, the PHS possessed "all of the authority" that it could be granted under the Constitution for "the investigation of the diseases of man and for the control of contagious and infectious diseases." The Lever bill would have helped the PHS to carry out its goals, but the absence of legislation did not mean that the service lacked the authority to act. The limitations that the PHS faced were not statutory or constitutional but rather financial. What the service needed, Warren argued, was "money and men."[56]

In July 1919, with the new fiscal year beginning, the Lever Rural Health bill a receding dream, and his funding dramatically scaled back, Lumsden began to build a new program out of the relationships with state and local officials that the PHS had developed during the war emergency. Rather than reverting to the "studies" of the prewar period, Lumsden devoted the first postwar appropriation for rural sanitation to funding county health work in thirty-one counties. Like the extracantonment zone effort itself, the regional tilt of the counties selected was unmistakable: all but one of the counties was located in the states of the former Confederacy or in the Border States. The exception was a county in southeastern Kansas that was made part of a tristate sanitary district encompassing an Ozark mining area that included parts of Kansas, Missouri, and Oklahoma.[57] The PHS's postwar plan had not become a reality, but Lumsden was determined to continue to build on the wartime effort even as the nation sought a return to normalcy.

CHAPTER FOUR

"SOME VERY DANGEROUS PRECEDENTS"

The fervor for change that seized the PHS's leadership in the aftermath of the war dissipated swiftly. In 1920, Treasury Secretary Carter Glass persuaded an ailing President Wilson to replace Surgeon General Rupert Blue with Hugh Cumming, a Virginian known for his reserved demeanor and political agility. Though Glass also considered Leslie Lumsden for the position, Cumming and Lumsden held distinctly different views about the role that the service should play in American life. In contrast to Lumsden and men such as Benjamin Warren and Edgar Sydenstricker, Cumming was satisfied with the status quo. Beyond this, he was highly attuned to the limitations imposed by the new political climate.[1] To a great extent, the ascendency of Cumming and election of Republican Warren G. Harding in 1920 signaled the end of the PHS's push for extended power and authority.

The PHS faced significant challenges in the postwar period. Placed in charge of the care of wounded veterans, the service found itself overwhelmed and publically criticized. In 1921, the service warned of a coming pellagra outbreak in the South, sparking an unexpected backlash from Southern politicians who took offense at the idea that the region was plagued by malnutrition. The same year, the Department of Labor's Children's Bureau won passage of the Sheppard–Towner Act, a program of federal assistance to states for improving the health of mothers and children. Officially opposed by the PHS and anathema to Surgeon General Cumming, Sheppard–Towner underlined the service's failure to achieve its own postwar aims and appeared likely to aggrandize the Children's Bureau at the expense of the service.

The service's rural sanitation initiative, however, gradually emerged as an unexpected area of success. Growing out of the wartime extracantonment effort and the failure of the Lever Rural Health bill, Leslie Lumsden's program steadily built on the service's relationships with local officials in the South. Embracing a broad vision of the role of the federal government in stimulating local health work, Lumsden was a fierce critic of the idea that health efforts should be strictly divided into separate realms dealing with public health and individual medicine. Although Surgeon General Cumming ultimately marginalized him, Lumsden's efforts during the 1920s would help to provide the framework for later federal expansion. The PHS's future leadership, meanwhile, would largely comprise men who at some point served under him.

When a massive flood overtook the lower Mississippi Valley in 1927, the PHS presented Lumsden's rural sanitation initiative as the solution to the area's mounting public health problems, leading to an extension of the program. When a severe drought hit the same area three years later, it grew even further. Although Lumsden had worked to move the rural sanitation program beyond its Southern origins, these disasters ensured that the region's severe health issues remained its central focus. The program itself remained relatively small scale, but the precedents it created had significant long-term implications. When Southern Democrats gained key leadership positions in Congress during the New Deal, their support would help place the proponents of expanding the PHS's role in a position to transform the rural sanitation program into a fully national program for stimulating and coordinating local-level public health work.

Postwar

The PHS faced a significant problem as the 1920s dawned: Congress had placed it in control of hospital care for wounded and injured war veterans. Writing immediately after the end of the war, Assistant Surgeon General Benjamin Warren suggested that this would prove a major benefit to the service, furnishing "wonderful opportunities for developing better methods of treatment and prevention of disease, especially tuberculosis and neuro-psychiatric."[2] Although the PHS remained at its core an organization that provided hospitalization services, it proved unprepared for the task. The funding provided, meanwhile, proved inadequate. As the PHS found itself overwhelmed, complaints from veterans about poor treatment and dangerous conditions in makeshift hospitals threated the service's growing reputation for competency. President Warren G. Harding transferred responsibility for the hospitalization of veterans to the newly created Veterans' Bureau in 1922. It was an embarrassing turn of events, but one that nearly everyone within the service greeted as a great relief.[3] The new Veterans' Bureau, meanwhile, developed its own problems. Charles Forbes, the man chosen by President Warren G. Harding to head it, ended up in prison after embezzling as much as $250 million.[4]

The service's struggles to provide adequate care to veterans were soon complemented by another major public relations problem. In the spring and summer of 1921, a postwar crash in cotton prices severely constrained the ability of rural Southerners to obtain meat and dairy products. With leading pellagra expert Joseph Goldberger concerned that the South faced a potential epidemic, the PHS released a public statement requesting that Congress appropriate funds to help stave off nutritional problems in the region. President Harding, alerted to the situation, wrote an open letter to Surgeon General Cumming.

Supportive of the PHS's request, the president used language that ended up backfiring spectacularly. "I have been greatly concerned," he wrote, "to note the public statement from the Public Health Service as to the menace of pellagra and condition of at least semi-famine in a large section of the cotton belt." The situation was similar to that faced in parts of Europe as a result of the war. "Famine and plague are words almost foreign to our American vocabulary, save as we have learned their meaning in connection with the afflictions of lands less favored and toward which our people have so many times displayed large and generous charity." The PHS and the Red Cross, Harding suggested, should work together to ease the danger that the collapse of cotton prices represented to Southern health.[5]

Southern political leaders responded bitterly. From Virginia to Texas, local officials, including some who had already publically backed the PHS's dire assessment of the situation, denounced Harding's statement, denying "any unusual number of cases of pellagra, or that 'semi-famine,' or any economic condition resembling it existed."[6] In Georgia, the state senate introduced and unanimously passed a resolution "denouncing the reports and asserting that Georgia was not affected by this disease to any appreciable extent." Both Alabama and Virginia asserted that incidence of pellagra had decreased in comparison with the previous year.[7]

The PHS's Goldberger-led pellagra research had long been a point of strength. Now it became something of a liability. In Congress, Southern representatives demanded an investigation into Goldberger's and the PHS's statements on the disease. South Carolina's James Byrnes wrote President Harding to assure him that the people of the South were not "menaced with famine and are not seeking charity," though he acknowledged that "pellagra may have increased in some one or in several States." When the president learned the facts, Byrnes hoped, he would rescind his earlier statement about "famine and plague" and "take appropriate action toward the officials who by misrepresenting conditions mislead you into making the statement."[8]

The enactment of the Sheppard–Towner Act in November 1921 further accentuated the sting of these struggles.[9] A federal grant-in-aid program, through which the federal government provided money to states on the condition that they offered matching funds and followed federal stipulations, Sheppard–Towner was aimed at improving the health of mothers and children. It was to be administered by the Children's Bureau, the Department of Labor–based agency that secured its passage.

For many within the PHS, the Children's Bureau and the issue of infant and maternal health were sensitive subjects. In 1911, advocates for improving infant and maternal health successfully pushed for the creation of a federal agency devoted to the issue. The Public Health and Marine Hospital Service was considered as a potential home for the agency, but Surgeon General Walter Wyman rejected the idea. As public health scholar Wilson Smillie later recounted it, Wyman was at his core "a gruff, grumpy Marine Hospital officer whose major concern was with the police powers of port quarantine and with the surgical treatment of sailors." When confronted with the possibility of overseeing what became the Children's Bureau, Wyman "was most emphatic in his refusal to complicate his life with the importunities of a group of sentimental women who were interested solely in the welfare of mothers and infants."[10] With Wyman opposed, the bureau ended up in the Department of Labor.[11]

Wyman's successor, Rupert Blue, was more open to the idea of cooperating with the Children's Bureau. New surgeon general Cumming, however, tended to view the bureau with disdain. For Cumming, it was an unqualified agency, largely comprising social workers infringing inappropriately into the field of health. If funding for maternal and child health was to be made available by Congress, it should be controlled by the PHS.[12] Like the AMA, which also opposed the bill, Cumming believed laypeople should not administer health-related programs. He opposed the Sheppard–Towner Act in 1921, and would continue to do so until 1929, when Congress ceased funding the program under pressure from the AMA. Sheppard–Towner represented a double blow to the PHS. Opposed by the PHS leadership, the act created a new federal health program that would be under the control of an agency unaffiliated with the service and perceived by many as antagonistic to its interests. In securing congressional support for a major federal grant-in-aid program, meanwhile, the Children's Bureau had succeeded where the PHS had failed.

While PHS leaders had initially imagined a central role for the service in postwar American health policy, most of the energy in health policy came instead from private foundations, which continued working to reshape medical education, research, and the organization of health services.[13] Still, the service's retrenchment was far from total. It remained engaged in a variety of activities, and continued strong in traditional areas of action such as the operation of marine hospitals, medical support for the Coast Guard, and quarantine efforts. In 1921, the service finished its long-standing program of fully nationalizing quarantine efforts. In the same year, it took control of the previously state-operated leprosarium in Carville, Louisiana.[14] The service also continued to expand its assistance to the Bureau of Indian Affairs in providing health services to Native Americans.

Edgar Sydenstricker, meanwhile, initiated serious improvements in the service's statistical capabilities as head of its office of statistical investigations.[15] In 1921, he began a major long-term study of illness and health conditions of the population of Hagerstown, Maryland. As part of its work in the realm of public health administration, the service detailed a small number of officers to assist state public health departments. Although Congress ceased being particularly interested in venereal disease, completely defunding the wartime Chamberlain–Kahn program by 1926, the service's new venereal disease division continued to function.[16] After 1926, the division would be taken over by future surgeon general Thomas Parran, who breathed new life into the service's efforts in this critical area. The PHS's Hygienic Laboratory continued to grow in stature during the postwar years, with the service focused on emerging issues such as water pollution. It also continued to work on problems such as malaria, collaborating briefly with the Rockefeller International Health Board on a project aimed at ridding the disease from Southern towns.[17] In 1930, the Hygienic Laboratory would be renamed the National Institute of Health, a sign of major changes to come.

Rural Sanitation

Disappointed with the $50,000 postwar appropriation for "studies of rural sanitation," Leslie Lumsden was committed to making the best of the situation. In the months after the end of the war, his men had continued to ask state and local governments to put up money for local health departments. Local civic organizations, the Red Cross, and the Rockefeller IHB also demonstrated a willingness to work with the PHS.[18] Now Lumsden's goal was straightforward: to continue stimulating the development of local health infrastructure and building relationships with state and local governments.[19]

From the summer of 1919 on, the office of rural sanitation would focus on providing the organizational resources and expertise necessary for the development of county health departments. The program had only limited funding to disperse. As a result, outreach was crucial: if PHS officers could persuade county and state officials to match their contributions, funding for the program would be effectively tripled. Money from private groups such as the Rockefeller Foundation and the Red Cross, which hoped to extend its expanded wartime work into the postwar period, would also be critical. Several future leaders of the PHS worked under Lumsden during this crucial early period, including future surgeon general Thomas Parran and future assistant surgeon general Joseph Mountin, founding father of the CDC.

County health work began with attempts by PHS officers, working with the approval of the state board of health, to secure local financial and political support. Officers visited a county and met with prominent citizens, women's groups, civic organizations such as the chamber of commerce, the local Red Cross, and physicians' groups. With the backing of such groups secured, the officer would appear before the county commissioners (or local equivalent) to attempt to persuade them of the importance of county health work and to secure an appropriation.[20]

Warren Draper, a future assistant surgeon general, was in charge of the effort in Virginia. As Draper explained, it was important "to discuss the matter with the more enlightened citizens, and get them to come up and appear before the [county board of] supervisors." Early in his work, Draper had attempted to drum up enthusiasm for a county health department by gaining the support of residents from a part of one rural county who he had been warned were "ignorant and are satisfied to remain so." After listening to Draper's pitch, during which he asked them to attend the next meeting of the county supervisors and tell them "just what you think of what I said," a number of these citizens ("the most disreputable looking specimens of humanity that I have ever seen") appeared at the meeting.

As Draper recounted it, they loudly opposed the creation of a county health department, informing the supervisors that they believed Draper was only interested in riding "up and down the county in an automobile while we are paying for it with the sweat of our brows." After this, Draper reported, his faith in democracy was weakened, and he began focusing on cultivating support among local elites.[21]

Once the support of a county government was secured, a PHS representative or representative of the state board of health would conduct a survey of local sanitary conditions. After assessing the situation, the nascent county health board began implementing health measures developed by the PHS in an order suited to the particular circumstances of the county.[22] A full-time county health officer, ideally recruited as locally as possible, headed each PHS-backed cooperative county effort. The officer's staff typically consisted of a full-time sanitary inspector and nurse.[23] As during the war, public health nursing would play a key role in the rural sanitation program. Following the precedent set during the war, county health officers were appointed to a position both under the existing state board of health and under the PHS. "Thus," Lumsden explained, "his position is an example of common-sense coordination of the administrative features of the activities of the properly constituted local, State, and National governmental health agencies."[24]

As field agents of the PHS, county health officers maintained routine contact with the service and enjoyed access to its publications and findings in areas such as malaria control. They also enjoyed franking privileges, allowing them to provide free postage for local residents or physicians to mail fecal or blood specimens, either to the county health board or to state laboratories. Often they used PHS stationery.[25] Under these arrangements, federal, state, and local public health authorities were brought together in new ways, and any uncertainty about the proper limits or constitutionality of federal intervention in local public health matters could be brushed aside.

"In every instance," Lumsden wrote, emphasizing the point that the program did not represent an intrusion on state police powers, "the cooperation of the Public Health Service is extended only in response to formal requests from the proper governmental authorities of the county and from the State health department." In addition, Lumsden contended, demanding that the county health officer meet federal standards—rather than simply enjoying the favor of county commissioners or other notables—ensured that the post was less likely to be used for the purposes of political patronage.[26]

Initially centered in the South and Border States, the rural sanitation program soon expanded into the rural Midwest and West. Where it was deemed necessary, the program encompassed smaller towns and cities, bridging the gap between rural and urban health work.[27] By 1927, when a massive flood of the Mississippi River led to a significant expansion of the program, PHS-backed rural health work was being carried out in eighteen states. Along with work in the South and Border States, efforts were underway in California (two counties and one health district), Iowa (one county), Kansas (three), Montana (two), and New Mexico (eight). In an attempt to determine how the county-based form of organization used by the PHS could be adapted to governing institutions in New England, the office of rural sanitation also helped, beginning in 1921, in the development of local public health capabilities on Cape Cod.[28]

Lumsden believed that health efforts should be based in permanent governing institutions; he was thus somewhat uneasy with the growing role of the Rockefeller Foundation in funding the development of county health departments. Nonetheless, he was well aware of the constraints of his position. With only a limited appropriation at their disposal, the men involved in the rural sanitation effort pursued any funding opportunities that they encountered. As it turned out, the Rockefeller IHB, which was also interested in stimulating local public health work, would prove a strong partner. Growing out of the Rockefeller-backed hookworm effort in the South, the IHB had taken on an increasingly large and international profile. During the 1910s, it embarked on efforts in British Guiana, the West Indies, India, and Ceylon. In France, it took on tuberculosis. By the 1920s, the board was engaged in efforts across a broad swath of the world. Nonetheless, the health problems of the rural South remained an important concern for IHB officials, and Rockefeller money continued to flow into the region.[29]

Throughout the postwar years, the rural sanitation program collaborated with the IHB, the Red Cross, various private philanthropies, and privately funded antituberculosis groups. At times, the lines between public and private authority and national and local authority were blurred. The rural sanitation program even collaborated with the Children's Bureau, an agency whose role in administering the Sheppard–Towner Act the PHS officially opposed, in twenty counties.[30] Health work, Lumsden believed, should not be divided up into a variety of different categories, such as tuberculosis control, malaria control, or child and maternal health. From his perspective, however, there was no reason not to pursue the Children's Bureau or any other agency focused on a single health issue as a potential partner and financial backer. Such organizations, Lumsden wrote, tended to realize "after practical experience, the advantage of dovetailing their specific activities with and making them a part of a well-rounded comprehensive program of local official health service under the immediate direction of a qualified, whole-time local health officer."[31]

Lumsden, Public Health, and Individual Medicine

In the years after the war, Leslie Lumsden took an aggressive stance on the question of the appropriate role of the federal government in backing local-level health efforts. Because diseases did not respect political boundaries, he asserted, federal action was necessary. Drawing sharp distinctions between public health and individual medical services, he maintained, was a serious mistake. County health departments backed by the rural sanitation program held clinics at which patients were diagnosed and given medical treatment. Offering vaccinations and providing treatment for venereal diseases were in many ways classic public health functions, but physicians were prone to viewing clinics that offered medical services as a potential threat to private practice. In urban areas where dispensaries offered medical care to the indigent, "dispensary abuse" was a growing concern of the increasingly cautious and conservative medical profession. Patients, it was feared, were going to free dispensaries rather than paying for private care.[32]

PHS-backed health departments engaged in other activities that potentially infringed on the private practice of medicine. Antituberculosis efforts aimed at both populations and individuals were typical of the county health work backed by the rural sanitation program. In addition, public health nurses were dispatched to the homes of those with communicable diseases. Inspections of schoolchildren, another area that organized medicine had expressed concern with, were followed up with "corrective" measures. Nurses also visited the homes of expectant mothers and mothers with infants.[33] For Lumsden, refraining from such activities would be a political choice, made with an eye toward the concerns of organized medicine rather than the best interests of the rural communities he hoped to serve.

Speaking in 1921, Lumsden condemned the growing attempts of physicians to erect a firm barrier between health efforts aimed at populations and those aimed at individuals. While there were those in the medical profession who sought to define "public" health as a strictly preventive endeavor, to be undertaken by government, and curative medicine as strictly "private," to be undertaken without government backing, dividing health policy in that manner was a misguided undertaking. "Health service," Lumsden asserted, "is essentially for the prevention of disease. Medical service is essentially for the cure of disease. Either may be conducted as a public or a private enterprise." Almost inevitably, questions of jurisdiction would emerge between public authorities concerned with health and private practitioners: "As a sharp line of demarcation cannot be drawn invariably between measures for prevention and those for cure, it is natural, at times, for some confusion or even conflict of opinion to occur as to the respective duties, rights, prerogatives, and prerequisites of the health service and of the medical service of a community."[34] Where the interests of the community ran up against the concerns of physicians in private practice, the community must win out.

In many cases, this would mean that individual medical services would have to be provided by public officials. The reason was clear: curing a disease in one individual was often the best means of preventing it in others. For Lumsden, the conclusion was "inescapable" that a wide variety of interventions, including "the treatment of diseased teeth, the removal of diseased tonsils and adenoids, the rendering of prenatal care, the treatment of venereal disease to remove dangerous foci of infection, the diagnosis and treatment of tuberculosis, and the correction of certain eye, ear and other physical defects," represented medical services that were of a "public health nature," whether they occurred "in the private office or the public clinic."[35] At the margins, public health and individual medicine would inescapably blur into one another. Rather than focusing on ensuring the autonomy of the medical profession and resisting the encroachments of public health, physicians should focus on the health of their patients and on the health of their communities.

Lumsden's description of a public health that crossed into the delivery of individual medical services was in keeping with the vanguard work of contemporary public health theorists such as C.-E. A. Winslow. "In the past," Winslow wrote in 1920, "a sharp line was drawn between the measures taken by public health authorities to check the spread of epidemic disease and the daily routine of the practitioner in the treatment of the individual case." The first "was public health, the second private medicine." Increasingly, however, it was becoming "harder to draw such a sharp line, more difficult to say where public health should end and private medicine begin."[36]

Highlighting the protean nature of the idea of public health, Winslow offered a capacious new definition. Public health, he asserted, was "the science and the art of preventing disease, prolonging life, and promoting physical health and efficiency through organized community efforts for the sanitation of the environment, the control of community infections, the education of the individual in principles of personal hygiene, the organization of medical and nursing service for the early diagnosis and preventive treatment of disease, and the development of the social machinery which will ensure to every individual in the community a standard of living adequate for the maintenance of health."[37]

Earlier, the PHS's Benjamin Warren and Edgar Sydenstricker had challenged conventional understandings of public health and of its relationship with individual medicine. As Paul Starr has argued, however, Winslow's definition was a particularly subversive one: "Public health cannot make all these activities its own without, sooner or later, violating private beliefs or private property or the prerogatives of other institutions."[38] Echoing and embracing Winslow's radical take on public health, Lumsden courted conflict with organized medicine, which was increasingly concerned with policing the boundary between public health and individual medical services.

Lumsden also embraced the controversial health center concept, associated with New York state commissioner of health Hermann Biggs. The Biggs health center plan was developed in the aftermath of World War I and the Spanish flu epidemic, which drew attention to the problem of access to medical care in rural communities.[39] Physicians could be drawn into practicing in rural areas and high-quality care provided, Biggs believed, if state governments worked with counties to provide publically funded medical facilities.

Under the Biggs plan, health centers would offer high-quality laboratory facilities, consultations from specialists paid with public money, and hospital facilities while also engaging in preventive and educational work.[40] They would house expensive diagnostic technology such as X-ray machines, which could be used by local physicians. "This plan," explained Biggs in 1920, "will in no way supersede the local physician, but rather furnish him with facilities which he does not now have." Health centers, in other words, would provide a publically supported context in which private physicians could practice. They would also provide a home for the local public health department and possibly social welfare agencies interested in health. In doing so, they would offer a framework for more effectively integrating public health and individual medical services.[41] Originally developed with rural areas in mind, the plan could be implemented in cities, where the dispensary system offered a model for delivering health services that might be built on.

Offered in the aftermath of the failed Progressive-Era push for health insurance, the Biggs plan suggested an alternative means of expanding access to individual medical services. When it was introduced in the New York state legislature, the *New York Times* described it as "compromise legislation" offered in place of health insurance. In the *Journal of the American Medical Association,* health centers were similarly described as a health insurance alternative. An article in the *American Labor Legislation Review,* meanwhile, described it as "a feeble compromise bill."[42] Biggs himself did not take a public position on health insurance, though he apparently viewed health centers as a superior approach.[43] Many within the medical profession, meanwhile, viewed the health center idea as comparably dangerous. Although Biggs stressed that the centers would offer publically funded facilities for use by private physicians, worried physicians maintained the plan might lead to "state medicine," with private physicians rendered government employees.

Defending the health center concept, Lumsden argued that a self-interested medical profession had maligned it unfairly. Opponents of health centers and other publically funded institutions offering individual medical services, Lumsden groused, "ruthlessly refer to them as manifestations of the old bugaboo of 'state medicine.'" Rather than an intrusive takeover, however, innovations such as the health center idea represented a means of bringing needed medical care to the nation's underserved rural populations.

The medical profession, Lumsden argued, should stop blocking progress and throw its weight behind community-minded proposals such as that of Biggs. Public health clinics, health centers, and community-oriented hospitals "should be encouraged and aided by governmental agencies—local, state, and national—concerned properly with the promotion of the general welfare." Commending the achievements of medicine and calling for physicians to cooperate with public health authorities, Lumsden warned that obstinacy in the face of change would ultimately hurt the medical profession. If, "because of erroneous ideas about his special rights and privileges," the private practitioner "gets in the way of progress for the general welfare, he will be run over by the procession—and that would be an unthinkably sorry place for him, with his glorious heritage, to take in these moving times."[44]

In adopting an antagonistic approach to organized medicine, Lumsden created serious problems for himself. As a general rule, Surgeon General Hugh Cumming allowed Lumsden a great deal of leeway in developing the rural sanitation effort. Nonetheless, he was a cautious man. Faced with a generally conservative Congress and political climate, a series of Republican presidents, and an increasingly inflexible AMA, Cumming sought conciliation wherever possible. Picking fights with the medical profession over the appropriate role of public health authorities in providing access to individual medical services, for Cumming, made little political sense. In time, Cumming's displeasure with Lumsden would lead the surgeon general to reassign him away from the rural sanitation program.[45] For the time being, however, Lumsden and his men went to work.

The 1927 Flood

In the spring of 1927, a massive flood overtook the lower Mississippi Valley. The flood covered 27,000 square miles, putting "as much as 30 feet of water over lands where 931,159 people" had previously lived.[46] In the aftermath of the flood, the knowledge, practical experience, and infrastructure that the PHS had developed over the preceding decade became of immediate and critical importance. Confronted with potential outbreaks of malaria and pellagra, the service translated its research into direct action on a wide scale. The rural sanitation program, meanwhile, emerged as the basis for federal efforts to tame the public health catastrophe resulting from the social and economic dislocations caused by the flood.

As the magnitude of the disaster in the lower Mississippi Valley became clear, the PHS coordinated its response with Secretary of Commerce Herbert Hoover, the American Red Cross, the Rockefeller IHB, and state and county boards of health. The Red Cross set up 149 camps for displaced individuals and families in Arkansas, Illinois, Kentucky, Louisiana, Mississippi, Missouri, and Tennessee, while state boards of health and the Rockefeller Foundation provided medical and other emergency relief personnel.[47] The PHS, meanwhile, assigned twenty-four medical officers, eight sanitary engineers, and five "scientific assistants" to the flood zone.[48]

PHS senior sanitary engineer Joseph A. LePrince, engaged in antimosquito work since the occupation of Cuba, was asked to formulate a plan for coping with the health threats emerging from the disaster. In an initial memo, he stressed the importance of clean water, sanitary privies, and effective screening. "Where homes are apparently unfit to screen," LePrince advised, "paste newspaper or other paper on inside walls. The negroes can do this work well and such homes can be made mosquito proof." Blood-engorged mosquitoes found inside homes in the morning should be swatted. Even within the context of a major natural disaster, LePrince emphasized the economic arguments about the need for public health work that the PHS had long made. The Lower Mississippi Valley's white elite, he emphasized, needed to be warned about the danger that disease posed to the area's economic livelihood. Plantation owners, he wrote, should be made to understand that "the situation is serious . . . Typhoid, Dysentery, and Malaria may so delay or prevent gathering of farm crops as to create a financial fiasco for farm tenant and plantation owner."[49]

The Red Cross financed the implementation of LePrince's plan, which centered on the screening of homes where malaria carriers lived. If female mosquitoes could not take blood meals from carriers, they could freely bite others without transmitting the disease.[50] It was a substantial undertaking. The "distance from the north to the south end of the entire project was about 320 miles, and the homes to be screened were scattered over 36 counties of four States."[51] Throughout the lower Mississippi Valley, in Arkansas, Louisiana, Mississippi, and Tennessee, teams of inspectors provided by the Red Cross and state health departments went door to door, attempting to establish where carriers of malaria were living. In around ninety days, PHS engineers under LePrince's supervision screened approximately 6,760 homes.[52]

Pellagra

The flood renewed national interest in the South's pellagra problem. In the words of popular science writer Paul DeKruif, the disaster "drove thousands of hidden, sick, pellagrous wretches—of whose existence our self-satisfied respectable citizens had no idea—out of their miserable cabins into Red Cross camps." The flood, DeKruif mused, "was really a high-powered advertising agent of neglected human misery."[53]

More than a decade before, Joseph Goldberger had established the role of diet in causing the disease. Recognizing that the South was unlikely to give up on the production of cotton and other major cash crops in order to produce more milk, vegetables, and lean meat for local consumption, Goldberger experimented with other means of preventing pellagra. By 1927, he had established that brewer's yeast contained the still-unidentified "pellagra-preventive" vitamin (later determined to be niacin).[54]

When Red Cross officials approached Goldberger about the thousands of afflicted Southerners showing up in the organization's camps, he informed them that the disease could be controlled for two cents a person per day. The Red Cross followed Goldberger's suggestions, distributing brewer's yeast in its camps and supplying it to state boards of health and county health departments in the flood zone. Funded by the Red Cross, USDA farm demonstration agents and volunteers from other organizations helped to distribute the yeast to people outside of the camps.[55]

In the aftermath of the disaster, Goldberger and his old colleague, Edgar Sydenstricker, traveled the affected area and attempted to document the flood's impact on pellagra incidence. Rates of pellagra, Goldberger and Sydenstricker noted, were extremely difficult to determine because the flood states were largely incapable of collecting information on disease morbidity.[56] Nonetheless, it was clear that pellagra—already a major problem in the lower Mississippi Valley—had become even more intense.[57] The provision of brewer's yeast, however, had apparently blunted the full force of the outbreak.[58]

Understanding the South's pellagra problem, Goldberger explained in his report on the aftermath of the flood, required an appreciation of its deep interconnections with the Southern system of monocrop agriculture. "Thus," he wrote, "it may appear at first glance that any attempt to remove the conditions which are fundamentally responsible for the prevalence of pellagra would involve a revolution of dietary habits and of the entire economic and financial system as it now exists."[59] His experiences since taking over as head of the PHS's pellagra effort in 1914, of course, suggested that an economic "revolution" was not on the immediate horizon.

Planting small gardens and owning milk cows offered some hope of weakening the grip of the disease, but plantation owners tended to discourage both. Gardens "use space which otherwise might be planted in cotton" and require "labor on the part of the tenant and his family during the season when all the labor possible is required in the cotton fields." Similarly, "because of the desire to use all the land for cotton, pasturage is not furnished" for cows. Along with concerns about land usage, landowners worried that tenants were "prone to divert feed destined for mules and horses to feeding their cows."[60]

Personally moved by the suffering of Southern victims of pellagra, Goldberger had no illusions about his own ability to alter the underlying causes of the disease. In an interview with DeKruif after the flood, Goldberger reflected on the poverty of the South and on the widespread lack of knowledge of pellagra and its causes. Monocrop agriculture, it appeared, would continue to play a dominant role in the region's economy for the foreseeable future. The economic factors driving the South's pellagra problem, Goldberger concluded, were beyond his reach: "I'm only a bum doctor."[61]

The distribution of brewer's yeast, however, offered the genuine prospect of a reduction in pellagra, and the response to the 1927 flood represented an initial demonstration of this approach's potential effectiveness. With increasingly conclusive proof that the disease could be combated without completely transforming the South, perhaps there was some hope. Indeed, brewer's yeast would be widely embraced by Southern health officials after the flood. The flood, DeKruif contended, "was a good disaster." Its aftermath had provided the opportunity for the "first field test, under practical conditions, under the worst possible scientific surroundings," of a means of confronting pellagra that proved supremely effective.[62]

In 1929, Goldberger died of cancer. Already, the transformative promise of his findings was on the verge of being fulfilled. His research, meanwhile, had significantly furthered the reputation of the service's Hygienic Laboratory. After Goldberger's death, Louisiana senator Joseph Ransdell secured the enactment of legislation granting his widow an increased pension on the basis of her participation in pellagra experiments during the 1910s.[63] A longtime PHS supporter, Ransdell had earlier helped secure Carville, Louisiana, as the site of the service's only leprosarium on the US mainland. In 1930, he sponsored a new law reorganizing the Hygienic Laboratory, Goldberger's institutional home, and renaming it the National Institute of Health. As it turned out, this was Ransdell's final achievement in Congress: Huey Long defeated him in that year's Democratic primary contest.

The Growth of County Health Departments

The crowning achievement of the PHS's intervention in the flood area was the rapid extension of the office of rural sanitation's cooperative plan for developing full-time county health departments throughout the flood zone. In spring 1927, only eighteen of the 103 flooded counties in six states had full-time county health departments. Their worth, however, appeared to have been proven by their performance in the aftermath of the flood. Leslie Lumsden, a far from a neutral observer, claimed that full-time county health officers, "as a rule, performed with remarkable promptness and efficiency in the organization of working forces and in the carrying out of measures for both immediate and post-flood sanitary protection of the stricken people." The difference between counties with and those without health departments with a full-time officer, he maintained, "stood out sharply."[64] Permanent county health departments, according to the PHS, were necessary "to carry on to a logical conclusion the preventive measures started" after the flood.[65] Because the affected states and counties were unable to fund the development of or provide the expertise necessary to build local public health infrastructure, the obvious solution was an expansion of the rural sanitation program.[66]

In June 1927, representatives from the PHS and the Rockefeller IHB, meeting in New Orleans, agreed to provide support for the development of county-level health infrastructure throughout the area devastated by the flood. By the end of October 1927, sixty-seven new counties had entered into cooperative agreements with either the PHS or the IHB. Within a year of the flood, seventy-eight counties, "or about 92 per cent of the total with which contact was made" by agents of the PHS and IHB, had signed on.[67]

Where county money was too scarce for even a small appropriation, the PHS and the IHB, along with state boards of health, wholly "financed the projects temporarily with a limited personnel. In many counties, the work was made possible by donations from the local Red Cross chapters, municipalities, chambers of commerce, and civic organizations."[68] In the short term, the PHS paid for the expansion of its county health efforts in the lower Mississippi Valley with money released from its "epidemic fund," designated for use in emergency situations.[69]

Congress, meanwhile, proved responsive to requests from the PHS for increased funding. Impressed with the service's response to the flood, and willing, given the emergency circumstances, to endorse its continued involvement, Congress more than quadrupled the annual appropriation for "special studies of and demonstration work in rural sanitation" in the following fiscal year. Beginning in the summer of 1928, Leslie Lumsden had a $347,000 appropriation at his disposal, up from an initial appropriation of $85,000 in the preceding fiscal year. A total of $85,000 was slated for general use, and the remaining $262,000 was earmarked for use in the flood zone.[70]

PHS officials could barely contain their excitement. "While deploring the frightful disaster of last spring," a PHS report asserted, "some comfort may be obtained in the knowledge that better communities are built on the ruins of those destroyed, and, as a rule, a better public-health regime may be inaugurated. Surely in this experience there has developed another flood—a flood of sanitation development which has placed us many years ahead of our old program of full-time county health service."[71]

Rather than endorsing the vision of the appropriate federal role in public health being articulated by Leslie Lumsden and other proponents of expanding the effort within the PHS, however, members of Congress were simply responding to an emergency situation as best they could. Convenience was a far greater factor in congressional approval than the arguments being made by PHS officers about the inherently interstate nature of disease or the economic impact of malaria. When Assistant Surgeon General Warren F. Draper, the former Lumsden subordinate who now oversaw Lumsden as head of the PHS's Division of Domestic Quarantine, appeared before a House appropriations subcommittee to discuss the flood effort, Representative William R. Wood (R-IN) highlighted the gap between PHS actions and reigning conceptions of the appropriate role of the federal government: "Have [the states in the flood zone] shown that they were unable to take care of the situation without Federal aid?" Told that they had, Wood wondered whether the states had given the PHS "an account of the money that they have available for state expenses, etc.?"

"Here is the trouble," Representative Wood told Dr. Draper: "When these disasters come, of course we help them in every instance, but they ought to understand that they ought not to abuse the generosity of the Government by using the Federal Government to do for them what they ought to do for themselves when the disaster is over."[72] For Wood, whatever benefits the PHS effort was bringing to the economically devastated flood region appeared outweighed by its significant risks, particularly the likelihood that the federal government was "establishing some very dangerous precedents by doing this sort of thing."[73] Wood was unwilling to endorse the vision of the federal government's role in ensuring the health of Americans that the rural sanitation effort represented. "You want to encourage these people," he concluded, "to help themselves and make them understand that the Government is not going to keep doing this for them forever. If we are, we are going to exhaust the Treasury before long."[74]

The Drought

Congressman Wood's concern about the precedent being set proved well placed. Previously an ignored and small-scale initiative, the PHS's rural sanitation program achieved a degree of national legitimacy after the Mississippi flood. During the spring of 1930, a massive drought, concentrated in Arkansas, overcame large parts of the South. The USDA described it as the "worst drought ever recorded in this country."[75] Particularly in the lower Mississippi Valley, the drought had severe effects for farm families counting on a decent harvest to pay back the debts they had incurred both to survive and to plant the year's cotton crop. After a substantial delay, during which President Herbert Hoover favored minimal federal intervention and reliance on the emergency efforts of the Red Cross, Congress began passing relief measures for the drought area.

Aware that the drought was exacerbating already poor health conditions, senators and members of Congress from the affected states began pushing for an expansion of the PHS's rural sanitation program as part of the federal response to the crisis. Leslie Lumsden, for his part, became increasingly confident that the rural sanitation program (still theoretically a demonstration program) would finally be formalized as a federal grant-in-aid program for the development of local public health efforts.[76]

Lumsden's lobbying, as well as the growing prominence of the program, put Surgeon General Hugh Cumming in a somewhat difficult position. It was clear that the rural sanitation effort was crucial to building a political coalition that would support the PHS. In particular, leading Southern

Democrats had embraced the idea of federal support for the development of local public health infrastructure. At the same time, the American Medical Association opposed Lumsden's program and increasingly signaled concern about its ongoing growth. Lumsden's expansive vision of the role of the federal government in promoting the health of Americans, long a sore spot, now appeared more problematic than ever.

In the midst of the drought crisis, Cumming decided to resolve the issue by promoting Lumsden out of his position in charge of the rural sanitation program. As 1931 began, Lumsden took on a new role as head of the PHS supervisory district headquartered in New Orleans.[77] It was, to put it mildly, not a promotion that Lumsden sought. By 1932, Lumsden's independence and unwillingness to take direction from Washington was viewed as a significant problem. C. E. Waller, head of the Division of Domestic Quarantine, found himself forced to write a somewhat harsh letter to Lumsden instructing him not to interfere with the operation of the rural sanitation program unless he was asked to do so. Displeased with his banishment to the Crescent City, Lumsden maintained that Cumming had acted in the hopes of avoiding any controversy that might compromise his goal of being elected to the AMA's presidency, a dream that Cumming would never achieve.[78]

Despite Lumsden's exile, supportive members of Congress continued working to enlarge the rural sanitation program. In making their case, proponents such as Senate minority leader Joseph Robinson (D-AR) and Senator Alben Barkley (D-KY) could now draw on evidence of the program's success in limiting disease, a growing base of local popular and political support, and, crucially, the example of 1927. As Arthur T. McCormack, Kentucky's state health officer, explained to the Senate agriculture committee, the precedent for federal intervention in public health in the drought area was unambiguous: "This proposal is based upon the action taken during the Mississippi flood under the leadership of President Coolidge and Secretary of Commerce Hoover."[79] Asked whether there was any local "opposition to Federal work of this kind," McCormack replied that "there is the general opposition to Federal aid of any kind. But there is no specific opposition, and so great was the improvement in the situation following this other work [in the aftermath of the 1927 flood] that in no county in the flood area during this period has there been any opposition to this work by anybody."[80]

As McCormack, Surgeon General Cumming, and Assistant Surgeon General Warren Draper testified before the Senate agriculture committee, their descriptions of the PHS's work in the South were met with knowing recognition. At one point, Senator Thaddeus Caraway (D-AR) interrupted

Draper to extol the virtues of federal public health efforts. Praising the service's work after the 1927 flood, Senator Caraway declared that he was "so thoroughly persuaded that there is no work the Government does which pays such a dividend as this in the matter of public health, that I feel there could be no objection to it, because a strong healthy population is most important. . . . It contributes more to the national welfare than otherwise could be contributed. I live in the valley of the Mississippi, and we know of what tremendous importance this is."[81]

A large collection of letters solicited by Arkansas state health officer C. W. Garrison underlined the growing interest in the PHS's cooperative program. In letter after letter, state and county officials testified to the urgency of local health problems and need for federal support. James M. Smith, a county judge from Desha County, Arkansas, explained that his home county needed money to continue to pay for a health officer, nurse, sanitary inspector, vaccines and antitoxins for typhoid and diphtheria, and brewer's yeast for the prevention of pellagra. The people of Desha County, Judge Smith wrote, "have begun to appreciate" the importance of the county's public health programs. "We feel sure that the death rate has been lowered considerably during the past three years." What advances had been made since the flood, Smith believed, would likely be lost if the county's public health board was discontinued.

Invoking the reasoning long used by federal public workers, Judge Smith highlighted the economic significance of disease. "I feel reasonably sure," he wrote, "that a continuation of the health program in this county would be worth $3 for every dollar it might cost. Well and healthful people are not only able to earn more money and produce a great deal more crops, but there is a great saving in doctor bills, medicine bills, and funeral expenses." Federal support was crucial to local well-being. "I cannot help but feel," he continued, "that our own Senator Robinson, with the able assistance of our other Senator and Congressmen, will be able to convince the Congress that the physical welfare of our people is a matter of grave and paramount importance."[82]

On February 6, 1931, President Hoover signed the drought relief package into law.[83] It contained an additional $2 million for the operation of the PHS's rural sanitation program in the drought-stricken areas. The existing appropriation for the 1931 fiscal year was only $338,000.[84] Acknowledging the weak economic condition of participating counties and states, the new authorization did not require local matching funds for "cooperative" projects.[85] When it came time to reauthorize the PHS effort in the drought area a year later, congressional enthusiasm was palpable. Senators Alben Barkley (D-KY) and Josiah Bailey (D-NC) testified to the need for the continuation and expansion of the rural sanitation program's federal–state–county cooperative projects, while Charles McNary (R-OR), chair of the Senate agriculture committee, wondered aloud whether the program should be expanded further.[86]

The growth of the rural sanitation program's efforts during 1930 and 1931 was substantial. In 1931, at the peak of the PHS's drought intervention, rural sanitation money supported work in 375 full-time county health departments, up from 69 in 1927. After the end of the drought, the program would continue at levels higher than those of the preflood and drought era. As of 1933, it supported work in 126 counties. In the aftermath of the flood and drought, the PHS now operated in more counties than the Rockefeller IHB.[87]

Precedents

After World War I, the PHS faced major challenges as a result of the trouble it encountered in administering a hospital program for veterans and poor public relations surrounding a major outbreak of pellagra in the South. Despite Congress's decision not to embrace the PHS's postwar program, Leslie Lumsden's rural sanitation initiative emerged out of the war as a means for the service to begin building a framework of cooperation with state and local governments. Aimed at ameliorating the health problems faced by rural America, the program was strongly tilted toward the Southern states, where diseases such as malaria and hookworm represented major and ongoing public health threats. After the 1927 flood of the lower Mississippi Valley and the 1930–1931 Southern drought, the effort was expanded and its Southern orientation strongly reinforced. Nonetheless, the rural sanitation program remained fairly small in scale. Indeed, the PHS's primary function continued to be its oldest one: the operation of marine hospitals. The base of political support that was being built for the rural sanitation effort and the precedents that it was setting, however, would prove to be of great importance.

CHAPTER FIVE

ECONOMIC SECURITY

Beginning with the collapse of the stock market in October 1929, the Great Depression settled in as an omnipresent social and economic fact during 1930. The Depression represented a substantial threat to the health of the American people and placed immense stress on the nation's health care delivery system. With their finances stretched past the breaking point, state and local governments found it difficult to fund public health work and to continue helping to finance individual medical services for the indigent. For physicians, the tradition of providing charity care became difficult to sustain as more and more patients became unable to pay. Hospitals faced similarly major sustainability issues. These pressures came on top of what by the late 1920s was already recognized as a looming crisis in the financing of American health care.

In 1932, after a more than decade-long lull, government-backed health insurance again emerged as a central issue in American health policy. The precipitating event was a report issued by the Committee on the Costs of Medical Care (CCMC), a privately funded group comprising physicians, public health workers, and social scientists. After the CCMC's majority proposal that the delivery of medical services be reorganized, with physicians working in groups connected to hospitals and payment financed through voluntary insurance, the AMA launched an all-out assault. The proposals, the AMA maintained, were the first step toward revolution. The divisions over health policy that reared their head in the aftermath of the CCMC report proved central in the development of the health provisions of what became the 1935 Social Security Act.

In November 1932, the month the CCMC report was issued, Democrat Franklin Roosevelt was elected president. Having claimed the House of Representatives in the 1930 midterm elections, Democrats also gained control of the Senate. In both chambers, the party's majorities were overwhelming. The federal government began funding the PHS's rural sanitation program through its Federal Emergency Relief Administration (FERA). FERA also began funding individual medical services for the indigent and, through its short-lived Civil Works Administration (CWA), large-scale public health interventions such as drainage projects aimed at Southern malaria.

The framework for the Social Security Act (originally called the Economic Security bill) was drafted by the Committee on Economic Security (CES), which was created by an executive order in June 1934. Edgar Sydenstricker, the longtime PHS statistician who now served as a chief researcher for the Milbank Memorial Fund, was put in charge of the committee's Technical Committee on Medical Care. In this role, Sydenstricker was in charge of drafting the report on risks to economic security arising out of ill health for the committee. Thomas Parran Jr., the prominent PHS officer, veteran of the extracantonment effort and rural sanitation program, and adherent of a broad vision of the appropriate role of the federal government in ensuring American health, was a key member of the CES's advisory committee on medical care. Already, it was widely known that President Roosevelt would soon appoint Parran surgeon general.

Ultimately, the CES's report to the president included a proposal that the PHS be granted a great deal of latitude in expanding the rural sanitation program into a nationwide system of assistance to states and localities for developing high-quality public health infrastructure. Public health, notably, was not among the areas that the CES originally instructed Sydenstricker's Technical Committee on Medical Care to investigate. Meanwhile, the CES did not endorse the Technical Committee on Medical Care's plan for federally funded but locally administered health insurance. Deemed too politically volatile, and potentially a threat to passing the entire economic security program, insurance was excluded from the CES's report to the president. The PHS's Thomas Parran proposed an alternative plan, centered around direct federal payments for indigent health services and for particularly expensive illnesses, treatments, and diagnostic facilities. Influenced by the earlier Hermann Biggs health center proposal, this plan was discussed favorably in the CES's medical advisory committee but was rejected by Sydenstricker.

The development of what became the Social Security Act's health provisions during 1934–1935 marked the beginning of a critical juncture in the political development of American health policy. At this point, a variety of approaches might have been taken to structuring the federal government's role in American health care, including the creation of a health policy regime that encompassed both public health and individual medicine. The decisions made beginning in 1934–1935, however, set federal policies dealing with public health and individual medicine off on divergent paths. Ultimately, a bifurcated policy regime would emerge and then become deeply entrenched.

Previous accounts of the development of the health-related provisions of the Social Security Act have tended to view the act's public health provisions as of little interest. As we will see, however, their inclusion was important in terms of both politics and policy. Hoping to defuse criticism that it was mindlessly obstructionist and position itself as being in favor of some sort of action in the field of health, the AMA adopted a posture of support for increased federal intervention in local-level public health work. With the strong support of Southern political leaders, who believed that expanded federal public health work would substantially benefit the region, and with the approval of the AMA, federal public health efforts gained a strong institutional base. Here, the often path-dependent nature of policy making proved critical. Building on the policies and institutions that its officers began forging during World War I and the reputation that it had secured for fighting Southern diseases such as malaria, pellagra, and hookworm, the PHS emerged as a genuinely national force in American public health.

Previous accounts have also paid little sustained attention to the proposals made by the PHS's Thomas Parran during the meetings of the CES's medical advisory committee.[1] Parran's plan, however, suggested a distinct path for health policy, and one that gained the approval of AMA-aligned members of the advisory committee. Under different conditions, it might have proved the basis for a new and more integrated federal health policy regime. In the policy debates that followed during the late 1930s and early 1940s, Parran and the PHS would continue to push publically funded medical services tied to health departments as an alternative to health insurance and as a means of more fully integrating public health and individual medicine. Tactical differences and substantive policy disputes between the PHS and the Social Security Board (created to implement most of the Social Security Act) would become an important feature of federal health policy. In contrast to the PHS, the Social Security Board would push hard for the adoption of compulsory health insurance.

The Committee on the Costs of Medical Care

The health policy debates of the 1930s began with the release of the Committee on the Costs of Medical Care's final report in 1932. Formed in 1926, the CCMC was funded by a group of private foundations, including the Milbank Memorial Fund, the Rockefeller Foundation, and the Julius Rosenwald Fund. The committee comprised individuals representing a variety of perspectives, including physicians in private practice, members of the public health community, social scientists, and representatives from the AMA and other interested professional groups. Edgar Sydenstricker was among the committee's members. Starting in 1925, Sydenstricker had worked as a research consultant with the Milbank Memorial Fund, an endowed organization focused on health and social welfare. In 1928, he joined the fund full time as its director of research. Despite this move, he retained a formal role as a consultant with the PHS.[2]

Other prominent committee members included C.-E. A. Winslow, the influential public health thinker. Michael M. Davis, the health policy reformer who had earlier headed the innovative Boston Dispensary, was also on the committee. Now he worked for the Julius Rosenwald Fund, one of the committee's funders and an organization particularly concerned with the issues facing black Southerners. In this role, Davis made important connections with the PHS. Isidore Falk, a former student of C.-E. A. Winslow, was asked to head the committee's technical staff after the research got off to a slow start. A social scientist deeply absorbed in health issues, Falk would forge a close bond and working relationship with Edgar Sydenstricker and emerge as a major force behind efforts to create a national health insurance system.

Between 1927 and 1932, the CCMC published a series of studies documenting the major shifts taking place in the practice and organization of American medicine. A number of factors fed the steady growth of medical costs. Stricter licensing laws, put in place during the Progressive Era, reduced the overall number of physicians while improving their overall quality. Advances in medical science and technology meant that physicians could provide far more effective treatments. Surgery and other medical procedures, meanwhile, were more likely to take place in hospitals, further increasing the costs that patients incurred. When an unexpected illness occurred, it could prove highly expensive.[3]

One highly influential response to these problems, group hospital insurance, was beginning to take hold on a small scale. Various forms of prepayment for medical services had long existed in a few industries, such as lumber, railroads, and coal mining. Faced with unfilled hospital beds and an uncertain supply of patients, Baylor University Hospital in Dallas, Texas, attempted to adapt existing prepayment models to its circumstances and stabilize its finances. Just before the October 1929 stock market crash, the hospital created a plan for Dallas schoolteachers, who would pay a fixed amount out of their salaries in return for a guarantee of 21 days of hospital coverage.[4]

The benefits of this approach proved significant. Because enrollees participated as a result of their employment status rather than as a result of their perceived health prospects, it created an insurance pool that was not disproportionally composed of the ill. In addition, deducting premiums from the paychecks of employees offered a reliable means of collecting them and lowering administrative costs.[5] Other hospitals, faced with an unsteady supply of paying patients as the Depression deepened, adopted the approach. County- and citywide plans followed, and in 1934, New York State would pass enabling legislation for nonprofit hospital insurance plans.[6] Under the New York legislation and laws passed in other states, so-called Blue Cross plans were exempted from many of the regulations placed on the private insurance industry, which only began to offer similar policies on a meaningful scale during the late 1930s.[7]

Group hospital coverage was only beginning to emerge when the CCMC released the final volume of its studies in November 1932. In a majority report, included in the volume, CCMC members recommended expanded public health efforts, improvements in medical education, and an increase in the supply of medical services and facilities. The organization and financing of individual medical services, however, was the central concern of the majority report. In a move that precipitated a major split among the CCMC's members, the majority report endorsed a reorganization of medicine along group practice lines, with teams of specialist physicians working in groups centered around hospitals. Medical care should be financed, it argued, through voluntary health insurance. The financing of care through insurance should be used to transform and rationalize the practice of medicine.[8] Edgar Sydenstricker, unwilling to endorse the claim that voluntary insurance would be an adequate means of setting in motion a reorganization of the practice of American medicine and addressing the nation's medical financing issues, wrote his own one-sentence statement, asserting the majority report's recommendations were incapable of fully confronting the problems at hand.[9]

A minority of the CCMC's members argued that the majority report's recommendations would both degrade the quality of American medical care and threaten the professional autonomy of physicians. The leadership of the AMA, which moved quickly to endorse the minority report, gave public voice to their concerns. *Journal of the American Medical Association* editor Morris Fishbein drafted a fierce response, painting the majority report as the product of a dangerous and insidious cabal. Group practice and voluntary insurance, he maintained, were entering wedges to revolution. On one side of the issue were "the forces representing the great foundations, public health officialdom, social theory—even socialism and communism—inciting to revolution." On the other was organized medicine, "urging an orderly evolution guided by controlled experimentation which will observe the principles that have been found through the centuries to be necessary to the sound practice of medicine."[10]

Fishbein's tone was caustic, but he and other AMA leaders acknowledged that there were growing problems with the financing of American medicine, and not just because of the Depression. As a means of addressing these problems, the AMA offered two recommendations. The first was that government funding of health services for the poor be both continued and enlarged, "with the ultimate object of relieving the medical profession of this burden."[11] From the AMA's perspective, there were clearly dangers in this approach. Nonetheless, continuing to provide charity care in the midst of an ongoing economic catastrophe was causing serious problems for the organization's members. Endorsing broad government payments was potentially risky, but the benefits for financially strapped physicians were obvious.

Second, the AMA offered its own perspective on insurance. Health insurance that did not seek to reorganize the practice of medicine, the AMA leadership suggested, would be acceptable. As Morris Fishbein wrote, the AMA-backed minority report did not oppose "any individual carrying insurance against the occurrence of a major illness or operation so that he might receive at such time funds sufficient to pay the hospital and the physician he might select." In contrast to insurance that covered routine expenses, insurance covering such catastrophic costs would not threaten the existing organization of medical practice or physician autonomy. Insuring against such costs, Fishbein wrote, was "foresighted, American, economical."[12]

For Edgar Sydenstricker and Isidore Falk, the AMA's vitriolic response to the CCMC majority report proved transformative. Both men regarded the AMA's counterrecommendations as calculating and disingenuous. Where they had previously viewed compromise with organized medicine as possible and even necessary, Sydenstricker and Falk emerged from the battle that followed the CCMC majority report convinced that the organization was intractable and reactionary. Falk had hoped that voluntary insurance could be a first step toward a broader compulsory system, and a step that might gain the backing of the AMA. Now he became increasingly convinced that pursuing an incremental approach in the hopes of gaining AMA support would prove futile.[13]

Roosevelt and the New Deal

The nation elected Franklin Roosevelt president just as the CCMC majority report revived the bitter debate over health insurance. Assuming office in March 1933, Roosevelt took a series of unprecedented actions. Within days of his inauguration, he ordered the nation's banks closed until Congress could pass emergency banking legislation. A barrage of legislation followed as part of Roosevelt's New Deal. In late March, Congress created the Civilian Conservation Corps, which would employ large numbers of young men in a variety of forestry, conservation, and flood control projects.[14] In May, it created the Tennessee Valley Authority, an ambitious endeavor aimed at fostering economic growth across a wide swath of land through the development of the Tennessee River's hydroelectric resources.[15] Among other major pieces of legislation, Congress passed the Emergency Farm Mortgage Act, the Truth in Securities Act, the Home Owner's Loan Act, and the Farm Credit Act.[16]

The Agricultural Adjustment Act (AAA), passed in May, was the centerpiece of the administration's plan to stabilize and reinvigorate American agriculture. Its core principle was straightforward: by inducing farmers to limit the size of their crops, the AAA would raise the prices of depressed commodities. As AAA administrator George Peek explained, "The sole aim and object of this act is to raise farm prices. . . . It is to enable [farmers] to do what all other producing social groups do, and that is . . . not to produce and send to market more goods than consumers at home and abroad want and have money to pay for."[17] AAA programs were developed for wheat, tobacco, cotton, corn, and other commodities.

In June, Congress passed the National Industrial Recovery Act, the administration's plan for addressing industry. The act created two new agencies: the National Recovery Administration (NRA) and the Public Works Administration. Under the control of the Interior Department, the Public Works Administration—which was charged with building large public projects—got off to a slow start. The NRA, however, embarked on a program intended to halt the downward spiral of wages and prices that had overcome industry. Headed by former brigadier general Hugh Johnson and broadly modeled on the World War I–era war industries board, the NRA was intended to allow businesses to cooperate with each other and with labor to design production codes and practices that would ensure that they did not price one another out of existence.

The NRA proved far less successful than the AAA.[18] Its attempts to allow American businesses to collude in stabilizing prices failed to create an industrial resurgence and were viewed with increasing skepticism. In 1934, after a tumultuous stint as the head of the NRA, Hugh Johnson resigned at the behest of the president. The next year, the Supreme Court found that, in allowing the executive branch to develop codes for regulating industry, the NRA was an unconstitutional delegation of legislative authority to the executive branch.[19]

Health and the New Deal

Roosevelt's views on health were somewhat opaque, even to those around him. As governor of New York, he had surrounded himself with progressive reformers, including Frances Perkins, commissioner of the state department of labor, and Harry Hopkins, formerly of the privately funded Anti-Tuberculosis Association. Both were close with the research staff of the Milbank Memorial Fund, which was working to develop an insurance plan that might be implemented in New York State.[20]

Roosevelt also forged a strong relationship with the PHS's Thomas Parran. After serving in the wartime extracantonment zones and in the rural sanitation program, Parran gained an increasingly national profile. Beginning in 1926, he headed the PHS's venereal disease division. In this role, he became involved in one of the most shameful actions undertaken by the PHS, the Tuskegee Syphilis Study. Working with the Julius Rosenwald Fund's Michael M. Davis in 1929, Parran helped to secure Rosenwald money for a PHS-led project aimed at studying the feasibility of treating syphilis among rural black Southerners. When the Julius Rosenwald Fund withdrew funding for the project, the PHS transformed it into a study of "untreated syphilis in the adult male negro." In effect, PHS officers watched for decades as black men in Macon County, Alabama, suffered the progressive effects of a terrible and painful disease that, after penicillin became available in the 1940s, was completely curable.[21]

Just as the Tuskegee study was getting underway, Parran took an important career detour. In 1930, at the recommendation of Edgar Sydenstricker and the New York–based Milbank Memorial Fund, Governor Roosevelt requested that Parran take a leave from the service to serve as the New York state commissioner of health.[22] After some discussion, the Treasury Department allowed Parran to both take the job and retain his PHS commission, on the assumption that the post would be temporary and with the condition that he forgo his federal salary and be paid by the state.

In New York, Parran worked on a plan for streamlining the state's complicated public health system. He collaborated regularly with Edgar Sydenstricker and the other reformers of the Milbank Memorial Fund.[23] He studied the public provision of medical care for the indigent, a growing issue as the Great Depression set in. In addition, Parran became engrossed in the health center plan articulated a decade before by state health commissioner Hermann Biggs, who had recently been the subject of a biography written by C.-E. A. Winslow.[24] Roosevelt asked Parran to come to Washington to serve as surgeon general after his election. Parran, however, "urged him to continue Dr. Cumming in office until the end of his term in 1936, unless Dr. Cumming wished to retire earlier." It was widely known during the early Roosevelt years that Parran would be the next surgeon general.[25]

Throughout his presidency, Roosevelt would maintain an ambiguous front on issues of health, particularly on insurance. Within months of his inauguration, however, the federal role in both public health and individual medicine began to grow. In May 1933, Congress passed the Federal Emergency Relief Act, creating a new Federal Emergency Relief Agency (FERA). Roosevelt placed his close associate and friend, Harry Hopkins, in control of the agency.[26] Soon FERA began funding the PHS's rural sanitation program, which had seen its funding drop since the end of the drought appropriation, at $1 million per year. FERA also put money toward projects such as a PHS-supervised "health inventory" of the nation and surveys of rat populations.[27]

In October 1933, FERA created the Civil Works Administration, an agency intended to shift able-bodied workers away from relief payments in favor of work relief. When the CWA requested that federal agencies submit proposals for how it might employ laborers, the PHS was happy to comply.[28] Soon, the CWA allocated $1.5 million toward a program for sealing abandoned mines, $5 million for a proposed privy-building project, and $4.5 million for an antimalaria drainage project. At its high point, the mine project employed "2,927 men and 24 women," mostly in Pennsylvania, West Virginia, and Alabama. The privy project employed "more than 35,000" at its peak.[29] By March 1934, the PHS estimated that the CWA had constructed more than 200,000 privies.[30]

The malaria project was even more ambitious. Loosely supervised by PHS officers, gangs of CWA workers embarked on drainage efforts that varied in quality from highly effective to clearly counterproductive. During January 1934, the PHS estimated that "the number at work on malaria drainage . . . was over 130,000 laborers," though the average for the period between December and March was likely around 64,000 workers.[31] As Louis L. Williams, head of the PHS's malaria research efforts, pointed out, the program had serious defects. "Many projects during their inception," Williams reported, "were improperly planned by supervisors of limited experience and some were constructed where work was unnecessary." Still, Williams reported that "the estimates of our most experienced men in the field who have visited a large number of projects indicate that at least 90 percent of the work has been good work."[32]

The CWA was discontinued in March 1934. Criticism of the agency, which was accused of patronage-based hiring, waste, and make-work efforts that made little practical sense, was widespread. The CWA's health-related efforts nonetheless set a precedent that another federal works program—the Works Progress Administration—would vastly expand on beginning in 1935. In the interim, FERA continued to provide funding for some PHS-supervised anti-malaria projects, including drainage and, in some areas, screening.[33]

Along with public health efforts, FERA helped to ensure access to individual medical services. In June 1933, FERA authorized payments, mediated through state and local governments, for physician services and medical supplies. In August, the agency laid out general rules for the provision of medical care using federal money. Following FERA's typical approach, the states retained authority "to formulate specific policies appropriate to local conditions." As a result, there was "wide variation in the scope of care considered permissible and possible within state and local budget limitations, ranging from the general medical attention provided in a few states, to emergency care only to which the medical program was limited in the states which interpreted the rules more strictly."[34] Following the CCMC's majority report a year before, the AMA had endorsed government payments for the care of the poor. Now with the active support of county medical societies, the federal government was involved in financing medical care for the indigent.[35]

Economic Security

On June 29, 1934, President Roosevelt issued an executive order creating the Committee on Economic Security. Charged with developing a comprehensive set of proposals to promote greater economic stability for Americans, the CES was given until December 1 to submit a report to the president. The CES's report would form the basis of the Social Security Act passed by Congress in 1935. Secretary of Labor Frances Perkins chaired the CES. Its executive board comprised Treasury Secretary Henry Morgenthau, Attorney General Homer Cummings, Agriculture Secretary Henry Wallace, and FERA administrator Harry Hopkins. Edwin Witte, a University of Wisconsin professor, was given an influential administrative role as the CES's executive director.[36]

The committee quickly became a sprawling affair. Along with the executive board, the CES included a technical board, which was headed by Assistant Secretary of Labor Arthur Altmeyer. After the Social Security Act was passed, Altmeyer would serve as head of the Social Security Board and its successor, the Social Security Administration. Holding this position through the late 1930s and the 1940s, Altmeyer would play a key role in the development of American social policy. The Altmeyer-helmed technical board comprised dozens policy specialists capable of studying the issues at hand and generating viable proposals for addressing them. The CES also included an advisory council (ultimately supplemented by various more specific advisory committees) intended to provide feedback on the proposals being considered.

Among the primary issues to be considered by the CES were old-age insurance, unemployment insurance, old-age assistance, and threats to economic security arising out of ill health.[37] The CES assumed that a health insurance proposal would be included in its report to the president. This intention was made clear by the appointment of Edgar Sydenstricker to head the CES's Technical Committee on Medical Care.[38]

For the AMA, Sydenstricker's selection appeared serious cause for alarm. Morris Fishbein, writing in the *Journal of the American Medical Association*, complained that Sydenstricker's views were "so completely antagonistic to the medical point of view that one wonders why he should have been among the first to be selected by the [CES] in developing its work."[39] State medical societies began sending telegrams, addressed to the president, protesting the potential inclusion of any health insurance provisions in the administration's planned Economic Security bill. "These attacks," CES executive secretary Edwin Witte wrote, "led the President to take a personal interest in the matter." Roosevelt did not ask, however, that Sydenstricker be replaced or that the CES avoid the issue of health insurance. Instead, he simply requested that the committee keep his personal physician, naval medical officer Ross McIntire, up to date on the development of its health plan.[40]

Sydenstricker, who had developed a serious heart problem, began working with Isidore Falk on a health insurance plan. Rather than a fully national program, Sydenstricker and Falk's plan would provide federal assistance to states for stimulating the creation of health insurance plans. The federal government would lay out a set of guidelines that states would have to follow in order to receive funding, but states would retain some flexibility and the option of participating or not. In late September, Sydenstricker met with Thomas Parran to discuss the substance of the plan as well as its politics. They also discussed who should sit on the CES's proposed medical advisory committee.

Parran, who knew Sydenstricker well, was surprised that Sydenstricker had been willing to go along with developing a plan that would encompass only health insurance. Although he felt uneasy with the insurance-only plan, Parran did not press the matter.[41] After mulling over their conversation, however, Parran became convinced that Sydenstricker needed to fight for a more comprehensive health plan that would include public health provisions. Writing to express his reservations, Parran told Sydenstricker that he had become "strongly impressed by the necessity of including a consideration of public health along with the problem of medical care."

Failing to include public health in the economic security program, Parran argued, would be a mistake with serious long-term implications. It "would be most unfortunate for a national program of medical care to be formulated," he wrote, "with the major emphasis on general medical care while the more important preventive needs are overlooked." Nearly twenty years before, Sydenstricker and Benjamin Warren had maintained that, if properly designed, health insurance would create strong incentives for expanded public health efforts. Now, however, Parran suggested that Sydenstricker's insurance plan might lead to a dramatically different outcome. "Once such a system of medical care procedure is entrenched," he warned, "it might be quite difficult to develop a constructive health program."[42] Directing its energies toward expanding access to individual medical services, federal policy might easily lose sight of the importance of preventive medicine, potentially fostering a highly inefficient health care regime.

For Parran, the implications were obvious. A combined federal program for increasing access to individual medical services and for stimulating the extension of public health capabilities, with significant resources devoted to public health, was necessary. The "expenditure of a reasonable part of the available funds for public health service," Parran wrote to Sydenstricker, "undoubtedly would produce a much larger return in terms of national vitality than consideration solely of the curative aspect."[43] If a medical program was to be included in the Roosevelt administration's plan for economic security, "it should be possible to have it embrace what you and I believe to be the basic and most important part, viz., prevention."[44]

Pressed by Parran, Sydenstricker asked Edwin Witte and the CES to allow him to expand the scope of his efforts.[45] Soon, the Julius Rosenwald Fund's Michael Davis also became involved in the push for a broader mandate. The PHS's rural sanitation program, Parran, Sydenstricker, and Davis believed, could form the basis for an expanded effort aimed at improving the nation's public health capabilities. Davis, writing to CES executive secretary Edwin Witte, argued that the "largest return for a given outlay" would come not from insurance but "from preventive work."[46]

The impact of public health work, Davis maintained, would be far more immediate. Detailing the evolution of the PHS's rural sanitation program, Davis explained that "administrative methods whereby such appropriations are made to stimulate, expand, and conduct local public health work upon a good standard have been fully and effectively demonstrated by the Service on a small scale. The policy pursued has, moreover, called forth from state and local funds amounts at least equal to the federal expenditures." Expanding the initiative was a clear means of achieving key national goals. "The time has come," Davis wrote, "to apply these methods on a scale which is commensurate with the size of the problem and the possibilities of public benefit." As an illustration of "the economy of prevention," he highlighted "the temporary Civil Works program in malaria control, carried out under the technical direction of the United States Public Health Service last year."[47]

In early November, Sydenstricker informed Parran that the CES would allow him to proceed along the lines that they had discussed. When the CES's medical advisory committee met, Sydenstricker wrote, it would be able to consider "not merely the examination, from the medical point of view, of certain proposals for health insurance, but also the extension of public medical facilities and services and, what I regard as most important, the development of the federal public health program including aid to states. In other words, the Committee on Economic Security has permitted me to enlarge the scope of the study that was first assigned to me from 'health insurance' to 'medical care and public health.'"[48]

Insurance, Public Health, and the AMA

At the beginning of October, the CES decided that it would hold a National Conference on Economic Security, at which the programs being developed under its auspices would be discussed publically.[49] The conference was held on November 14. As a prelude, the CES announced the formation of a variety of advisory committees, each of which would offer input on the policies that the CES's technical groups were working on. Among these committees was the medical advisory committee that Sydenstricker and Thomas Parran had discussed. Sydenstricker, Edwin Witte, and presidential physician Ross McIntire selected the members of the medical advisory committee with the goal of addressing the concerns of the AMA. Its members included Parran, AMA president Walter Bierring, the Cleveland Clinic's George Crile, Emory University's Stewart Roberts, and Harvey Cushing, the eminent Yale neurologist whose daughter had married Franklin Roosevelt's son.[50]

As in the choice of Sydenstricker to head the technical medical committee, the announcement of the medical advisory committee provoked a firestorm of criticism. "Despite the care with which [the committee] was selected," Edwin Witte recalled, "it drew instant fire from groups close to the inner circle of the American Medical Association." Telegrams "poured in," complaining, among other things, that the CES was being unfair in its attitude toward organized medicine, that no general practitioners were included, and that the advisory committee was not geographically diverse enough. The National Medical Association, the professional organization for black physicians, protested its exclusion, as did groups representing chiropractors, osteopaths, and homeopaths. "None of these groups," Witte commented, "could be included without seriously offending the major medical associations."[51]

When the National Conference on Economic Security was held, its roundtable discussion of health insurance proved a fiasco for Edgar Sydenstricker and other insurance proponents. In a surprise turn of events, Michigan physician Henry Luce, who was to speak in favor of insurance along with Michael M. Davis, publically disavowed his previous support for compulsory insurance.[52] Luce, it soon emerged, was cajoled into changing his position by a last-minute visit from AMA representatives. The AMA, he was told, would lift the informal but effective boycott imposed on him after he had written a proinsurance report for the Michigan State Medical association if he came out against insurance at the conference.[53] Michael Davis, the only nonphysician participating in the discussion, also proved the only defender of Sydenstricker's insurance plan.[54]

On the evening of November 14, immediately after the conference's conclusion, the CES's medical advisory committee met to begin considering the Sydenstricker-helmed technical committee's working plan. In introductory remarks to the advisory committee, Labor Secretary Frances Perkins informed its members that the technical committee would not be required to submit its report in December as originally planned. If the advisory committee needed more time to consider the technical committee's proposals, she explained, both committees would be granted an extension.[55] Conciliatory in tone and forthright about the concerns of organized medicine, the speech hinted at the growing concern of the CES about physician opposition to insurance.

As the advisory committee met, it became evident that its members were sharply divided. Health insurance, its members informed Perkins and the CES after the conclusion of its meetings, was a complex issue, requiring "the study of a considerable body of facts, some of which are now available and others which will shortly be secured." Given the circumstances, the advisory committee's members asked "to avail ourselves of the suggestions which you made, that we might have more time for this survey than has been available during these few days."[56]

Sydenstricker and Isidore Falk had held out hope that portions of organized medicine might support an insurance plan that states could opt in or out of. Both men believed that the medical profession was substantially less monolithic than the AMA leadership would have the public and political leaders believe. This conviction was bolstered by events in October, when the AMA's House of Delegates endorsed experimental voluntary insurance plans. Such plans were acceptable, according to the AMA, as long as they were physician controlled and followed a set of guidelines intended to ensure that they would not affect the practice of medicine.[57]

This endorsement, however, was largely the result of an attempt by the AMA leadership to appear reasonable and open to change while simultaneously portraying Sydenstricker and Falk as dangerous proponents of policies that would damage American medicine. The AMA endorsement was also clearly not consistent with Sydenstricker and Falk's goal of using insurance to remake the day-to-day practice of medicine. For Sydenstricker and Falk, reorganizing the delivery of medical services continued to be a central concern, in many ways trumping the concerns about economic well-being that underpinned the creation of the CES.

Split on insurance, the medical advisory committee reached consensus on the issue of continuing FERA's foray into the financing of individual medical services. Without controversy, it endorsed "the use of federal relief funds to supplement local funds" to pay for physician services and hospital visits. An endorsement of existing policy and broadly consistent with the AMA's public position on charity medicine, this statement did not represent a proposal for new legislation.[58]

Notably, the medical advisory committee expressed support for Sydenstricker and Falk's proposal that federal support for the development of local public health infrastructure be expanded under the auspices of the PHS.[59] Both Sydenstricker and Falk recognized this as an important development. The AMA had long been skeptical of the PHS's rural sanitation program and its efforts to stimulate the development of local public health infrastructure. Now, however, the AMA-aligned members of the advisory committee hinted at a new stance: organized medicine would support federal public health efforts as a means of attempting to head off the threat of health insurance.[60]

This was a shrewd move. The growth of medical costs, the strain of the Depression, and the ascendency of the New Deal coalition had placed the AMA in a precarious position. Given the context, wholesale obstructionism was a potentially dangerous approach to take. As Isidore Falk explained it, the "more the AMA and related groups were finding themselves in the position of building up opposition to the expected health insurance proposals, the more anxious they were to be in a position of supporting something, or being for something constructive." The politics of insurance and public health, meanwhile, differed in important ways. While compulsory health insurance had no strong base of support, the PHS could call on the backing of the Southern political representatives with whom it had forged a strong bond since World War I. With the Democrats in control in Washington, Southerners now held a key role in the national government, controlling influential committees in Congress and shaping the contours of national policy.[61] By accepting an expansion of federal public health efforts, the AMA could align itself with a potentially popular issue and ward off criticism that it blindly opposed all federal action.

For public health in the United States, the AMA's shift proved an important development. "The more the opposition against our health insurance program crystalized and the harder the opposition jelled," Isidore Falk later pointed out, "the stronger and warmer came the support of the AMA for public health work."[62] Over time, opposition to federal intervention in health insurance would help to drive the formation of a new federal policy regime in the realm of public health.

Health and Economic Security

The CES delivered its report to the president on January 15, more than a month after the original December deadline. With the medical advisory committee divided and requesting more time, Sydenstricker and Falk's insurance plan was quietly excluded.[63] Instead, the report on health focused largely on the issue of public health. Asserting that the "development of more adequate public-health services is the first and most inexpensive step in furnishing economic security against illness," the CES report endorsed a large-scale federal program of aid for the development of local public health work.[64] It was careful to note that this was not a new innovation but rather the expansion of an existing program. "What we recommend," it asserted, "involves no departure from previous practices, but an extension of policies that have long been followed and are of proven worth."[65] The PHS's rural sanitation initiative, if the CES report was translated into law, would become the basis for a nationwide program.

Health insurance was another matter altogether. With further study clearly needed, the CES reported, it was impossible to "present a specific plan of health insurance." Still, the report laid out eleven "broad principles and general observations" regarding health insurance.[66] These principles did not constitute a health insurance recommendation, but their inclusion was something of a victory for Sydenstricker and Falk, implying that a future for government-backed insurance might exist.[67]

The report's insurance section brought on a new wave of condemnation. It aroused, in the words of Edwin Witte, "a great furor in the official circles of the American Medical Association. In the medical journals, the committee's recommendations were described as an endorsement of health insurance and many doctors got the impression that the economic security bill included health insurance." On January 17, the Economic Security bill—embodying the CES report's proposals—was introduced in Congress. The bill's only mention of health insurance was a statement that studying health insurance would be among the duties of the Social Security Board, which was to administer the law. Nonetheless, wrote Witte, "this was sufficient, plus the discussion of the subject in the report of the committee, to once more bring down upon it the full wrath of the opposition to health insurance." With the AMA vehemently opposed, Congress swiftly dropped even this bare mention of insurance.[68]

The Catastrophic Option

Arthur Altmeyer, the chairman of the CES's technical board, emphasized that the CES did not want the Economic Security bill "to be hung up because of any big row on health insurance." There was little public interest in the issue, and President Roosevelt was unwilling to throw his weight behind it. Nonetheless, the CES and its staff remained somewhat optimistic that a compromise might be worked out even after the bill was introduced in Congress. "We were hoping," Altmeyer explained, "that we'd get agreement on the part of the medical advisory committee for some sort of a beginning on health insurance." In particular, it appeared possible that a plan for fostering state-level catastrophic insurance plans might be worked out.[69] The AMA had endorsed catastrophic insurance in responding to the CCMC's majority report only two years before, and it dispatched R. G. LeLand and A. M. Simmons from its Bureau of Medical Economics to assist Sydenstricker and Falk's technical committee in the hopes of shifting their attention toward catastrophic insurance.

In late January 1935, the medical advisory committee reconvened to continue its discussion of insurance. During the late January meetings, the AMA's LeLand and Simmons offered a skeletal proposal for catastrophic health insurance. Insurance, they argued, should be aimed at pooling risk for particularly high and unexpected medical costs, rather than for routine services. Designed in such a manner, health insurance would not impact the practice or even most of the financing of medicine. Many members of the advisory committee were open to these arguments, although there were some concerns about how they could be applied in practice.[70]

The plan did not get a particularly fair hearing. According to Sydenstricker, the catastrophic plan would demand close monitoring of physicians and of patients and would be too administratively complex to bring into practice.[71] Others on the committee agreed that it might require close monitoring of physicians and patients by some sort of government authority. The underlying reality, however, was that Sydenstricker's vision of what insurance should accomplish was vastly different than that favored by proponents of catastrophic insurance.

For both Sydenstricker and Isidore Falk, insurance was important as a means of helping to ward off the threat of economic ruin to individuals and families as a result of unexpected and expensive medical bills. This, however, was only part of the picture. Far more important for both men was the role that insurance could play in reorienting the practice of medicine and shifting physicians toward working in groups linked to hospitals. Catastrophic insurance, designed to allow the prevailing arrangements in American medicine to remain intact, was of little interest to them. The likelihood that insurance would be used to transform the practice of medicine, of course, was precisely why the AMA was opposed to Sydenstricker and Falk's plan.[72] It is impossible to know whether any insurance plan could have gained the support of the AMA in practice. Nonetheless, the catastrophic option provided a potential path toward compromise. This path, however, would have embraced and reinforced the existing system rather than challenging and attempting to transform it.

The Parran Plan

In addition to discussing Sydenstricker and Falk's plan and the catastrophic plan, the medical advisory committee considered a proposal from Thomas Parran. Parran's plan has received little scholarly attention, but its reception makes clear the fluid nature of the options available to health policy makers during this period.[73] Framed in conciliatory and pragmatic terms, the Parran plan succeeded in garnering the support of the AMA-aligned members of the medical advisory committee.

Parran introduced his plan by pointing out the obvious: it was unlikely that Sydenstricker and Falk's insurance proposal would be adopted in the near future. Despite the potential advantages of insurance, the attention of physicians had been "repeatedly called to the faults and defects of health insurance as utilized in other countries."[74] Many American physicians viewed insurance as a dangerous and foreign concept, threatening outside control of the medical profession and almost certain reduction in the quality of medical services. Were Congress to enact a health insurance program, parts of the nation might embrace it. In many areas, however, physician opposition would mean that health insurance "would not have the guidance and cooperation necessary to insure its success."[75] The signals from the president and the leaders of the CES were clear by this point: no health plan was going to be introduced in Congress that threatened to create a backlash against the entire economic security program.[76]

As Parran noted, there was also a general lack of popular interest in or support for health insurance. Americans cared about health and about the costs of accessing medical services, but few viewed insurance as a solution to their problems. Most were unfamiliar with insurance as a means of financing health services. For the majority of Americans, proposals for unemployment insurance and old-age assistance appeared far more important.[77]

Physician opposition and a lack of popular support were crucial factors working against the Sydenstricker and Falk plan, but Parran was more concerned by something else: his belief that insurance would not prove an effective mechanism for improving the overall health of Americans. Like the authors of the Social Security Act's provisions for old-age pensions,

Sydenstricker and Falk assumed that their program would cover a distinct category of wage-earning workers.[78] Although later scholars have often suggested that farm workers and domestic servants were excluded from the Social Security Act's old-age pension program as passed in 1935 at the behest of Southern members of Congress who wished to deny benefits to black Southerners, this was not the cause of the exclusion.[79]

Farm workers and domestic servants were excluded during the development of the old-age pension provisions because collecting payroll taxes from these categories of workers (whose compensation was not necessarily in the form of regular cash payments) was viewed as prohibitively difficult. The CES's leaders asked that such workers be included in the legislation when it was introduced, and they initially were. Nonetheless, they were quickly excluded at the behest of the Treasury Department, where officials continued to believe that the contributory model of social insurance could not be applied effectively to farm workers and domestics.[80]

The members of the medical advisory committee did not believe that a contributory health insurance plan could be extended to most Americans living in rural areas or working in agriculture, and their exclusion was an important point of concern for both Thomas Parran and Stewart Roberts, of Emory University. It was crucial, Roberts argued during the meetings, that a plan be devised for extending protection to black Southerners. Although Roberts thought that some sort of insurance plan might be devised, Parran looked instead to the health center model proposed fifteen years before by New York state health commissioner Hermann Biggs.[81] Building on the AMA's expressed support for catastrophic health insurance, Parran reframed the health center proposal as a form of insurance against particularly expensive medical costs that would not threaten physician autonomy.

After detailing the political obstacles to insurance and suggesting that Sydenstricker's plan would not fully address the issue of economic insecurity arising out of ill health, Parran proposed a new federally backed system, to comprise two categories of beneficiaries. The first category would consist of the unemployed, those on work relief at "less than industrial wages," the indigent, and dependent children. For this group, general medical care, specialist services, hospital care, some dental care, home nursing, and drugs would be paid for using federal tax revenues and state matching funds.[82] The size of the group that Parran proposed to cover was huge: around 20 million Americans were currently on relief. Nonetheless, the proposal was broadly consistent with principles that had already been agreed to by the AMA in both theory and practice.

The second group of beneficiaries would encompass those making up to $2,500 annually. In lieu of the Sydenstricker plan or the catastrophic insurance approach endorsed by the AMA, the government would directly finance medical care in catastrophic cases for this category of beneficiaries. The nation, Parran explained, had "a background of experience on providing for certain expensive illnesses, tuberculosis and mental diseases, crippled children, upon which we might readily extend the system to include persons who are in the low income group but not paupers."[83]

The services covered for these beneficiaries would include expensive diagnostic testing, treatment for diseases such as cancer, syphilis, tuberculosis, and arthritis, major surgery, and childbirth. While noncatastrophic hospital care might be covered, Parran suggested, routine physician fees for working beneficiaries would continue to be paid for out of pocket: "full payment on our present basis would be made for the ordinary illness treated in the home or the doctor's office."[84] This was a crucial point. For the medical profession, the key appeal of catastrophic coverage was that it would not affect routine care. As a result, it was believed, catastrophic coverage would not affect the patient–physician relationship or compromise the autonomy of the medical profession.

As in the health center plan proposed by Hermann Biggs, the Parran plan suggested that government would help to pay for the facilities that physicians used, for laboratory work and expensive diagnostic tests, and for particularly expensive specialist services. Now, however, the federal government would back the entire system. In effect, the federal government would help to fund the framework in which private physicians operated. When the cost of services passed a certain point or when certain expensive diseases or procedures were involved, federal and state money, collected through general taxation rather than through payroll deductions, would kick in.

In embracing general revenues as a means of funding health services, Parran's plan diverged from the social insurance model that underpinned old-age pensions. As he explained in a speech in May 1935, Parran believed that general taxation was a fairer means of funding health programs than individual contributions. Although both were acceptable means of spreading the risk of high medical costs, contributory health insurance as proposed by Sydenstricker was less equitable. "From one point of view," Parran explained, "even the weekly contribution of the wage earner can be considered as taxation. There is this important difference however: The cost of health insurance is borne chiefly by the low-income group of the population." The cost, Parran continued, fell "most heavily upon those least able to pay. In this way it differs from general taxation which, in theory at least, assumes payment of taxes in proportion to ability to pay."[85] The idea of earned benefits, so crucial to those who designed both Social Security's old-age pensions (and later the Medicare program), held little appeal for Parran.

If states wished to adopt contributory insurance plans, they could be given the option to do so, but Parran clearly believed that his own approach would prove more effective and less politically treacherous. Apparently he believed that the pressures being created by the growing costs of medical care and by the decline in paying patients resulting from the Depression would lead the AMA to accept his plan as a compromise option. Administratively, he suggested that such a direct approach would prove easier than the catastrophic insurance approach, which some believed would prove too complicated. Like Hermann Biggs, Parran viewed the issue of individual medical services from the perspective of the health of the population as a whole. By placing state and local health departments in charge of administering the program, he hoped, his plan would provide an avenue for more effectively integrating public health and individual medicine.[86]

The Road Not Taken

Parran's plan pushed at the boundaries of what organized medicine might be expected to agree to. Parran himself acknowledged that the system of publically provided medical service for the indigent that he proposed "might conceivably be extended in a socialist state to include the whole population," though he "personally would oppose in my own philosophy any such extension."[87] At first, it appeared that his proposal might be regarded as dangerous and revolutionary rather than conciliatory and pragmatic, as he suggested it was. California physician Rexwald Brown, who was particularly concerned about maintaining the autonomy of the medical profession, almost immediately suggested that Parran's plan might "put the whole matter under the control of politicians." The plan, he worried, might lead to "state medicine." Robert Greenough, president of the American College of Surgeons, was highly skeptical of the idea that the medical profession would actually embrace Parran's plan, suggesting only half-jokingly that the advisory committee's "own lives would be somewhat at stake" if they voted for it. Virginia's Shelton Horsley, meanwhile, suggested that health insurance might be a simpler proposition. He mused that Parran's plan, "however excellent it may be, would be almost impossible to execute."[88]

The tide began to turn, however, when AMA president Walter Bierring spoke up. "Taken in its general principles," Bierring told the committee, "this appeals to me very strongly and I believe that if it is regarded purely as an extension of public medical services, that it furnishes a solution." The Parran plan, he asserted, was "practical and can be carried out." The nation already "had some experience with public medical services, particularly during the depression period, and I believe that this will meet with more favor and accomplish more than will the special system of insurance." The plan contained no more state medicine, he asserted, than insurance did, and would meet "with more favor in the organized profession than a definite plan of national health insurance, which I do not believe medical men of this country are prepared for at this time."[89]

Coming from Bierring, this was an important assessment. After further discussion, it became clear that key committee members viewed Parran's proposal as acceptable. The Cleveland Clinic's George Crile, who believed that health insurance would create a dangerously high degree of government control and make it difficult to recruit talented young men into the field of medicine, expressed his support. "This appeals to me greatly," he told his fellow advisory committee members. "I don't know how it will work out as a practical measure, but I can see how it equalizes the existing professional feeling, supplementing the incomes of a great many men all over the country, in the cities and in the rural communities, and it seems to me to have a very broad application. I like it."[90]

Harvey Cushing, important both for his standing in the medical profession and for his personal relationship with the president, also expressed support. For Cushing, the key was the idea that the plan would not attempt to transform the practice of medicine. Parran's plan, he asserted, was both unique and promising: "We can call it the American plan versus what so many people have gradually come to believe is a very undesirable foreign plan which we must introduce just because a lot of other countries have already done it, and we see the evils of it." Evils might also develop out of the new proposal, he acknowledged, "but at least it is a new proposition."[91] Later in the committee's deliberations, Cushing came back to the importance of framing the Parran proposal as different from European approaches. "If we could call it the American plan," he maintained, it would almost certainly be sellable. The "psychology of the American citizen being such as it is, he would say, 'that is the plan I want.'"[92]

There was a general consensus that Parran's plan would be more effective than insurance in rural areas. For some members of the medical advisory committee, the Saskatchewan plan, under which the heavily rural Canadian province allowed localities to recruit and hire physicians to be paid using tax dollars, appeared to be a worthy model. Similar provisions, AMA president Walter Bierring suggested, could be included in a fully fleshed-out Parran plan. Parran did not favor the Saskatchewan approach, which was more limited than the government-backed network of medical facilities and technology that he envisioned, but Bierring's openness is a good indication of how fluid the options still remained from the perspective of the men involved in the advisory committee meetings.

Gradually, it became evident that the members of the medical advisory committee were willing to back the Parran plan. Sydenstricker, however, remained committed to his own insurance plan, a stance that greatly irritated CES executive director Edwin Witte. Throughout Sydenstricker and Falk's efforts, Witte had attempted to persuade the AMA to hold back on its assaults, even briefly securing something of a truce after the tumultuous National Conference on Economic Security in November. Sydenstricker's unwillingness to compromise during the second round of advisory committee meetings, however, enraged many of the AMA-aligned physicians involved. Witte, who by this point had given up on the idea that any insurance plan would prove politically viable, found himself subject to an avalanche of angry letters from advisory committee members who felt that Sydenstricker had conducted the meetings in an unfair and biased manner.[93]

In its final report to the CES, Sydenstricker's technical medical committee proposed a health insurance plan along the lines that he had favored all along. Despite all of the work that Sydenstricker and Falk had put into it, the Roosevelt administration viewed the plan as politically explosive and decided to not release it publically.

There are strong reasons to believe that things might have gone differently had Sydenstricker been more open to compromise and had the CES not been operating under such significant time constraints. Sydenstricker and Falk were largely concerned with the problems confronting wage earners, but it is highly likely that a formal legislative proposal aimed at improving access to individual medical services for the indigent could have gained the approval of the AMA. For lower-income individuals and workers, either the catastrophic insurance option or the Parran plan might have offered a starting point for compromise. Of the two, the Parran plan was far more warmly received by the advisory committee, and was viewed as more administratively plausible.

Even a heavily scaled-back version of the Parran plan might have set American health policy on a dramatically different path. In other nations, comprehensive health systems have tended to emerge through an evolutionary process rather than through one legislative act. As Parran himself noted during the advisory committee's meetings, paying the health costs of the indigent—already a massive portion of the population—might easily have led to direct payments for other groups. Financing particularly expensive services for the employed and funding new infrastructure, meanwhile, would have created an additional platform through which federal involvement in the financing of medical services might have been expanded.

Harvey Cushing praised Parran's plan for its noninterference in the practice of medicine, but federal support for physician-controlled medicine for millions and payments for expensive medical treatments and diagnostic services would over time have almost certainly led to an ever more expansive federal role in the provision of individual medical services. Rather than a "big bang," however, the process would have been an incremental one, with an uncertain conclusion. With the federal government deeply involved in financing individual medical services, issues of both cost control and quality might soon have become an important feature of public policy debates. Conversations about these issues might plausibly have led to a discussion about how the delivery of medical services should be organized.

Economic Security

Rather than proposing an integrated system encompassing both public health and individual medical services, the Economic Security Act introduced in Congress included only provisions for public health efforts. Where health insurance provoked controversy and possessed no significant political constituency, the bill's public health provisions were deemed an acceptable concession by the AMA. In addition, they possessed a deep well of support, particularly among the Southern Democrats who played key roles in the congressional leadership. As Edwin Witte wrote, the proposed expansion of federal support for local-level public health efforts was "throughout the congressional consideration of this measure a source of strength for the bill."[94]

As Daniel Carpenter has argued, organizational reputation is a key component of a bureaucracy's ability to shape the development of new policies.[95] Beginning during World War I, the PHS generated a strong reputation for itself as an organization committed to fighting the diseases that plagued the rural South. Rather than acting as an outside force, its officers had worked to embed the organization in the governing structures of the region. Developing effective techniques for combating disease, they also forged relationships with local civic leaders, landowners, and state and local political officials. These bonds, as well as the belief among Southern officials that the PHS was an agency that supported the economic interests of both localities and the region, placed the proponents of an expanded role for the PHS in a strong position once Southern Democrats became key players in the national government under the New Deal.

During the debate over the proposals that became the Social Security Act, vocal proponents of expanding federal public health efforts included, among others, Senate Finance Committee chairman Pat Harrison of Mississippi, and House Ways and Means Committee chairman Robert Doughton of North Carolina. In line with the geographical origins of federal involvement in the development of local public health efforts, the Economic Security bill's public health provisions (which were eventually codified as Title VI of the Social Security Act) were aimed to a great extent at addressing the health needs of the South.

"The aids provided in this title," Edwin Witte noted, "were understood to be primarily for states in which public health work had been backward, due largely to state poverty. These were particularly the southern states, and the heads of the state departments of health in nearly all these states appeared before the congressional committees to endorse this part of the bill."[96] Malaria, pellagra, and hookworm would be key targets of the proposed program, and the South would be its most obvious and immediate beneficiary. Southern state health officers, Witte explained, "gave very strong testimony regarding the need for additional public health work in the South and these arguments strongly appealed to members of Congress from this section, many of whom were very influential in the two committees considering this legislation."[97]

Surgeon General Hugh Cumming was initially cool to the idea of expanding the rural sanitation initiative into a nationwide program aimed at the development of local public health infrastructure. Once the legislation was introduced, however, he offered consistent support. The Economic Security bill's public health provisions were also strongly supported by new assistant treasury secretary, Josephine Roche. Formerly a staff member at the Children's Bureau, Roche was now the assistant secretary with oversight of the PHS.[98] Her ascendency, some believed, would hasten the demise of Cumming and ascent of Thomas Parran to the position of surgeon general.[99] Out of loyalty to Roosevelt and also perhaps because of a desire to gain favor with Roche, Cumming also embraced provisions of the Economic Security bill that essentially recreated on a large scale the 1920s Sheppard–Towner program of grants-in-aid to states for the health and well-being of mothers and children, a program that he had long opposed and indeed had helped to destroy.

Testifying before the House Ways and Means Committee and the Senate Finance Committee, representatives of the PHS and the Treasury Department portrayed the Economic Security bill's public health provisions as an unobjectionable and logical expansion of existing federal activities. As Surgeon General Cumming explained, the proposal was "treading no new ground; it is an extension of an attempt on the part of the Federal Government many years ago which has been eminently successful. It is not a problematical thing."[100]

The PHS had expanded its reach significantly in the preceding decades, but the service's single biggest expenditure continued to be for the operation of marine hospitals, which consumed around $5 million of the PHS's $10 million budget. Most of its other work was in the area of scientific research, undertaken through the service's National Institute of Health. For members of Congress familiar with the PHS's rural sanitation work, the service's ongoing focus on marine hospitals appeared to come as something of a surprise. "In other words," Kentucky congressman and ardent PHS supporter Fred Vinson exclaimed during Assistant Treasury Secretary Roche's testimony before the House Ways and Means Committee, "half of the sum total that is generally said to be for public health went to the marine-hospital activity. Is there any connection between the marine hospitals and the public health services?"[101]

Assistant Surgeon General Clifford E. Waller, who oversaw the rural sanitation program as head of the Division of Domestic Quarantine, began his testimony by attempting to respond to Vinson's concerns about "what percentage of our total appropriation goes for health work." It was, he explained, only a small portion of the service's appropriation: "I may say that it is slightly over a million dollars [the rural sanitation program was at the time allotted $1,000,000 annually through FERA], or a little over one-tenth of the total appropriation to the Public Health Service."[102]

Briefly allowing Waller to explain the proposed expansion of the PHS's support for local-level public health efforts, Vinson interrupted him in an attempt to further "paint the picture that I want to present to the committee." After describing PHS efforts to vaccinate schoolchildren in Kentucky, he professed to his fellow committee members that he was "perfectly willing to testify, because I have had personal observations and knowledge of how those things work, in my own country. It is the hardest-working crowd I know . . . they carry this preventive medicine into the roots of our rural society and, to my mind, it is the most splendid work that the Federal Government participates in."[103]

And so it went. Public health was used to generate support for the Economic Security bill where health insurance would likely have mobilized a concerted opposition. Southern support for and experience with the PHS ensured that the service would be given substantial latitude in implementing the provisions of the Economic Security Act that granted it expanded authority. The president signed the legislation, now called the Social Security Act, on August 14, 1935. Title VI of the Social Security Act authorized $8 million in grants-in-aid for the development of state and local public health infrastructure and training of public health workers. Another $2 million was authorized for the expansion of the PHS's research activities.

The formula for the allocation of Title VI funds strongly favored the PHS's Southern constituency, taking into account "special health problems," economic need, and the need for trained public health personnel.[104] The enabling language, Edwin Witte noted, was "drafted to suit the wishes of the United States Public Health Service."[105] Reaping the benefits of a reputation developed through the efforts of PHS workers to develop local public health capabilities and control diseases such as malaria beginning during World War I, the PHS received "broader discretionary power . . . than is conferred upon any federal agency in any other title."[106]

CHAPTER SIX

"THE RELIGION OF MANKIND'S FUTURE"

Thomas Parran was sworn in as surgeon general of the PHS in April 1936. The organization he now headed was significantly more powerful than the one he joined on the eve of World War I. The centerpiece of its new authority, Title VI of the Social Security Act, was built on the foundation of the rural sanitation program that he had worked to build during his early years in the service. Energetic, experienced, and highly regarded by his peers, Parran was committed to further expanding the scope of the PHS's power. Over the next twelve years, he would push for an approach to national health policy that encompassed public health, individual medicine, biomedical research, and the construction of new medical facilities.

Parran assumed his new role in time to oversee the implementation of Title VI. After the passage of the Social Security Act, Louisiana senator Huey Long, who viewed it as inferior to his own Share Our Wealth program, blocked appropriations for the new legislation. After Long's assassination in Baton Rouge, however, an appropriation was made for the Social Security Act, including Title VI. In the interim, Rockefeller philanthropy, which had discontinued its assistance after FERA began funding the rural sanitation program, stepped in to help fund county health work.[1]

During the summer of 1936, the service began distributing the first of the funds made available through the Social Security Act. The money was directed toward creating new health departments, sustaining and improving existing departments, and initiating an array of training efforts. In the West, the PHS expanded its efforts to monitor plague, still regarded as a potential threat. In the urban North, new funding was put toward efforts at ameliorating occupational diseases in industrial areas. In the South, the PHS focused strongly on malaria, hookworm, and pellagra. Throughout the nation, the PHS strengthened its ties with state and local governments and worked to stimulate high-quality public health work.

For Parran and other PHS leaders, the Social Security Act unmistakably signaled the beginning of a new era in American health policy. "Under the public health provisions of the Social Security Act," Parran wrote in October 1936, "a national health program has been made possible for the first time in the history of the Public Health Service."[2] Within the next year, the PHS developed and put in place new programs for assisting state efforts in the realms of nutrition, dental hygiene, and laboratory methods. The PHS also began offering support to states for devising effective accounting systems.[3]

Parran proved effective at gaining additional congressional support and funding. During 1937, Parran and the PHS worked with members of Congress to secure passage of the National Cancer Institute Act, which created a National Cancer Institute under the umbrella of the PHS's National Institute of Health. The National Cancer Institute became the first NIH program to distribute grants for extramural research, an innovation that foreshadowed a much larger expansion of federally supported biomedical research to come.[4] In 1938, Parran and the PHS persuaded Congress to back a new Venereal Disease Control Act.[5]

Parran had long been concerned with the issue of venereal disease, and he made a point of highlighting its widespread and often ignored presence in the United States in an open and frank manner. In 1937, he published an influential book on syphilis, *Shadow on the Land*. It was also in this area that Parran made a series of callous decisions that, when revealed decades later, greatly injured his reputation. Since 1932, the PHS had observed the course of untreated syphilis in a group of black men living around Tuskegee, Alabama.[6] The study became even more unconscionable as the PHS launched a new antisyphilis campaign under Parran's leadership. With Parran's support, Tuskegee study participants were purposefully denied treatment. While the PHS's late 1930s antisyphilis campaign led to a 30 percent reduction of the incidence of syphilis among blacks living in Macon County, Alabama (where Tuskegee is located), the men involved in the Tuskegee study remained untreated.[7]

This chapter deals with the impact of New Deal–era public health as well as the shifting dynamics of the New Deal coalition. Although the PHS's outlook expanded far beyond the rural South during the late 1930s, the Southern diseases that drove its expansion into local-level public health efforts beginning with World War I remained a key concern. For the Southern Democrats who represented the PHS's core base of support, the service's ability to control the diseases that had long plagued the region continued to be of great importance. In the years after the passage of the Social Security Act, the federal government attacked malaria, pellagra, and hookworm on an unprecedented scale. At the same time, however, the emergence of the conservative coalition of Southern Democrats and northern Republicans significantly altered the domestic policy landscape. During 1937, Franklin Roosevelt's ill-fated Supreme Court–packing plan and the economic decline termed the Roosevelt Recession placed the president in a newly defensive posture. As the PHS pushed for an expanded mandate, to include action in the realm of individual medical services, the political climate became increasingly less hospitable.

Southern Maladies

Despite more than two decades of outside intervention, health conditions in much of the South remained dire. In the summer of 1936, just as the PHS began distributing Social Security funds, journalist James Agee and Farm Security Administration (FSA) photographer Walker Evans traveled to rural Alabama. Exploring the circumstances of three white tenant families living in Hale County, Agee and Evans found conditions only somewhat improved from those of previous decades. The deaths of infants and young children, Agee wrote, were an expected aspect of life, painful but ubiquitous. Malaria was pervasive. "Nobody escapes malaria and its returns; and in its milder forms, such as diarrhea, nausea, headache, dizziness, sudden departures of strength, and retching of bile, everyone takes it for granted. Every so often, though, you get such a bad spell of it you mighty nigh have to quit work."[8]

One of the mothers was stricken with pellagra for the past decade. "Three years ago," Agee wrote, "she was out of her head for a long time." Suffering from dementia, she at one point attempted to kill her baby daughter "with a chunk of stovewood." Recently, the woman had started taking brewer's yeast and was improving. "She is better now and thinks it must be the powders, that is to say, the yeast. For the past year and a half she has been taking Brewer's Yeast stirred up in molasses, milk, and water." Still, she continued to have "nervous spells . . . and they are bad. She can feel them coming on like something terrifying sneaking up behind her and then all of a sudden she sees black and yellow lights busting all around and after that she doesn't know anything for a while."[9]

There were some signs of hookworm among the tenants' children, but Agee was not sure whether they had the disease or not. Instead, the parasite melted into a more general and all-encompassing sickliness. "Charles's anemic pallor may be a symptom of [hookworm], but Charles has been very sick. The halting of Squeaky's growth may be a result of it; and on the other hand may be some glandular sprain. . . . None of the children were dirt-eaters, outside the normal course of getting down their meals."[10]

Agee offered only a fleeting assessment of the situation of the local black population, but again he highlighted their poor health. "Venereal disease," he wrote, "is thick among them." Although the state had at one point subsidized the purchase of the antisyphilis drug Salvarsan, it was now being sold at $1.50 per shot, "which is prohibitive to most Negroes and to many whites. Malaria flowers as richly on their blood as on white. The skins of many are rusty with what can be merely ill health, and what can be pellagra." Pneumonia was a major issue during the winter, while infant mortality was staggeringly routine. "Their babies," Agee wrote, "die off like flies in autumn."[11]

The Decline of Southern Malaria

As Agee and Evans traveled to Alabama, the South was on the verge of a major and permanent transformation. The overall malaria death rate in the states where the disease was historically endemic hit its last peak in 1933, at twelve deaths per 100,000 residents.[12] Variation among the endemic states, importantly, was substantial, with the 1933 death rate ranging from 0.4 in Virginia to 46.4 in Arkansas. Within the states themselves, some areas were largely free of malaria deaths, while others faced an extreme malaria burden. Six counties in Arkansas, for instance, had malaria death rates of over 100 per 100,000 residents in 1933.[13]

Mortality statistics are an imperfect means of gauging the extent of both malaria's reach and its impact on Southern society, which came largely in the form of sickness rather than death. Deaths from malaria came almost exclusively from *Plasmodium falciparum*, rather than from *P. vivax*, which was also endemic but largely caused only illness. Reliable morbidity statistics, however, are not available. As a result, deaths rates represent the only workable and consistent proxy for the disease's presence.

Despite these limitations, the overall trend of malaria's demise in the Southern United States is clear. Beginning in 1934, the first malaria season after New Deal public works drainage efforts began, regionwide deaths from the disease entered a marked and permanent decline. From twelve deaths per 100,000 in 1933, the malaria death rate in endemic states declined to 10.9 in 1934. A more dramatic decline occurred between 1936 and 1937, when deaths dropped from 9.5 per 100,000 residents to 5.6. Notably, this was the first year of the PHS's expanded public health efforts under the Social Security Act. By 1940, the death rate had declined to 3.3 deaths per 100,000. By 1945 it stood at 0.9 per 100,000 (Figure 6.1).

From any perspective, the decline of malaria during the 1930s is sur-

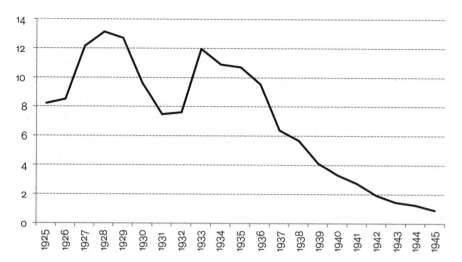

Figure 6.1. Malaria deaths per 100,000 residents in historically endemic states, 1925–1945. *Source:* Census Bureau Mortality Reports, 1925–1945. Data for mortality, 1925–1938, http://www.cdc.gov/nchs/products/vsus/vsus_1890_1938.htm; data for 1939–1945, http://www.cdc.gov/nchs/products/vsus/vsus_1939_1964.htm. The decline in deaths during 1930–1931 was a result of the drought conditions that prevailed in much of the South. States included are those of the former Confederacy plus Kentucky, Missouri, and Oklahoma.

prising. Malaria is a disease of poverty, and the Depression hit the rural South hard. Severe economic dislocation, along with the increase in potential mosquito breeding grounds in areas where the Agricultural Adjustment Act and its successor, the Soil Conservation and Domestic Allotment Act, had reduced the amount of acreage planted in cotton or other cash crops, might also be expected to have increased the extent of malaria's reach in the region.

Margaret Humphreys, a leading scholar of the history of science, has argued that social change was the primary factor in the elimination of malaria in the South. Public health interventions, Humphreys maintains, did not play a central role in elimination of the disease. "Although New Deal programs included drainage projects to combat malaria," she writes, "these were poorly planned and likely had little impact. More important were agricultural programs that paid landowners to take land out of production and other measures that resulted in the depopulation of the southern countryside."[14]

After the AAA, Humphreys argues, malaria victims began to move away from endemic areas: "Once the sharecroppers moved away from the densest clouds of anopheles, the critical links in the continual malaria chain began to break down, one community at a time. Certainly other factors such as returning prosperity, drainage, pyrethrum sprays, and screening played their roles. But it was this removal of the malaria carrier/victim from the vicinity of the anopheles mosquito that probably had the largest effect on the decline in the plasmodium's presence."[15]

This analysis, however, is not consistent with the chronology of malaria's decline. The long-term implications of the AAA and the Soil Conservation Act, passed as a substitute after the Supreme Court found the AAA unconstitutional, were of course substantial. Indeed, they helped to set in motion the end of the sharecropping system and an almost complete reorganization of the Southern political economy. For the time being, however, out-migration from the region on anything approaching the scale suggested by Humphreys did not occur.

As James N. Gregory suggests in a careful and data-driven study of Southern out-migration, the 1930s are best understood as an "interlude" between two phases of migration, one starting near the beginning of the twentieth century and another beginning with World War II.[16] During the Depression, there were few jobs outside of the region or in Southern cities for rural Southerners to migrate toward. Only the far western portion of the malaria-endemic United States experienced large-scale rural out-migration during the 1930s. In parts of Oklahoma and Texas, drought and soil erosion led to the Dust Bowl migration that caught the attention of journalists and was described in popular works such as John Steinbeck's *Grapes of Wrath*. That the rural South was not depopulated during the Depression is made clear in data collected by the US Census Bureau. In the malaria-endemic states as a whole, the rural population increased from 24,715,971 in 1930 to 25,965,678 in 1940.

It was World War II and its economic aftermath that led to significant declines in the population of the rural Southern counties where malaria was endemic. By that point, malaria had largely been banished from the region. Throughout the Depression, Southern agriculture remained unmechanized, guaranteeing a strong demand for workers to pick cotton at the end of the growing season and limiting the ability of landowners to get rid of tenants despite reduced acreage. Federal relief agencies helped to ensure the availability of this labor supply, regularly releasing workers from the relief rolls in order to provide landowners with labor at harvest time.[17]

Rather than out-migration, it was the combination of public works efforts aimed at malaria and the development of local-level public health infrastructure under the auspices of the Social Security Act's Title VI that led to malaria's demise.[18] The federal CWA began putting unemployed Southerners to work on drainage projects during the winter of 1933–1934. Loosely supervised by the PHS, these early efforts appear to have at times been ineffective and even counterproductive.[19] The CWA was dissolved in early 1934, and the drainage program was continued by the Federal Emergency Relief Agency. In 1935, the federal Works Progress Administration began providing labor for drainage projects, and continued to do so throughout the 1930s. By the end of the decade, public health workers were increasingly focused on the development of methods of lining ditches to make them more permanent.[20]

After 1936, when Title VI funds became available, drainage efforts became increasingly effective.[21] Title VI money was tied to requirements that states increase spending on public health, and was allocated under a formula that took into account special health problems (including malaria), economic need, and the need for trained personnel. By providing a more permanent basis for malaria control through greater federal–state–county coordination, fully staffed county health departments, and money for the training of state and local public health workers, Title VI helped to both advance and solidify the gains in malaria control being made by the public works agencies.

The new Social Security–funded program, fully operational by the end of 1936, marked a turning point in the elimination of Southern malaria.[22] The scope of the drainage work now underpinned by increasingly high-quality public health infrastructure was massive. Overall, the works projects "involved a daily average of 211,000 men for 6.5 years working on malaria control drainage in an average of 250 counties." In the malaria-endemic South as a whole, it was estimated that, by the time the nation entered World War II, 544,414 acres of mosquito breeding sites had been drained through the construction of 33,655 miles of ditches.[23] Although comprehensive data are not available, local health departments pursued a variety of other measures, including screening windows and dusting stagnant water with the chemical Paris green.

Wisely, contemporary public health workers expressed only a restrained optimism about the decline of malaria during the late 1930s. For some, the decline of malaria appeared consistent with a broader cyclical pattern of malaria incidence. In 1938, Tulane University malariologist Ernest Carroll Faust suggested that the national malaria death rate, "which developed to a peak so suddenly in 1933," had "apparently reached its trough, and that, unless unusual circumstances supervene, an average rise in the rate may again be anticipated in 1938 or 1939." That malaria remained an ongoing threat in the face of substantial federal efforts also suggested a resurgence might occur when spending was reined in.[24]

The Decline of Pellagra

Despite extremely the unfavorable economic conditions, pellagra deaths also declined throughout the 1930s (Figure 6.2). In retrospect, it was clear that the 1927 Mississippi flood was a crucial turning point. Joseph Goldberger's discovery that brewer's yeast would prevent and cure pellagra meant that the disease could be confronted head-on even in the context of the Depression. Knowledge of the cure, meanwhile, could be spread through the growing system of county health departments, and in particular through educational meetings and the efforts of public health nurses. Because yeast was a commercially distributed product, there were also incentives for private companies, such as Fleischmann's, to advertise its health benefits. The spread of knowledge about the pellagra-preventative qualities of brewer's yeast was complemented by the changing face of the Southern countryside: reduction

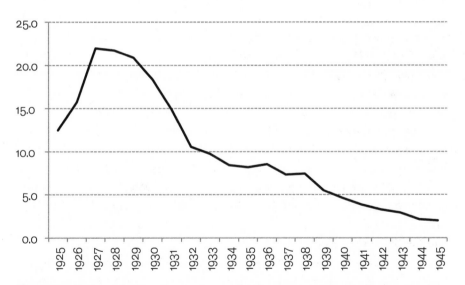

Figure 6.2. Pellagra deaths per 100,000, endemic states, 1925–1945. *Source:* Census Bureau Mortality Statistics. Data for mortality, 1925–1938, http://www.cdc.gov /nchs/products/vsus/vsus_1890_1938.htm; data for 1939–1945, http://www.cdc.gov /nchs/products/vsus/vsus_1939_1964.htm. States included are those of the former Confederacy plus Kentucky, Missouri, and Oklahoma.

of the cotton crop after the AAA meant that families could grow small gardens. The confluence of brewer's yeast, county health departments, and new opportunities to plant vegetables signaled the onset of pellagra's retreat.

Following up on his earlier writings on Goldberger's pellagra research, science writer Paul DeKruif traveled to Sunflower County, Mississippi, in May 1937 with officers from the PHS. With financial support from the Red Cross and the help of community groups, the PHS officers hoped to identify pellagra victims in a select group of Mississippi Delta counties. Within these model counties, the PHS planned to wholly eliminate the disease by administering brewer's yeast and persuading residents to grow their own gardens.

Aware of the decline of pellagra over the course of the preceding decade, DeKruif was nonetheless shocked by what he saw in Sunflower County. The county, he wrote, was "supposed the blackest pellagra spot remaining in Mississippi. This was where over thirteen hundred had been found pellagrous in 1931, and though the sickness had been since then on the downgrade, yet the number suffering in 1935 was formidable." By the time of DeKruif's visit in 1937, pellagra had nearly vanished. The disease "had become so no-account that it was not mentioned as a public health menace in County Health Officer Hugh Cottrell's report for 1936."[25]

The residents of Sunflower County, DeKruif found, were well informed of the menace of pellagra and of proper methods of warding off the disease: "Did the Negro sharecroppers know about pellagra? Oh, yas, suh, we know pellagracy. Did they know about yeast? In leaky cabin after ramshackle shanty the dark people, mammies, aunties, told how 'east was mighty good for the pellagracy." In addition to consuming tablespoons of yeast mixed with water, sharecroppers were now growing vegetables in home gardens. Ten years before, Joseph Goldberger had noted that Southern landowners, insisting that as much land as possible be dedicated to cotton, often prohibited tenants from planting gardens. Now, DeKruif wrote, "it was astounding to find so few cabins without their fenced-in patch of green. Here was Aunt Lyra, in her garden patch on a big plantation near Indianola. Yas, suh, she'd had the pellagracy. Not no more."[26]

Having spent the day driving throughout Sunflower County looking for pellagra victims, DeKruif and the PHS officers found only one case, that of a white tenant farmer. Mississippi state epidemiologist H. C. Ricks, Sunflower County health officer Hugh Cottrell, and a local public health nurse each offered DeKruif a similar explanation for pellagra's decline, which was seconded by local planters and black sharecroppers: "Pellagra was bad business, in the literal sense of the word business." Working to generate political support for public health interventions and for the development of local public health infrastructure, PHS officials had long portrayed the diseases that plagued the South as above all an issue of economic development. Unleashing the region's potential, they had argued, would require freeing both white and black Southerners of the diseases that ensured low productivity in both agriculture and industry. As DeKruif traveled Sunflower County, it became obvious that the economic logic of confronting disease had made a significant impact on local patterns of thought. In blunt language that captured much of the reasoning long used by public health workers in the South, Dr. Ricks explained to DeKruif that white landowners would cooperate with antipellagra efforts "because your planter wants his nigger to work."[27]

The changes observed by DeKruif had a clear basis in the development of local public health capabilities. Before 1927, Sunflower County did not have a full-time county health department. The Rockefeller Sanitary Commission recorded treatment of only twenty-eight cases of hookworm between 1910 and 1914 in the lightly infected county, which also fell outside the jurisdiction of the PHS's efforts in the wartime extracantonment zones.[28] Beset by both pellagra and malaria in average years, the county was hit hard by the 1927 Mississippi flood.[29] A full-time county health department was created in July 1927 as emergency funds from the PHS and the Rockefeller Foundation became available. By the end of the year, the PHS had spent $2,063 in the county and the Rockefeller Foundation $987. Meanwhile, the state government contributed $1,375 and the county government allocated an impressive $1,825. By 1933, in the depths of the Depression, the health department's annual budget stood at $10,480.[30]

DeKruif was impressed by the health department's efforts at community outreach. Using techniques developed by visiting nurse pioneers such as Lillian Wald, local public health nurses made public health an important concern for rural women and an aspect of daily life. At a black church in Inverness, Mississippi, he observed a health clinic put on by county health officer Hugh Cottrell and the department's public health nurses. The mothers and children present, he wrote, were "participants in a service that was—to this reporter—prophetic of the religion of mankind's future." The children were given diphtheria antitoxin and vaccinations for smallpox and typhoid, while the mothers were instructed in "how to care for themselves before their babies came" and "the latest in the science of the feeding of their children, in little words that all could understand."

From DeKruif's perspective, "there was something the opposite of conde-scending or paternalistic in the atmosphere of that church clinic." Instead, he asserted that "Cottrell and his nurses, white people, highly educated, were exactly like older brothers and sisters teaching the great power of sci-ence—not the book knowledge of it but the actual use of it—to these child-like dark mothers." White scientific expertise, in the form of practical public health measures, represented a gateway to racial uplift and modernity: "It was plain that these present descendants of a people, benighted and savage two hundred years ago, were now beginning to understand this new magic, and to depend upon its life-giving power."[31]

Lingering Hookworm

By the 1930s, hookworm was far less of a problem than two decades before. Indeed, there was a growing sense among the public that the dis-ease no longer represented a significant threat. Rather than being fully eliminated, it seemed, the parasite would continue to persist but with a sig-nificantly reduced prevalence and impact. In 1927, the Rockefeller Interna-tional Health Board announced that hookworm had "almost disappeared from the United States."

The announcement dismayed hookworm pioneer Charles Wardell Stiles. When publicized, he complained, it "had the effect of still further decreas-ing the school interest in hookworm disease and, very unfortunately, in inducing many mothers to refuse to accept the diagnosis by physicians and consequently to decline to permit the children to be treated." Nonetheless, Stiles believed, few Southern physicians took the announcement seriously.[32] Writing in 1930, he presented data collected from state health departments and intended to demonstrate that the IHB was wrong. The information on hookworm was compiled through a variety of techniques and was, as he pointed out "not strictly comparable" either across states or with informa-tion from the Rockefeller hookworm surveys of the 1910s. At best, it was a hodgepodge of surveys sent to him by state health officers eager to assist in highlighting the ongoing presence of the disease. While 46,036 people were examined in the numbers presented for Alabama, resulting in a 36.9 percent infection rate, West Virginia's supposed rate of 55.7 percent was based on only 209 examinations. It is impossible to draw meaningful con-clusions based on the data Stiles compiled, but it is clear that the disease remained an ongoing problem. "What the figures for 1929 mean to the 'old timer,'" Stiles wrote, "the one point they are intended to illustrate, is that hookworm infection is still widespread geographically in the Southern States."[33] Despite their best efforts, the RSC, the IHB, the PHS, and state and local health departments had not fully conquered hookworm by the 1930s. A study of hookworm infection in schoolchildren living in five East Texas counties during 1933 and 1934, for instance, found that 33.9 percent of students were infected.[34]

Beginning in late 1933, the Civil Works Administration embarked on a large-scale privy-building campaign. The effort was continued first by FERA and then by the Works Progress Administration. Over the course of the 1930s, the works programs constructed and distributed hundreds of thousands of sanitary privies.[35] Quantifying the impact of this program, however, is difficult. As a cause of death, hookworm disease was minor. Reliable information on cases or infection rates is not available. The best available evidence suggests that the prevalence of hookworm disease was greatly diminished by the end of the 1930s, but also that the disease persisted on a small scale. As late as 1969, South Carolina senator Ernest "Fritz" Hollings would receive condemnation and the epithet "Hookworm Hollings" when he brought attention the presence of hookworm in the South Carolina low country during a "hunger tour" of the state.[36]

The Shifting Politics of the New Deal Coalition

Just as Title VI of the Social Security Act was beginning to bear fruit, the political context in which the PHS operated in and in which national health policy developed shifted dramatically. In a series of cases decided during Franklin Roosevelt's first term as president, the Supreme Court had declared key legislative components of the New Deal to be unconstitutional. The Court's 1935 decision in *Schechter Poultry Corp. v. United States,* striking down parts of the National Industrial Recovery Act, called into question the expansive interpretation of the Constitution's Interstate Commerce Clause that underpinned much of the New Deal's efforts to regulate the American economy. In 1936, its ruling in *United States v. Butler* invalidated the AAA, forcing Congress to replace this key component of the Roosevelt program with the Soil Conservation and Allotment Act.

Roosevelt and other administration officials worried that the Court might dismantle the bulk of Roosevelt's legislative accomplishments, including potentially the 1935 Social Security Act.[37] These fears led to a serious misstep, which augured a precipitous decline in the president's ability to push forward new domestic programs. Reelected with 60.8 percent of the popular vote in November 1936, Roosevelt began his second term by proposing that he be allowed to appoint one additional judge to the Supreme Court for every sitting judge over the age of seventy. The president cited easing the burden of excessive workloads for older judges as the rationale for his plan, which was transparently aimed at shifting the ideological makeup of the Court in favor of the New Deal.[38]

A handful of congressional Democrats offered early public support for the president's plan, though most remained silent. In a sign of what was to come, Virginia senators Carter Glass and Harry F. Bird quickly "indicated fundamental opposition." North Carolina senator Josiah Bailey, the most vocal early Democratic opponent of plan, announced that he would "do all that I can to preserve the independence of the judiciary and that respect for the judicial branch of the Government which always has been and always will be indispensable to the national stability."[39] In the House of Representatives, judiciary committee chairman Hatton Sumners of Texas soon announced that he would not support the proposal.[40]

Almost unflinchingly supportive of Roosevelt during his first term, most congressional Democrats were at best skeptical of the president's plan to pack the Court with New Deal supporters. The disingenuous manner in which the president framed the proposal further accentuated the unease felt by many. For some Southern Democrats, already wary of the implications of growing federal government power and of the strength of the executive branch, Roosevelt's clumsy proposal represented an opportunity to speak out against a president who remained intensely popular within the region. Previously quiet in their criticisms, key Southern politicians began to voice concerns about federal encroachment.[41]

The Supreme Court, for its part, moved decisively away from the philosophy that had provoked the president in the first place. In late March 1937, the Court ruled state minimum wage laws constitutional in *West Coast Hotel v. Parish*, signaling a major shift in its attitude toward government regulation of contracts. In April, the Court upheld the constitutionality of the 1935 National Labor Relations Act, inaugurating a trend of Supreme Court deference to legislative claims about the extent of Congress's power to regulate interstate commerce that soon placed the New Deal on solid constitutional ground. Over the course of a few short months, the threat to the Social Security Act and other New Deal legislation from Court essentially disappeared.[42]

Roosevelt's problems, however, were just beginning. As the court-packing battle continued over the spring, his legislative agenda stalled. During the late summer, a new recession overtook the nation, further worsening the president's political situation. In November, hoping to make up for the wasted first months of his second term, the president called Congress into a special session.[43] The session proved a disaster for the Roosevelt administration, marking the clear emergence of an inter-party "conservative coalition." In a "conservative manifesto" made public in December 1937, a group largely comprising Southern Democrats and Northern Republicans criticized the growth of the welfare state and increasing strength of unions while calling for a balanced budget, lower taxes, and a reinvigoration of states' rights and local rule.[44]

With the ongoing recession and the emerging conservative coalition sapping his political strength, Roosevelt decided to openly back the primary challenges of pro–New Deal candidates against conservative Democrats during the 1938 midterm elections. Southern Democrats were among his key targets, and as part of his planned purge of conservatives, the president created a group—the Conference on Economic Conditions in the South—charged with compiling a report on the roots of Southern economic underdevelopment. In detailing the region's problems, he hoped to strengthen the case for federal action through the New Deal.[45] The South, Roosevelt maintained in a widely publicized speech to the group, was "the Nation's No. 1 economic problem." There was, he continued "an economic unbalance in the Nation as a whole, due to this very condition of the South. It is an unbalance that can and must be righted, for the sake of the South and of the Nation."[46]

Issued in July 1938, the committee's report painted a devastating picture of life in the South. It drew heavily on the work of the PHS. Health, the report found, was among the primary obstacles to Southern economic development. "The low-income belt of the South," it concluded, "is a belt of sickness, misery, and unnecessary death." Malaria, it reported, "infects annually more than 2,000,000 people" and was "estimated to have reduced the industrial output of the South one-third." Its impact was widespread and increasingly well documented: "One of the most striking examples of the effect of malaria on industry was revealed by the PHS in studies among employees of a cotton mill in eastern North Carolina. Previous to the attempts to control malaria, the records of the mill one month showed 66 looms were idle as a result of ill-health. After completion of control work, no looms were idle."[47]

The report also pointed out the high rate of syphilis among black Southerners and high rates of both pneumonia and tuberculosis. Its section on health concluded by noting that the "scourge of pellagra, that affects the South almost exclusively, is a disease chiefly due to inadequate diet; it responds to rather simple preventive measures, including suitable nourishing food."[48] A fundamentally political document, the *Report on Economic Conditions in the South* was intended to make clear the ways in which the region was benefiting from expanded national government action under the New Deal.[49]

In August, Roosevelt spoke out against sitting Democratic members of Congress in their home states. Appearing in Georgia, the president deemed incumbent senator Walter George "a dyed-in-the-wool conservative" and endorsed his opponent in the upcoming Democratic primary, Lawrence Camp.[50] En route back to Washington, Roosevelt addressed a crowd of around 15,000 from the platform of his railroad car in Greenville, South Carolina. "If you believe in the principles for which we are striving," the president said, in a speech aimed at Senator Ellison "Cotton Ed" Smith, "then I hope you will send representatives to the National Legislature who will work toward those ends." Alluding to Smith's claim that a man could support a family in the "lap of luxury" on 50 cents a day in South Carolina, the president ended his remarks by noting that he didn't "believe any family or any man in South Carolina can live on 50 cents a day."[51]

Backlash

Roosevelt's attempted purge was a failure. His preferred candidates were defeated. The purge also further accelerated the backlash against the New Deal among some Southern Democrats and made explicit its undercurrents of racism and antilabor sentiment. Both Walter George in Georgia and "Cotton Ed" Smith in South Carolina responded to Roosevelt's attempts to interject himself into local politics by raising the specter of federal intervention in Southern race relations. Always a potentially effective campaign tactic, the appeal to concerns about race had an added air of urgency given the recent passage of a federal antilynching law in the House of Representatives and mounting fears about the potentially leveling role of labor unions in Southern life.

"This is the one time," Smith told voters in South Carolina, "whether you like Ed Smith or not every red-blooded white man should vote for Smith, because outside organizations are seeking to defeat me because of my stand for white supremacy."[52]

North Carolina senator Josiah Bailey told a convention of young Democrats that the South would "not permit Northern Democrats to frame a race policy or any social policy for us, no more than we would permit Northern Republicans to do so." The Macon *Telegraph,* in a statement that gained national notice, editorialized that the "people of the South have been definitively warned that it is the purpose of the New Deal strategists to destroy the Democracy of the South by exploitation of the Negro vote." First through a federal antilynching law and then through the abolition of the poll tax, the paper alleged, the Democratic Party would gain the support of both Northern and Southern blacks, helping to form the base for a new party, shorn of the conservatives who were the president's targets during the midterm elections.[53]

Expansion and Constraint

The Social Security Act led to a major expansion of the PHS's role in the development of local public health infrastructure and in fighting major diseases such as malaria, pellagra, and hookworm. Working with the Works Progress Administration, the PHS oversaw a dramatic decline in malaria. Fully controlling the diseases that had long driven the PHS's expansion, it appeared, was a goal within reach. Extending its work in both the West and the North, the PHS also embarked on major new initiatives such as the creation of the National Cancer Institute.

Despite its growing success, the PHS faced major challenges as its leaders articulated an increasingly broad vision of the appropriate role of the federal government in ensuring the health of Americans. Almost from the beginning of Roosevelt's second term, the political context began to look bleak for the proponents of an expanded federal health role. In the wake of the 1937 court-packing plan and the so-called Roosevelt Recession, substantial opposition to the Roosevelt administration's domestic agenda emerged among conservative Democrats in Congress, particularly among those from the South. In the 1938 midterm elections, the Republican Party regained an important role in Congress. In a few short years, Roosevelt's political power had been substantially diminished. For those who believed that the federal government should play a larger role in attempting to ensure access to individual medical services, and for those who sought to create a federal policy regime that would integrate public health and individual medicine, this would prove a key turn of events.

CHAPTER SEVEN

AN INTEGRATED APPROACH

After the enactment of the Social Security Act in 1935, President Roosevelt created an Interdepartmental Committee to Coordinate Health and Welfare Activities. The inelegantly named committee was headed by Josephine Roche of the Treasury Department. It was given the important role of facilitating communication among the various federal departments and agencies dealing with issues of health and welfare. Under the auspices of the Interdepartmental Committee, the PHS, the Social Security Board, and the Children's Bureau worked together to develop a plan for future federal efforts in the realm of health. During 1938, the Interdepartmental Committee introduced and pushed for the adoption of a new National Health Program.

Presented at a presidentially sponsored National Health Conference, the National Health Program embodied the goal of linking public health and individual medical services now being articulated by the PHS under Thomas Parran's leadership. It also embraced the goals of the Social Security Board, which administered much of the social security program. Though interested in the broader program, the Social Security Board was particularly committed to the creation of a federally backed health insurance system. Many of the participants in the 1938 National Health Conference believed the comprehensive plan introduced at it might soon lead to a new set of additions to the Social Security program.

This chapter deals with the politics of the 1938 National Health Program and the 1939 Wagner Health bill that followed on its heels. For scholars focused on national health insurance, the National Health Program and the Wagner bill have largely been of interest because of their insurance components, which received strong opposition from the AMA. Although the insurance provisions were the most important aspects of these proposals from the perspective of the Social Security Board, they were the least important aspects from the perspective of the PHS. For the PHS, the National Health Program represented a framework for bringing together public health and individual medical services. Rather than insurance, Thomas Parran and other PHS leaders continued to hope that economic insecurity arising out of ill health could be confronted through a comprehensive system. This system, they hoped, would include government payment for medical services, funding for biomedical research, and funding for facilities construction.

Despite hopes that the conference had created the momentum for a major policy breakthrough, a set of interlocking factors ensured that the plan would not become law. Primary among them were the pushback against the New Deal manifested in the emergence of the conservative coalition and in the 1938 midterm elections, the response of the AMA, divisions within the Interdepartmental Committee, and the gathering likelihood of war in Europe. Nonetheless, there was room for compromise.

As in 1934 and 1935, the AMA's leaders worried that the president and his allies in Congress might successfully push for health insurance. Meeting with members of the Interdepartmental Committee after the National Health Conference, representatives from the AMA offered a deal: they would support the health program if the committee would agree to drop the provisions that allowed for federally backed insurance plans at the state level. Interdepartmental Committee chair Josephine Roche, pushed by the Social Security Board's Isidore Falk and Arthur Altmeyer, rejected this compromise.

The reasons for this decision were both substantive and political. Both Roche and the Social Security Board strongly supported health insurance, which they viewed as a critical next step in American social policy. Abandoning it in order to pursue compromise with the obstructionist AMA did not appear an appealing option. The AMA, they believed, was offering to endorse aspects of the health program that it would have accepted regardless. Isidore Falk and Arthur Altmeyer recognized that insurance was the aspect of the National Health Program with the least support. For the board, it appeared that the prospects for an insurance program would be much improved if it was part of a broader plan that included more popular and less controversial proposals for expanded maternal and child health programs, public health, and hospital construction.[1]

The decision not to compromise with the AMA in the aftermath of the National Health Conference was a critical one. Already during the development of the Social Security Act, President Roosevelt had indicated his commitment to avoiding a clash with the organization over insurance. With the political context now far less favorable, AMA support was a necessary condition for legislative progress. Even had the Interdepartmental Committee and the AMA reached a compromise, however, Roosevelt might not have backed the plan. With his political capital in serious decline, the president was not in a strong position to push for a major new domestic initiative in the realm of health.

Whatever room for making a deal existing in the aftermath of the National Health Conference was gone by 1939, when New York senator Robert Wagner introduced a bill based on the health program. Increasingly, the situation in Europe demanded the attention of Roosevelt and other national leaders. During 1938, Nazi Germany annexed Austria and the Czechoslovakian Sudetenland. In 1939, the Nazis invaded first the remainder of Czechoslovakia and then Poland, an action that marked the beginning of World War II in Europe. With the outbreak of war, the National Health Program and Wagner Health bill were quickly swept from the national policy agenda. In the years that followed, federal policies dealing with public health and individual medicine would diverge even further.

The National Health Program

After signing the Social Security Act in 1935, President Roosevelt created the Interdepartmental Committee to Coordinate Health and Welfare Activities. Given the expansion of federal involvement in health and welfare under the Social Security Act, it appeared that some effort should be made to harmonize the work of the various federal agencies operating in these fields. The committee would also have a policy-making role. In his statement announcing the Interdepartmental Committee, Roosevelt noted that creating a special subcommittee "to study and make recommendations concerning specific aspects of the government's health activities" would be among the Interdepartmental Committee's immediate tasks.[2]

Josephine Roche, an adept leader who was the assistant treasury secretary with jurisdiction over the PHS, was made head of the Interdepartmental Committee.[3] In 1937, Roche left the Treasury Department to return to her home state of Colorado and deal with the affairs of the Rocky Mountain Fuel Company, a coal mining operation that she had inherited a decade before. Despite her departure from the Treasury Department and from Washington, Roosevelt continued to value Roche's skills. At his request, she continued to serve as head of the Interdepartmental Committee, which included representatives from the departments of the Interior, Agriculture, and Labor as well as from the Social Security Board.

After the passage of the Social Security Act, the newly created Social Security Board continued to refine the insurance plan developed by Edgar Sydenstricker and Isidore Falk during 1934–1935.[4] Sydenstricker, a central player in the development of American health policy beginning in the 1910s, died suddenly of a heart attack in 1936. His close ally, Falk, however, continued to advocate for health insurance as a Social Security Board staffer. Pressed forward by Falk and strongly supported by Social Security Board chairman Arthur Altmeyer, health insurance would remain at the heart of the board's legislative program for years to come.[5]

Leading PHS officers, meanwhile, focused their hopes on the creation of a federal health program that would encompass both public health and individual medicine. C. E. Waller, the assistant surgeon general who oversaw the transformation of the rural sanitation program into the new Title VI under the Social Security Act, publically expressed dismay at the act's lack of provisions for individual medical care only months after it was signed. The problem of medical care for the poor and for lower-income families that "can pay something but not the whole cost of medical and hospital service," Waller asserted in October 1935, would remain a serious one until some form of action was taken.

Speaking before members of American Public Health Association, Waller highlighted the importance of access to individual medical services, noting that he was "personally unable to hold with some others to the doctrine that the working out of some solution of this problem is not a part of the public health problem." Continuing, he used language that captured the feelings of an important and ascendant faction within the PHS: "I have been unable to see the soundness of the distinction some of us have maintained between what we have called 'public health work' and the responsibility for seeing that adequate medical care is provided for those who cannot afford it."[6] While Waller was delighted at the expansion of the PHS's program for stimulating the development of local public health infrastructure, he understood it as only a partial beginning.

In 1936, the Interdepartmental Committee created a new Technical Committee on Medical Care, charged with developing proposals that might address the ongoing health needs of the nation.[7] The Technical Committee on Medical Care was, by its nature, a consensus-seeking endeavor. It brought together the Children's Bureau, which controlled new funds for promoting maternal and child health under the Social Security Act, the Social Security Board, and the PHS.

The PHS and the Children's Bureau were often at odds during the preceding decades, with PHS officials such as Surgeon General Hugh Cumming at times expressing disdain for the bureau and its work. After former Children's Bureau staffer Josephine Roche became assistant treasury secretary with oversight of the PHS in late 1934, however, Cumming endorsed the revival of the Children's Bureau's grant-in-aid program. After the enactment of the Social Security Act, the two agencies reached an explicit understanding on the importance of cooperation.[8] After Thomas Parran became surgeon general in 1936, relations improved even further.

Dr. Martha Eliot, who also chaired the technical medical committee, represented the Children's Bureau. A pediatrician, Eliot was an accomplished researcher and advocate who would later become the first female president of the American Public Health Association. The indefatigable Isidore Falk represented the Social Security Board. Assistant Surgeon General C. E. Waller, Joseph Mountin, and George St. John Perrott represented the PHS. The head of the PHS's Division of Domestic Quarantine, Waller, remained in charge of the new grant-in-aid program being implemented under Title VI of the Social Security Act.

Joseph Mountin, who would later assume Waller's position and then oversee the creation of the PHS's Communicable Disease Center, began his career working in the wartime extracantonment effort. Afterward, he served in the rural sanitation program, where he formed what would prove a lifelong bond with his immediate superior, Thomas Parran.[9] By the late 1930s, Mountin had emerged as a leading thinker in the field of public health administration and a strong proponent of a public health program that would encompass individual medical services.[10]

George St. John Perrott, who began his career as a chemical engineer, became involved in health-related research after the Depression sank the company he worked for. Recruited by Edgar Sydenstricker, who was his brother-in-law, he worked for the Milbank Memorial Fund before joining the PHS as a statistician.[11] As of the 1936, Mountin and Perrott were in the process of wrapping up the PHS's National Health Survey. Undertaken during 1935 and 1936 with funding and personnel from the Works Progress Administration, the survey was originally proposed and designed by Sydenstricker and Falk.[12]

Working to develop a comprehensive National Health Program, the new technical committee relied heavily on the National Health Survey, which detailed the need for expanded health work. By early 1938, the committee had produced a proposal consisting of five recommendations: (1) expansion of the public health and maternal and child health programs created by the Social Security Act; (2) federal support for the construction of hospital facilities; (3) grants-in-aid for the public provision of medical care to the indigent and the "medically needy"; (4) a flexible "general program of medical care," grounded in federal assistance to the states for either publically supported medical services or health insurance; and (5) disability insurance.[13] Heavily influenced by the PHS, the proposal encompassed both the PHS leadership's vision of publically provided and supported medical services, paid for through general revenue, and the Social Security Board's preference for contributory health insurance for workers.

The National Health Conference

On July 18, 1938, with the midterm elections looming, the Interdepartmental Committee presented the National Health Program at a presidentially sponsored National Health Conference. By this point, the Interdepartmental Committee comprised Josephine Roche, who still headed it, Assistant Interior Secretary Oscar Chapman; Undersecretary of Agriculture Milburn Wilson; Assistant Labor Secretary Charles V. McLaughlin (the Labor Department housed the Children's Bureau); and Arthur J. Altmeyer, chairman of the Social Security Board. The PHS had played a key role in the development of the National Health Program. Roche's departure from the Treasury Department, however, meant that the service did not have formal representation on the Interdepartmental Committee. This omission was corrected in October 1938, when Surgeon General Parran was made a member.[14]

President Roosevelt was on a cruise during the National Health Conference, an absence that did not bode well for the National Health Program's prospects.[15] Nonetheless, most of the participants in the conference believed it represented the beginning of a new wave of innovation in health policy.[16] Throughout the conference, the program's proponents presented it as an evolutionary approach to health policy, to be fully put into practice over a period of ten years.[17]

Speaking at the conference, Surgeon General Parran portrayed the health program as a means of shifting national health policy toward a more comprehensive approach, capable of confronting the nation's health needs in a flexible manner. Americans, Parran maintained, were beginning to demand that government provide not just a healthful environment but also a means for accessing medical care. Shifts in public opinion and a growing recognition of the deficiencies of the nation's health care system meant that the political prospects of the new program were greater than those of past proposals. Indeed, it appeared that "people in general are beginning to take it for granted that an equal opportunity for health is a basic American right." In typical PHS fashion, Parran presented health as an economic issue. Public interest in a comprehensive health program, he maintained, was driven not just by an individual desire to be well or from "humanitarian and charitable motives." It was fueled also by "an economic urge—the money waste of preventable sickness."[18]

Health was an individual right, and one that could only be guaranteed through collective public action. Ultimately, government responsibility would have to encompass both public health and individual medical services. "Just as the community tries to protect itself against burglaries, embezzlement, arson, and murder," Parran argued, "so it is beginning to concern itself with the prevention, alleviation, and cure of sickness, disability, and premature death."[19] Generally accepted understandings of responsibility for individual health would have to be reconsidered. "When a man's house is burning down," Parran remarked, "the city does not fail to call out the fire department because he cannot pay for its services; yet if the man's family is ravaged by sickness, there is rarely provided as swift and efficient a means of assisting him; and this in spite of the fact that the damage done to him and the danger and expense to the community may be greater from sickness than from fire."[20]

Extolling the virtues of the National Health Program, Parran emphasized its flexibility and the opportunities it contained for experimentation. Under the plan, individual states would be able to implement an approach best suited to local circumstances. Crucially, the National Health Program also provided a framework for integrating public health and individual medical services. Government involvement in ensuring access to individual medical services was essential, but it was only part of the equation. "The ideal traffic plan," Parran told the conference, "is not that which provides a first aid station at all intersections and stream-lined ambulances to carry away the victims of traffic accidents. Both doctors and drainage are needed to save the inhabitants of a malarious swamp."[21]

It was, Parran continued, "as important to reduce the number and seriousness of industrial hazards as it is to provide hospitalization for the unlucky worker who breathes rock dust from the drill or loses a hand under the trip hammer." The point, he explained, was that the nation's disparate health-related activities needed to be integrated. Health policy makers "should not continue to think in terms of the separateness of public, private, and voluntary efforts or of the separateness of preventive or curative efforts to reduce death and disease. Each contributes to the health of the individual and the nation. All are parts of the same entity." Though they were often "not smoothly functioning parts," it was the job of those assembled to "make them mesh."[22]

The influence of such thinking was clear in the National Health Program's approach to individual medical services. Expanding on Parran's proposal during the development of the Social Security Act, the health program included grants-in-aid to directly cover medical services for a broad swath of the population, including those without income and receiving general relief, those receiving aid to families with dependent children, those on work relief, and lower-income families who qualified as medically needy, meaning that they were generally self-supporting but unable to afford the costs of medical care. Notably, the costs of medical care would also be covered for those receiving old-age assistance. This massive new program "would be developed around and would be based upon the existing preventive health services." Health departments would be responsible for both public health and "the provision of public medical care."[23]

Large-scale federal involvement in guaranteeing access to individual medical services for the poor, other indigent or borderline categories of the population, and the elderly needy would by itself have represented a monumental policy development and entering wedge for federal intervention. If it proved effective and popular, the program might plausibly be expanded to include all of the elderly population. This, however, was only the beginning. The National Health Program also contained two proposals for dealing with "self-sustaining" lower-income and middle-class families. One was based on the Parran plan for catastrophic care introduced during the meetings of the Economic Security Committee's medical advisory committee. The other was the Social Security Board–backed plan for health insurance. States might elect to pursue either approach or some mix of the two. While framed as flexible, the PHS-backed program of public medical care would open the door to federal backing for state and local investments in medical technology, facilities such as laboratories, and payments for services provided to self-supporting citizens for expensive illnesses.[24]

Under the National Health Program, individual medical services for self-supporting Americans would be connected to existing public health efforts. Tied to the proposed program for the indigent, the medically needy, beneficiaries of various assistance programs, and the elderly needy, the "public medical care" program would operate through state and local health departments.[25] By their nature, the plan asserted, a number of health issues could only be addressed through an integrated approach to health. Confronting sexually transmitted diseases and diseases such as tuberculosis and malaria, for instance, would require both the treatment of specific individuals and a population-based approach. Other illnesses that would need to be addressed through a general program of publically funded medical care, either because of their expensive nature or because of their impact on public health, included pneumonia, cancer, mental illness, and diseases related to industrial work.[26] Like Parran's earlier proposal, the public medical care program would have a broader scope than health insurance because it would encompass those who were not included in the Social Security Act's old-age pension program, such as agricultural and domestic workers.[27]

Crucially, federal funding for a "general program of medical care" might also be used to create state-based insurance programs. The plan for insurance included in the program was an updated version of the plan developed by Sydenstricker and Falk during 1934–1935. The Social Security Board favored this approach, which its members viewed as critical to funding individual medical services and to reorganizing medicine along group practice lines. Far less committed to insurance, PHS leaders were nonetheless increasingly prone to viewing it as a potentially valuable piece of the broader puzzle of federal health policy. The PHS's growing appreciation of the virtues of insurance was fueled in large part by its experiences in helping to create insurance plans for clients of the Farm Security Administration (FSA).

Originally known as the Resettlement Administration, the FSA was engaged in an extensive program of providing loans to small farmers. Early on, the Resettlement Administration recognized that one of the primary causes of farmers becoming unable to pay back their loans was poor health. In 1936, the PHS assigned Ralph C. Williams to head up the Resettlement Administration's new medical services program. Williams, one of the many PHS leaders who had served under Leslie Lumsden as part of the rural sanitation program during the 1920s, took eagerly to the challenge.[28]

During 1936, Surgeon General Parran personally traveled to the Dakotas to help negotiate an agreement between the Resettlement Administration and local medical societies aimed at paying physicians to treat farmers hit hard by drought.[29] The emergency situation in the Dakotas aided the swift growth of local prepayment plans. Coordinating with and often relying on the expertise of the PHS, the FSA negotiated county-level prepayment agreements with physicians in rural counties throughout the nation. By the time the United States entered World War II, more than 600,000 individuals were enrolled in some form of FSA-backed health plan. In addition, the FSA set up a program for providing health care to migrant workers. The rationale offered by the FSA for its foray into health was a straightforward one, consistent with the PHS's long-standing emphasis on economics: farmers in poor health were far less likely to be able to pay back government loans than those in good health.[30]

Though still championing direct payment for services and federal support for high-cost medical technology, procedures, treatments, and facilities, the FSA experience made Parran and other PHS leaders more open to insurance. The PHS was also open to the idea that states with diverse economies might adopt some mix of publically provided care and health insurance as a means of expanding services to groups living under differing circumstances.[31]

The AMA and the National Health Program

The National Health Conference was held over the course of three days, and it succeeded in generating a great deal of positive press for the proposed National Health Program. From the perspective of the AMA, the threat represented by the National Health Program was clear. The Social Security Board, Children's Bureau, and PHS, it appeared, were all on board with the idea of compulsory insurance. The growing FSA program, like the earlier payment of physicians through the Federal Emergency Security Administration, demonstrated the willingness of physicians with their backs against the wall to work with federal officials. The AMA was also on alert as a result of the mild insurgency that it faced in the form of the Committee of Physicians for the Improvement of Medical Care, a group of prominent physicians who believed that the organization's leadership had adopted an unnecessarily harsh line against government involvement in health insurance.[32]

Days after the conference, Josephine Roche, Social Security Board chair Arthur Altmeyer, Isidore Falk, and members of the Interdepartmental Committee met with representatives from the AMA. The AMA's representatives arrived willing to make a deal. The organization, they announced, would openly endorse almost all of the proposed National Health Program. The section that included provisions allowing for the creation of state-level health insurance plans along the lines favored by the Social Security Board, however, would have to go.[33] Given the strong drift of the political agenda away from new domestic reform programs and emergence of the conservative coalition in Congress, the AMA's willingness to make these concessions was highly noteworthy. Its demand that provisions relating to health insurance be dropped, meanwhile, was far from surprising.

Nonetheless, the representatives of the Interdepartmental Committee rejected the AMA's offer.[34] Roche, Altmeyer, and Isidore Falk were all strongly committed to health insurance, and they apparently believed that the National Health Conference had turned the tide in their favor. The offer of compromise, from their perspective, was an empty one. As Altmeyer pointed out, the AMA had never actually opposed any of the points that it now proposed to endorse.[35] Falk, adamantly opposed to the compromise proposal, would later describe "the kind of a floozy bargain they offered us. What we were going to get anyhow, they were prepared to support." All the proponents of insurance would have to do in return was "dump the things that [the AMA] didn't like. That was the sum and substance of that."[36] The AMA, he believed, viewed him, Roche, Altmeyer, and other insurance proponents as politically naive.

The proponents of insurance had other reasons for rejecting the AMA's compromise. While Falk and Altmeyer hoped that the National Health Conference had expanded public support for insurance, the reality was that the public remained far less than fully engaged. It was difficult to gauge whether a majority of Americans would have supported or opposed the proposal, and the experience of the Progressive Era suggested that interest group mobilization could prove decisive.

Clearly, insurance would be the most problematic aspect of the health program. Translating the program into legislation, meanwhile, would require difficult choices. Insurance proponents, Falk explained, were confronted with the question of whether to "gain support for, say, the highly controversial elements, like the health insurance one, by interlocking it in the same bill with other proposals which have largely noncontroversial support to bring to them." For Falk, this was a key consideration, as there was "a very strong lobby, say, for the maternal and child health program, a moderately strong lobby for the public health program, another very strong lobby clamoring for money for the hospital world." By tying everything together, insurance supporters could put their own preferred proposals on far firmer ground. In effect, support for the other components of the program could be used to bolster the prospects for insurance.[37]

In rejecting the AMA's overtures, the Interdepartmental Committee ensured that whatever small window of opportunity had been opened up by the National Health Conference was closed. Without clear AMA support, the likelihood of presidential support or any progress in Congress approached zero. When President Roosevelt returned from his cruise, Roche and Altmeyer met with him to discuss the prospects for the National Health Program going forward. Although Roche and Altmeyer remained optimistic, the president presented an ambiguous front. Even during 1934–1935, when

Roosevelt's political power was at its zenith, he directed the Committee on Economic Security to avoid a clash with the AMA. With his party divided, there was little reason for the president to pick a new fight with organized medicine over the issue of health insurance.

During his meeting with Roche and Altmeyer, Roosevelt indicated his support for the National Health Program, including its insurance components. Altmeyer left the meeting with the impression that the president would back the full health program at some point in the near future. Later, he recalled that the president "was so enthusiastic about the public response to the proposed National Health Program that his first inclination was to make it an issue in the congressional campaign which was then under way." This burst of apparent enthusiasm, however, was followed immediately by a correction. Drawing back, Roosevelt told Roche and Altmeyer that it would "be better to make it an issue in the 1940 presidential campaign."[38] Roosevelt was clearly sympathetic toward the Interdepartmental Committee's proposal. As a matter of politics, however, he recognized the dangers inherent in the National Health Program, and particularly in an insurance push that would result in a negative response from the AMA. Despite his suggestion of support to Roche and Altmeyer, Roosevelt remained distinctly silent on the issue of the health program.

The Potential for Compromise

The AMA, for its part, continued working to present its positions in the best possible light. In response to the National Health Conference, its leaders called a special session of the AMA House of Delegates, which met in September. At the conference, the AMA endorsed its own significantly modified versions of the Interdepartmental Committee's proposals for public health, hospital construction, grants-in-aid to states for the care of the indigent, and disability insurance. Altered in tone and substance to better coincide with the interests of physicians as perceived by the AMA, these endorsements suggested that compromise was possible, even in the realm of individual medical services. The plan for grants-in-aid to the states for covering services for the indigent, recipients of relief, and for the elderly needy, for instance, was important to the Interdepartmental Committee and not opposed by the AMA.[39]

The AMA's endorsements also highlighted its continued focus on the threat of government-backed health insurance.[40] As in 1934–1935, the idea that insurance might be used to transform the practice of medicine continued to animate the organization's approach to health policy. In addition to their gestures toward compromise, the AMA's publicists offered characteristically harsh condemnations of the National Health Program's insurance components. The proposal, according to *Journal of the American Medical Association* editor Morris Fishbein, would prove disastrous both to the nation's health and to its system of government. The AMA's "chief opposition to compulsory sickness insurance," Fishbein wrote, "is not so much that it deteriorates the nation." The AMA did not object just because health insurance "degrades the quality of medical service," nor "only because it enslaves the medical profession of the country."

Instead, Fishbein professed, the AMA opposed government-backed health insurance primarily because "it is the first insidious approach to the breakdown of the democratic system of government." The issue at hand, he asserted, went far beyond medicine. "Give anybody the right to interfere thus intimately with the lives of the people, to pay for them the physician, whether or not the physician is selected by the patient, and you have the first step toward totalitarianism." The Interdepartmental Committee's health insurance plan, he suggested, would set the United States on the path of Nazi Germany and the Soviet Union. "Personally," Fishbein commented, "I hate and fear totalitarianism, whether it be under the name of Fascism or Communism. America is the greatest refuge for a free people existing in the world today."[41]

Condemning the Interdepartmental Committee's health insurance plan in the harshest possible terms, the AMA did not denounce the PHS-backed proposal for a general program of medical care aimed at covering catastrophic costs, illnesses, and expensive diagnostics.[42] Later scholars focused on the development of health insurance have overlooked this point. Even at the time, it was largely ignored in the furor surrounding insurance. Nonetheless, the AMA's decision not to take on the PHS-backed proposal for publically provided medical care was potentially quite significant. As the University of Chicago's *Social Service Review* pointed out in a rare acknowledgment of the AMA's omission, "The House of Delegates has at least left the way open for future approval of the use of public medical care to provide for the self-supporting members of the population as well as the medically needy." The benefits of such an approach, it continued, might be significant: "No other type of service or combination of types of service, not even a health insurance scheme in which the contributions for the medically needy were paid by the government, would eliminate the means test nor meet equally the rural as well as urban needs."[43]

It is impossible to know whether the PHS-backed plan for public medical care covering catastrophic diseases and procedures for "self-sustaining" groups could have been included in an agreement with the AMA. The organization's decision not to condemn the program, however, is telling. Framed as a means of insuring against the costs of catastrophic care, the PHS proposal might have been accepted as consistent with the AMA's insistence that medical care programs not interfere with the day-to-day practices of physicians. During the development of the Social Security Act a few years before, AMA-affiliated leaders had embraced the approach when proposed by Thomas Parran.[44]

Immediately after the National Health Conference, the Interdepartmental Committee had the option of pursuing compromise with the AMA. According to its representatives, the AMA would have embraced substantially expanded public health efforts, hospital construction, a federally backed program of health care for the indigent, medically needy, those on assistance, the elderly needy, and disability insurance. The organization might even have backed the PHS's program for publically funded catastrophic care. For Interdepartmental Committee head Josephine Roche, Arthur Altmeyer, and Isidore Falk, however, the AMA's proposed "deal" was an empty one. In return for gaining AMA support in areas that the AMA had already signaled it was open to working with the federal government in, the committee would have to give up on the issue of health insurance. Both practically and politically, Roche, Altmeyer, and Falk believed that this was a bad approach.

The fate of the National Health Program, already under fire from organized medicine and lacking presidential backing, was sealed by the midterm elections held in November. For Roosevelt and other proponents of the New Deal, the elections were a disaster. Marginalized for years, the Republican Party made significant gains in both the House and the Senate. The conservative coalition of Southern Democrats and Northern Republicans, born of the court-packing plan and the recession of 1937, would grow stronger in the years that followed.[45]

When Roche and Altmeyer met with the president to discuss the National Health Program again after the elections, he stated clearly that a presidential endorsement for insurance would not be forthcoming. As the year came to a close, the PHS pushed for an approach that would jettison health insurance and embrace compromise with the AMA. The Social Security Board, however, viewed this concession as unacceptable. The lines of communication between the Interdepartmental Committee, the AMA, and the president would remain open in the months to follow. It was obvious, however, that a major breakthrough would not come in the short term. In a slight concession, the president indicated that he would back a limited proposal for hospital construction. The rest of the program, including both insurance and those aspects where the AMA might have accepted a compromise, would not receive presidential support.[46]

In January 1939, the president forwarded the Interdepartmental Committee's report to Congress. In a special message on the National Health Program, Roosevelt offered the vague suggestion that it might ultimately lead to healthier lives for Americans and increase national efficiency, then called for "careful study" of the issue.[47] The administration's attention, however, was directed increasingly toward Europe. In September, as the midterm elections approached, Great Britain and France signed the Munich agreement, allowing the Nazis to annex the Czechoslovakian Sudetenland. In March 1939, Germany acted on the agreement.

The Wagner Health Bill

In February 1939, New York senator Robert Wagner introduced a bill intended to embody the National Health Program. Largely drafted by the Social Security Board, the legislation included both provisions for federal support to states for the creation of "general medical programs" or for health insurance.[48] With the conservative coalition on strong footing in the new Congress, the president silent on the issue, and the situation in Europe escalating, there was little reason to believe that the bill would move forward.[49]

From the perspective of PHS, the introduction of the Wagner bill suggested trouble. It clearly reflected the priorities of the Social Security Board, which was given a controlling role in administering much of the proposed health plan. Although the service played a central role in drafting the 1938 National Health Program, its leaders remained unaware of the Wagner bill's contents until it was introduced in Congress.[50]

Writing to Thomas Parran, longtime ally Michael M. Davis of the Julius Rosenwald Fund attempted to underline the severity of the situation. The Wagner bill, Davis wrote, was undeniably a mess, with responsibility for the administration of its components divided among the Social Security Board, PHS, and Children's Bureau. As written, it "would be administratively unworkable on either federal or state levels."[51] Confident that the bill would not become law, Davis was nonetheless worried about the "underlying situation." It seemed, Davis wrote to Parran, that "many important people in public life, labor circles and elsewhere, feel that the Public Health Service is too much under the control of organized medicine to be trusted with a general program of medical care, and that the public health officers generally do not seek this responsibility."[52]

By seeking compromise with the AMA and signaling a willingness to back down on the insurance issue, Parran was courting trouble with the Social Security Board and with its supporters in Congress. For Parran, it made short-term sense to focus on the issue of health for the indigent, an area where the AMA had indicated a willingness to accept expanded federal action. Integrating publically funded individual health services for the indigent with public health work, he believed, represented a strong first step toward a more effective health system. Davis, however, argued that limiting proposals to the indigent would ensure their failure. "No important law concerning medical care," he admonished the surgeon general, "will be passed unless it includes self-supporting people of small means. Wage earners and farmers will not push large measures for the indigent." If Parran highlighted only the needs of the worst off in advocating for health legislation, Davis warned, the outcome would be something that both men viewed as undesirable: a constrained health program administered by welfare agencies rather than by local health departments.[53]

Almost immediately after the introduction of the Wagner bill, the AMA announced its opposition to the entirety of the proposed health program.[54] Left out of the development of the Wagner bill and recognizing the political danger in a battle over insurance, the leaders of the PHS were not excited about the new legislation. Nonetheless, Parran and other prominent PHS officers continued to back the National Health Program. During the summer of 1939, the Senate's Education and Labor Committee held hearings on the Wagner Health bill. PHS officials, along with representatives from the other agencies involved in developing the National Health Program, offered support for the concepts represented in the Wagner bill. In his testimony, Surgeon General Parran argued that the plan was "not a measure to socialize medicine, but one that will free medical practice."[55]

Organized medicine took an opposing view. Appearing before the committee, its representatives denounced the bill's cost and its "socialistic" and "dictatorial" content.[56] Already AMA representatives had demonstrated an unabashed willingness to connect the Interdepartmental Committee's health insurance proposal with the threat of Nazism. Now, in an echo of the Progressive-Era battle over a state-level health insurance plan, the opponents of the Wagner bill once again tied government-backed health insurance to the encroaching danger of German authoritarianism. Senator Wagner, some pointed out, had himself been born in Germany.[57]

Battle Lines

The Interdepartmental Committee's National Health Program represented a significant step in terms of the development of a more comprehensive federal approach to the issue of health. For a brief period, it appeared possible that progress might be made on some aspects of the National Health Program. The obstacles that the program's proponents faced, however, were substantial. Internally, they were divided. Though they presented a unified front at the 1938 National Health Conference, the PHS and the Social Security Board in reality had very different views on the question of what national health policy should look like. Where leading PHS officers were focused on integrating public health and individual medicine, the Social Security Board was focused on insurance. Their strategic approaches, meanwhile, diverged in ways that appeared to be irreconcilable. Where the PHS embraced compromise and half measures, the Social Security Board rejected both bargaining and incrementalism.

By 1939, the proponents of the health program faced the opposition of the AMA, a domestic political context that was highly unfavorable, and the mounting threat of war in Europe. The factors arrayed against the Wagner bill, which had only tepid support from the PHS, were too numerous and the well of support for it far too shallow. Already battered by Senate hearings in which it was portrayed as a threat to the American way of life, the Wagner Health bill became a moot issue on September 1, 1939, when Nazi Germany invaded Poland.

CHAPTER EIGHT

DIVERGENT PATHS

World War II further accelerated the divergence of federal policies dealing with public health and individual medical services. Over the course of the 1930s, strong Southern political support, grounded in the region's experiences with the PHS, helped the PHS secure an expanded role in American public health. A variety of factors worked against federal intervention in individual medicine. Plans for federally backed health insurance for workers stalled as a result of the opposition of the AMA, the lack of a strong base of popular or political support, and the unwillingness of President Roosevelt to push forward on the issue. Compromise or incremental approaches—including catastrophic insurance, direct payments for the indigent, and the PHS's plan for publically funded catastrophic services, infrastructure, and diagnostic facilities—might have been pursued during the 1930s. Internal divisions among policy makers, both over the substance of policies and over political strategy, ensured that they were not.

When the United States mobilized once again for war, the window of opportunity that opened beginning in 1933 was closed. During the war and in its aftermath, the bifurcated federal health policy regime that began to emerge during the 1930s was further reinforced. Pushed forward by the PHS and by the need to ensure that Southern diseases such as malaria would not threaten the war effort, the federal government asserted an increasingly central and direct role in American public health. In Atlanta, the PHS created the Malaria Control in War Areas (MCWA) program, which became the basis for the postwar CDC. Its National Institute of Health began funding biomedical research on an increasingly large scale. In the realm of individual medicine, federal tax policy helped foster a system in which most Americans accessed medical services through employer-sponsored health insurance. Federal money, meanwhile, began pouring into states and localities for the construction of hospitals.

During the 1940s, the PHS continued to push for a health policy regime that would encompass both public health and individual medicine. Ultimately, PHS leaders found common ground with the leaders of the Social

Security Board on the importance of insurance. Beginning in 1945, President Harry S. Truman offered strong support for a comprehensive health program and for insurance. The bifurcated policy regime that emerged from the war, however, would become locked in during the years and decades that followed. While health policy makers had confronted a variety of alternatives during the 1930s, their choices were now significantly constrained. The creation of federal policies dealing with both public health and individual medicine fostered a new political and policy environment in which the options available during the pivotal period from 1933 through mobilization for World War II were foreclosed.

Mobilization

After occupying Norway during the spring of 1940, the German Wehrmacht moved swiftly into Belgium, Luxembourg, and then France, taking Paris in June. With the Nazis overcoming much of Europe and Britain under siege, the United States moved toward a war footing. In September 1940, Congress passed legislation creating the nation's first peacetime draft. In March 1941, it approved the lend-lease program, granting President Roosevelt a great deal of leeway in supplying war matériel to support the British effort to withstand the Nazis.

The PHS, which was transferred out of the Treasury Department and into the newly created Federal Security Agency in 1939, was prepared. As the army began training maneuvers in the South, the service engaged in preliminary surveys of local disease conditions.[1] The PHS's venereal disease division, meanwhile, mapped out a plan for working with the military, states and localities, and private groups to deal with the threats of syphilis and gonorrhea.[2] In May 1941, the service secured an emergency appropriation to create a new Mosquito Control in Defense Areas program within the States Relations Division (previously known as the Division of Domestic Quarantine).[3] The division was now under the control of Assistant Surgeon General Joseph Mountin, a close associate of Thomas Parran, veteran of the World War I extracantonment effort and the rural sanitation program, as well as an outspoken advocate of an increased federal role in public health and individual medical services.[4]

An onslaught of appropriations followed the Pearl Harbor bombing on December 7, 1941.[5] As in the previous war, venereal disease and malaria were viewed as major threats to troops and to war-related industries. In both areas, the PHS took an aggressive stance. Men found to have venereal diseases, the PHS argued, should not be excluded from the draft. Once inducted, they could be treated.[6]

PHS officials rejected the idea, pushed by some in the military, that venereal disease could be controlled through the creation of regulated brothels. Instead, Surgeon General Parran and venereal disease division head R. A. Vonderlehr endorsed a clampdown on prostitution, aimed at the middlemen and pimps who sought to profit from the sex trade. A "consistent policy of repression," Parran argued, "will take the profits out of the business of prostitution, render the women less accessible, and reduce the total number of patrons of any one woman." The women involved, he continued, "must be encouraged and aided to find other occupations and to establish their own houses."[7]

The measures taken against women suspected of being involved of prostitution near military installations or defense industries were often harsh. If found to be infected with a venereal disease, they were typically detained and then confined to "rapid treatment centers," funded with federal money. Although the PHS operated some of the centers, most were controlled by states and localities.[8] Men who sought out prostitutes, meanwhile, were said to need "the counteracting influence of recreation, interesting leisure-time activities, opportunity for wholesome friendships with women, and participation in community life."[9]

Venereal disease was a major concern for the PHS, but malaria represented a crucial opportunity for the service to build on its New Deal–era growth. Throughout 1940 and 1941, the service worked with the military to survey areas where troops would be stationed in order to ensure that they would not be prone to the disease. After Pearl Harbor, the issue became critical. After considering an expanded antimalaria operation based in Washington, DC, Assistant Surgeon General Joseph Mountin elected to headquarter the PHS's new Malaria Control in War Areas program in Atlanta, near the heart of the nation's malaria belt. All PHS antimalaria work, it was soon decided, would be centered in the new program, which operated under the umbrella of Mountin's States Relations Division.[10]

By late March 1942, expanded malaria control operations were under way in the field. Following the established pattern of the States Relations Division, which administered the PHS's Social Security funding, MCWA "carried on its malaria control activities largely within the framework of the State health departments."[11] Reminiscent of the service's extracantonment zone efforts during World War I, MCWA could draw on a vastly increased budget, improved malaria control techniques, strong existing relations with local communities and political leaders in many areas, and increasingly sophisticated public health capabilities at the state and local levels.[12]

Altogether, New Deal works programs drained an estimated 544,414 acres of mosquito breeding grounds in the years preceding the war.[13] In a report written for the Army Medical Department, the PHS's Justin Andrews and Jean Grant highlighted the importance of these efforts, as well as the impact of the Social Security Act's Title VI, in ridding the region of much of its malaria burden. The Social Security Act, they noted, had provided "for malaria survey and control personnel to be added to State health departments and for an increase in the number of local health departments through which antimalaria activities could be promoted and administered. This stimulated the interest of States and counties in malaria control which, with operational assistance from the Works Progress Administration (renamed Work Projects Administration on 1 July 1939), advanced environmental control until late 1941."[14] As a result of already existing public health infrastructure, another PHS report concluded, "There was no loss of time in acquiring a background of knowledge of the malaria problem and of previous malaria control activities, such as malaria surveys and drainage and larviciding projects, and prompt advantage could be taken to permit institution or expansion of control measures where needed."[15]

The Threat and Challenge of Malaria

Malaria incidence was at an all-time low in the United States.[16] Still, MCWA confronted significant challenges. During 1942, around 2 million men went through camps located in the South. In 1943, the figure was 3.6 million.[17] Often composed of tenant farmers, sharecroppers, and itinerant laborers, the surrounding populations could be extremely unhealthy: "Many were undernourished and chronically ailing from secondary anemias due to their limited diet but frequently compounded by malaria and, in sandy coastal areas, by heavy hookworm infestation."[18] Civilians regularly engaged in activities, such as "sitting out in front of their homes in the hot summer evenings, fishing at night, and an occasional sociable which brought groups of all ages together after dark at country churches or schoolhouses," that allowed for easy malaria transmission. Their homes, meanwhile, were often "rude, ramshackle hovels, unscreened and with gaping holes in floors, sidewalls, and roofs, providing easy access by nocturnally active, blood-hungry anophelines."[19] Massive population movements might easily lead to outbreaks of the disease if control measures were not undertaken.

In describing the problem, PHS officers portrayed poor health among blacks as a threat to both white health and to national defense. In particular, the PHS viewed black Southerners as a potential reservoir of *Plasmodium falciparum*, the form of malaria most likely to result in death. The "location of military camps in the Southeast where the adjacent Negro population frequently outnumber the white," PHS officials wrote in explaining the need for MCWA, "could have resulted in an enhanced exposure of training troops to the more deadly type of malaria, unless active measures had been taken to forestall it."[20]

Because of the emergency nature of the effort, larvicide operations were MCWA's first line of defense. Fuel oil and Paris green were applied to water surfaces by men wielding hand dusters and sprayers or from airplanes to limit *Anopheles* breeding in rivers, streams, lakes, and swampland.[21] Drainage efforts, meanwhile, continued on a significant scale. A variety of ditching techniques, employing dynamite, hand-digging, and heavy construction equipment, were used to drain mosquito breeding grounds.[22]

This work was complemented by increased disease surveillance and community education campaigns aimed at giving people the information necessary to avoid infection. Schoolteachers taught lessons about malaria transmission and sent students home with questionnaires soliciting information on cases of malaria within their families. Public health workers went house to house, held public meetings, placed articles in newspapers, and appeared on local radio broadcasts in an effort to prompt community members to engage in preventative measures such as the screening of windows, doors, and front porches.[23]

The 1943 Wagner–Murray–Dingell Bill

Largely off of the national political agenda since 1939, health insurance emerged again as an important issue after 1942, when the British government published William Beveridge's proposal for a revamped and expanded welfare state. The Beveridge report, which became the framework for postwar social policy in the United Kingdom, included a proposal for the direct provision of hospital and medical services under government auspices. Like Britain's 1911 adoption of compulsory health insurance for workers, the wartime report influenced debates over health and insurance within the United States.[24]

After its publication, Beveridge traveled to the United States to give a series of talks, a visit paid for by the Rockefeller Foundation.[25] Speaking with Labor Secretary Frances Perkins, President Roosevelt jokingly suggested that Beveridge was only copying his own plans for "cradle to grave" social insurance.[26] Although the administration's National Resources Planning Board issued a set of recommendations for the postwar period in 1943 that suggested a health insurance plan, the program was quickly shelved. Roosevelt would never formally endorse such a plan. [27]

Instead, action on insurance came from within Congress, with assistance from the Social Security Board. In June 1943, New York's Robert Wagner joined with Senator James Murray (D-MT) and Representative John Dingell (D-MI) to introduce a bill proposing a sweeping series of amendments to the Social Security Act.[28] Already well under development before the Beveridge report was published, the 1943 Wagner–Murray–Dingell bill was intended as an opening salvo and statement of principles. Its sponsors did not expect it to become law in the immediate future. It proposed extending old-age pensions to an additional 15,000 to 20,000 people, including farm workers and domestics. The bill would also centralize key programs that had been operating on a federal–state cooperative basis. Unemployment insurance, under the bill, would become the sole responsibility of the national government, as would support for families with dependent children.[29]

The Wagner–Murray–Dingell bill included a health insurance plan, designed by Isidore Falk and other staffers from the Social Security Board and strongly supported by organized labor.[30] Where the 1939 Wagner bill included health insurance as an option for states, to be operated locally with financial support from the federal government, the 1943 Wagner–Murray–Dingell bill proposed a contributory national system that would operate on the model of Social Security's old-age pensions.[31] In 1939, the Wagner Health bill was introduced without its contents being shared with the PHS. This time, the Social Security Board's Arthur Altmeyer sent Surgeon General Parran the plan as a courtesy before the bill was introduced.[32]

The PHS was far from impressed. Focused heavily on insurance, the Wagner–Murray–Dingell bill was, from the perspective of Parran and PHS leaders, something far less than a proposal for actually improving the health of Americans. Indeed, it paid little heed to the preventive health work, integration of public health and individual medicine, and facilities construction that PHS leaders viewed as critical.[33] The bill's approach, from the perspective of the PHS, was far too narrow. Individual medical services, PHS officials continued to insist, needed to be addressed as part of a broader and comprehensive health program.

The PHS leadership also disliked the bill's proposal that insurance be nationally administered. Surgeon General Parran and Assistant Surgeon General Joseph Mountin believed health systems should be both flexible and grounded in local governing institutions. The PHS, which gained much of its power from its relationships with local governments, was far from alone in this assessment. Prominent public health figure C.-E. A. Winslow, for instance, explained to Senator Wagner that he was "in favor of the administration of health insurance through local arrangements, utilizing available facilities and local advisory bodies representing interested groups."[34] While old-age pensions might be distributed effectively through a centralized system, health insurance should be tailored to the differing health care contexts that prevailed in various parts of the nation. The leaders of the PHS believed that the federal government should play a coordinating role, should offer support and expertise, and should back local institutions financially. They also believed, however, that nationally administered insurance would prove cumbersome and inflexible.

The proposed role of the service in the program was further cause for concern. The Social Security Board drafted the bill without meaningful input from the PHS, but the surgeon general was made formal administrator of the proposed system. The Social Security Board, however, would also be deeply involved in its administration. This arrangement, it was reasonable to conclude, might prove cumbersome.[35] If things went poorly, the surgeon general might shoulder most of the blame despite possessing only limited authority.[36]

The AMA swiftly announced its opposition to the Wagner–Murray–Dingell bill, with *Journal of the American Medical Association* editor Morris Fishbein offering a typically scathing denunciation. Ironically, given the PHS's misgivings, Fishbein condemned the bill as giving dictatorial power over American medicine to the surgeon general. The bill, he maintained, "apparently attempts to avoid the innumerable difficulties involved in developing a government controlled medical service by making the Surgeon General of the Public Health Service, whoever he might, a virtual 'gauleiter' of American medicine." It was doubtful, he continued, "if even Nazidom confers on its 'gauleiter' Conti the powers which this measure would confer on the Surgeon General of the US Public Health Service."[37] AMA opposition to a proposal for national health insurance was to be expected, but the harshness of Fishbein's attack was notable. The wartime comparison of the Wagner–Murray–Dingell bill's insurance plan with the political structures of Nazi Germany was a brutal reminder of the no-holds-barred approach that organized medicine took when confronted with the prospect of government-backed health insurance.

The American Public Health Association also expressed unease with the bill. Since the defeat of state-level health insurance proposals during the Progressive Era, the association had adopted a cautious approach to the issue of insurance. Internally, it remained split on the proper role of health departments in providing access to individual medical services. Within the association, the PHS's Joseph Mountin had emerged as the key voice pushing for a more expansive definition of public health. Divided on the issue of the appropriate relationship between efforts aimed at populations and services for individuals, members of the APHA also worried that endorsing insurance would put the association at odds with the far more powerful AMA.[38]

In an editorial published in the *American Journal of Public Health,* the association's leaders expressed concern that compulsory insurance might direct money toward an increasingly expensive system of individual medical services while underfunding critical public health efforts. Sympathetic to the goal of expanding access to individual medical services, the editorial offered a critical appraisal of the Wagner–Murray–Dingell bill. "Most of those who are not emotionally prejudiced in favor of or against this bill see in it provisions that seem reasonable and necessary and implications that may be dangerous." Nationalization of insurance appeared to be a particularly bad idea. While "care would be more nearly assured to the population at large," the editorial suggested, "that care would inevitably be burdened with the by-products of red tape, perfunctoriness and mediocrity inherent in most civil services, and possibly with some politics."[39]

The bill's strongest support came from organized labor, a constituency that was closely aligned with Senator Wagner and the Social Security Board. It lacked support, however, from President Roosevelt. Offered during a period in which few domestic policy proposals went anywhere, greeted without enthusiasm by the PHS, and strongly opposed by the AMA, the 1943 Wagner–Murray–Dingell bill represented a first step toward a postwar push for national health insurance. It had no immediate chance, however, of becoming law.

"Two Facets of a Unit Problem"

While the Social Security Board and Wagner, Murray, and Dingell pushed their bill as the basis for postwar health planning, PHS leaders outlined their own expansive vision of the federal government's postwar role in health. Building on the PHS proposals of the 1930s and the earlier ideas of men such as New York state health commissioner Hermann Biggs, Surgeon General Parran, and Assistant Surgeon General Joseph Mountin imagined a postwar system in which private medical practice would be integrated with public health work and nested in a federally funded system, based in large research hospitals and smaller affiliated hospitals and health centers.[40]

Speaking at a postwar planning session held by the American Hospital Association in September 1943, Parran outlined his thoughts on the "Public Health of Tomorrow." Public health, he argued, should move decisively beyond population-based efforts and prevention. While classic functions such as "the provision of safe water supplies and the control of communicable diseases" were essential to guaranteeing the health of the public, they were only part of the story. "It is not possible to insure good health for a whole population merely by preventing disease, even though this be done to the fullest. It is necessary also that all should have an opportunity for the best possible medical care." Linking public health and individual medicine was key to the future success of health efforts: "Public health and medical care," he asserted, "are two facets of a unit problem."[41]

For Parran, there were strong reasons for optimism. The "tremendous energies" unleashed by the war, he maintained, "will spur us to build soundly for the health and happiness of our people in the postwar years." The path of progress was obvious. Venereal disease was being attacked as never before, with rapid treatment centers throughout the nation. Malaria, "a number one health problem" in much of the South, was in sharp decline as "a result of persistent control work during the past decade" and might well be banished from the United States within the next ten years. Progress in the field of cancer was slower, but important strides were being made.

Health insurance in some form was inevitable. Serious illness, Parran noted, was "an unpredictable risk," and becoming increasingly expensive with the advance of technology. "Against other comparable risks of life," Parran asserted, "the American people have adopted a policy of social insurance. We are insurance minded, and I believe there will be a growing sentiment for extending the prepayment principle, through compulsory insurance or otherwise, to include the hazards of illness." The "generally accepted meaning" of the term "health insurance," however, was wrong. "Standing alone," he argued, "it is not a service of health. It should be a part of a more comprehensive national health service, concerned also with prevention, research, the physical structures, scientific equipment, and trained personnel needed for health."[42] Rather than simply funding the existing system, the federal government needed to help build a more integrated and effective one. This was Parran's strongest endorsement yet of insurance, and his inclusion of it among his own postwar priorities marked an important shift in direction.

Assistant Surgeon General Joseph Mountin, meanwhile, pointed out that the health threats confronting the nation had changed dramatically in the preceding decades as a result of the achievements of public health. The "whole group of acute communicable diseases toward which so much public health effort is directed," Mountin noted in October 1943, "accounts for less than 3 percent of general mortality." In the years to come, chronic disease would pose an increasingly greater threat. Preserving existing gains while combating the nation's emerging health problems, Mountin noted, would prove a difficult task. Health efforts would have to be reoriented, and a successful transition would require changes "in social attitudes, improvements in methods of finance, and relocation of both professional personnel and physical facilities."[43]

Future public health work, Mountin maintained, would have to move beyond population-based efforts such as water chlorination and attempts to halt the spread of communicable diseases. Instead, broadening "the definition of public health service to include essential elements of general medical care" should be among the primary concerns of public health professionals.[44] The public, he was convinced, was open to a more expansive definition of public health. In the past, "a man's illnesses have been regarded as his personal affair—something he may endure if he prefers, or from which he may obtain relief if he is both willing and financially able to do so."

Now this was changing: "Gradually, as society has increased its investment in the training and security of the individual, this point of view has become a subject of serious debate. There are signs which clearly suggest that a complete reversal of attitude is in the offing." Changes in public philosophy would have to be matched by changes in practical capability. "With such a shift in viewpoint," Mountin continued, it was important to begin considering the specifics of "implementing an enlarged program of medical care."[45] Adequately addressing the nation's health needs would require a comprehensive system. This system would have to encompass public health, individual medical care, and ongoing improvements in biomedical science. The nation would have to build the infrastructure to bring advancements in science and in applied medicine to Americans wherever they lived and whatever their economic circumstances.

Divergent Paths

By 1944, the growing divergence of federal policies dealing with public health and individual medical services was evident. In that year, Parran and the PHS persuaded Congress to pass a new Public Health Service Act, streamlining the haphazardly organized PHS and expanding its powers.[46] As part of the act, the PHS's program of assistance for the development of local public health infrastructure was moved out of the Social Security Act and given a new statutory basis.[47] The new legislation also allowed individuals from a variety of health professions, including nursing, to be commissioned as PHS officers.[48]

In addition, it gave the service authorization to "make grants in aid to universities, hospitals, laboratories, and other public or private institutions and individuals."[49] First through its Hygienic Laboratory and then through the National Institute of Health, the PHS had established itself as a force to be reckoned with in scientific research. The National Cancer Institute, created in 1937, was authorized to distribute research grants to universities and other institutions. During the war, Congress expanded such extramural research grants to other areas of concern.[50] Now the Public Health Service Act laid out the framework for a postwar explosion in biomedical research funded by the federal government and implemented through the PHS's National Institute of Health (later renamed the National Institutes of Health).[51] In the years to come, NIH would build a strong relationship with Congress, strengthened by the support and lobbying of lay supporters of biomedical research such the philanthropists Mary and Albert Lasker.[52]

The service actively pursued other areas of expansion. Working with the American Hospital Association and congressional allies such as Alabama senator Lister Hill, the PHS promoted a plan for constructing a series of hospitals that could provide the backbone for a new American health system. If access to medical services were to be extended, both the PHS and the Social Security Board agreed, physicians would need modern facilities. This was a proposition that could both gain the support of the hospital industry and avoid the wrath of the AMA, which did not view hospital construction as a threat to professional autonomy.[53]

By 1944, MCWA had developed into something far more than a simple resurrection of the World War I–era extracantonment effort. Assistant Surgeon General Joseph Mountin, for his part, viewed the program as an ideal means of centralizing the service's efforts to stimulate public health work and coordinate public health work across the nation's varied political jurisdictions. The NIH could focus on pure scientific research, while a reoriented and presumably renamed MCWA could support disease control efforts by states and localities.[54]

Planning for the postwar period, the PHS continued to emphasize the threat of malaria and engaged in a series of studies dealing with the possibility that soldiers and sailors returning from malarial areas might spark outbreaks.[55] Malaria remained a key area of concern and research for federal officials, as well as for private organizations such as the Rockefeller Foundation.[56] In experiments that took place at the National Institute of Health's Malaria Research Laboratory in Columbia, South Carolina, the Public Health Service, the army, and the navy studied the problem of malaria imported from abroad.[57] During World War I, the Austrian psychiatrist Julius Wagner von Jauregg had demonstrated that exposing patients to malaria and inducing a high fever could treat neurosyphilis.[58] In the years that followed, *Plasmodium vivax* malaria was used to treat syphilis patients consigned to mental hospitals. Hoping to test the virulence of foreign strains of malaria, PHS researchers infected South Carolina syphilis patients with malaria from recently returned US soldiers. American mosquitoes, they found, could transmit foreign strains of malaria. In addition, these strains often resulted in higher rates of relapse than those present already in the United States.[59]

The PHS had a long history of experimenting on vulnerable populations. In the 1910s, Joseph Goldberger had made his name inducing pellagra in prison inmate "volunteers."[60] In Tuskegee, Alabama, the service's venereal disease division continued to observe the course of untreated syphilis among a group of black men, a project initiated more than a decade before. In Atlanta, meanwhile, the service was working with the Bureau of Prisons to test antimalaria drugs, including chloroquine.[61] Such experimentation would continue into the postwar period, perhaps most notably in the PHS's syphilis experiments on vulnerable human subjects in Guatemala.[62]

The South Carolina study appeared to underline the need for continued vigilance. "Military demobilization," the PHS's Louis L. Williams argued in November 1944, "will introduce a large number of malaria carriers into the civil population. Some of the new strains will be more virulent than those we now have and will present a more difficult therapeutic problem. The greater relapse of Mediterranean and South Pacific strains will make these soldiers more dangerous carriers, as they will be more frequently infectious to the mosquito."[63]

Postwar malaria outbreaks could cost lives. They could also injure the service's reputation. In addition, the malaria threat could be used to help secure support for extending the wartime expansion of the PHS's role. In January 1945, the PHS announced an Extended Malaria Control Program, administered by MCWA. The program would continue controlling the disease around military installations, defense-related industries, and would work to ensure that returning military personnel would not reintroduce malaria.[64]

As the war in Europe came to an end, MCWA embraced the new insecticide, DDT, already being used in the South Pacific to fight malaria and in Europe to kill typhus-carrying fleas. Large-scale application of DDT within Southern homes began in March 1945.[65] Working closely with state and local agencies, MCWA's Extended Malaria Control Program sprayed approximately 400,000 homes with DDT during the 1945 malaria season.[66]

DDT was not an important factor in the demise of malaria in the United States, where by this point the disease persisted only in a few lingering pockets.[67] Nonetheless, it was of great political value. Effective and versatile, the insecticide could, in addition to killing mosquitoes, be used to kill houseflies, cockroaches, and bedbugs. DDT was also used on a large scale to confront typhus, resulting in significant improvements in the lives of many Americans. Interest in DDT helped to ensure a high level of support for ongoing MCWA activities in the months after August 1945, when the United States dropped atomic bombs on Hiroshima and Nagasaki.

Health Services Revisited

Federal involvement in individual medical services expanded in important ways during the war years. American soldiers and sailors became accustomed to receiving medical services directly from federal authorities, while their wives and children became eligible for a new Emergency Maternity and Infant Care program, operated by the Children's Bureau. The program gave free medical care to the wives and children of service men in the lowest four pay grades.[68] In 1943, the PHS was placed in charge of the new US Cadet Nurse Corps program, which funded nurse training in return for a two-year service commitment. Lucile Petry Leone, who headed the effort, became an assistant surgeon general after the 1944 Public Health Service Act, making her the first woman to achieve flag rank in an American uniformed service.[69] The PHS also worked with the War Food Administration to provide both preventive and curative services to migratory farm workers. Under the program, federally funded clinics, typically staffed by local physicians, offered services to low-income farm laborers who did not meet local residency requirements for welfare.[70]

Crucially, wartime federal policies helped to foster the development of a new health insurance regime. In the 1930s, the growth of Blue Cross plans demonstrated that issues of adverse selection and administrative cost could be overcome by linking health insurance to employment-based groups. If individuals were enrolled in insurance programs on the basis of their employment, rather than their health status, insurance plans would not be dominated by sick enrollees who expected to use health services. If premiums were paid automatically, administrative expenses could be limited. During the late 1930s, physician-controlled Blue Shield plans emerged, complementing hospital insurance with insurance for physicians' services. Private insurers, previously unconvinced that health insurance could prove profitable, also became involved. While growing, the number of individuals covered by insurance plans remained fairly small during the 1930s. In 1940, only 11.96 million Americans were covered by hospital insurance. Three million, meanwhile, had insurance for physicians' services.[71]

During World War II, wage controls forced employers to seek out innovative means of attracting employees. Given the growth of the costs of medical care, offering health insurance emerged as an effective strategy for attracting high-quality employees in a tight labor market. The Internal Revenue Service, meanwhile, elected to treat employer contributions to health insurance premiums as a nontaxable fringe benefit. With employer contributions being made on a pretax basis and large groups spreading out risk, employees enrolled in group health insurance plans could enjoy greater benefits at lower cost.[72] By 1945, slightly more than 32 million Americans had hospital insurance; 4.7 million had insurance that covered physicians' services.[73] The impact of these developments on health politics and policy making would prove significant, though their full meaning was not yet evident.

President Roosevelt, for his part, hinted that he might be open to an expanded postwar federal role in individual health services, calling for a "second bill of rights" in his January 1944 State of the Union speech. The wartime resurgence of American power and prosperity, he argued, was leaving many behind, and the rights guaranteed to Americans by the existing Bill of Rights were "inadequate to assure us equality in the pursuit of happiness." In the speech, Roosevelt called for a national commitment to ensuring a broad new array of rights, including "the right to adequate medical care and the opportunity to achieve and enjoy good health" and the "right to adequate protection from the economic fears of old age, sickness, accident, and unemployment."[74]

It is impossible to know whether Roosevelt would have pursued a new health program after the war, or what form such a program might have taken.[75] According to Michael Davis, who was in contact with key Roosevelt advisor Harry Hopkins on the issue of health insurance, Roosevelt's "private position seems to have been that sufficient political support was not yet available for a broad health insurance program." After Roosevelt's reelection in November 1944, however, Hopkins informed Davis that the president was prepared to move forward with a new health program. Roosevelt's death in April 1945 meant that the plan that Davis was beginning to conceptualize would come to nothing.[76] New president Harry Truman, however, signaled his strong interest in pursuing a health program.[77]

In Congress, Senator Wagner, Senator Murray, and Representative Dingell began to shift gears, embracing a health program more in line with the program being advocated by the PHS. While the PHS had not been consulted on the substance of the 1943 Wagner–Murray–Dingell bill, Thomas Parran and other PHS officials were now asked to work on a new Wagner–Murray–Dingell bill. The product that emerged was heavily shaped by the Social Security Board, and in particular by Isidore Falk, but it embraced a far broader approach than that of the 1943 bill.[78]

Federal funding for constructing hospitals and other medical facilities, a key goal of both the PHS and the Social Security Board, was included in the bill. It also included provisions for expanded public health efforts, maternal and child health services, and disability insurance. Like the 1943 Wagner–Murray–Dingell bill, the new legislation proposed a system of compulsory health insurance. As Thomas Parran noted, insurance would include "agricultural and domestic workers, seamen, and employees of non-profit institutions, such as hospitals, who are not now protected" by the Social Security Act.[79] The new version of the Wagner–Murray–Dingell bill also allowed for a stronger local role in administering the system. In addition, although the Social Security Board and Children's Bureau would play key roles in its implementation, it appeared that the PHS would be able to shape much of the program to fit its own goals. As drafted, the service would play a crucial role in the program's operation, administering the hospital construction program, health insurance, and new funding for public health.

President Truman, while not explicitly endorsing the Wagner–Murray–Dingell bill, called on Congress to adopt a program along the lines it proposed. Less involved in the policy-making process than they would have liked, Surgeon General Parran and other high-ranking PHS officers were nonetheless ecstatic.[80] In a series of speeches, Parran argued that a health insurance system was necessary and that Truman's approach would allow the PHS to implement the program he had advocated in increasingly expansive terms since the late 1930s. "The President," Parran happily noted, "has recommended the greatest possible decentralization of services and administration." The American people were growing accustomed to voluntary hospital insurance and to publically funded medical services such as those that had emerged during the New Deal and the war. Now "we must seek to pool these experiences in the development of services on a much vaster scale than either our voluntary insurance plans or our public medical care programs have ever provided."[81]

Parran had long worked to maintain positive relations with the AMA, an approach that made some health insurance proponents skeptical of both him and the PHS. Nonetheless, he had already been dragged into the fight over insurance.[82] Though the service sat on the sidelines during the debate over the 1943 Wagner–Murray–Dingell bill, *Journal of the American Medical Association* editor Morris Fishbein had asserted that the bill would make the surgeon general "gauleiter" of American medicine. Now, with a bill he could back offered in Congress and the president supporting a push for a new health program, Parran broke decisively with organized medicine. On December 10, 1945, he distributed copies of the president's address on health to the PHS's commissioned corps, with instructions to treat the program, including its health insurance aspects, as official service policy.[83]

Speaking at Dartmouth six days later, Parran called on the experiences of the Mayo Clinic, the Kaiser Permanente Health System, and the controversial Ross-Loos Clinic as examples of how prepayment for health services could be combined with group practice, centered in hospitals and clinics. Such programs included preventive services and emphasized early detection of disease through periodic exams. Highly attentive to both the preventive and the curative aspects of medicine, they appeared to Parran to offer an avenue toward better integrating public health and individual medicine.

Parran argued that hospitals and health centers, funded in part by the federal government, should form the backbone of an integrated postwar American health system.[84] "What is needed today," he explained, "is the application of this principle of 'group medicine' on a much wider scale— so that its benefits—and therefore the benefits of the best modern medicine can offer—may reach down into the smallest community, even into the lonely farm house." Physicians, working together in groups coordinated by primary care doctors and including members from different specialties, should be paid through an insurance system funded with both contributory payroll taxes and general revenues and should operate out of hospitals constructed in part with federal dollars. Larger hospitals within the system, Parran explained, would be "linked administratively" with "smaller rural hospitals or health centers." When patients from remote areas had serious problems, they would be sent to larger hospitals.

Despite his increased enthusiasm for insurance and broad description of what American health care should look like, Parran's approach remained consistent with the ideas he had long embraced. Local physicians, he suggested in language that evoked the Biggs health center plan of the 1920s, "would have access to the consultive, laboratory, and educational facilities of the center; the center would send teams to the smaller groups to conduct refresher courses and teaching clinics, possibly also students for clinical and administrative internships." Particularly in rural areas, hospitals and health centers "may well become the base of operations for the local health department and the private physician. A common laboratory, space for community clinics and offices for the doctors would be under one roof—or on the same grounds." A strong federal commitment to funding both medical education and ongoing medical research would underpin the entire system.[85] Imagining prepayment for services as a means of reorienting the practice of medicine and delivery of medical services, Parran embraced the Wagner–Murray–Dingell approach as a plausible means of furthering the PHS's goal of creating a health policy regime encompassing both public health and individual medical care.

Postwar

The immediate postwar period was in many respects a triumphant one for the PHS. With authorization for extramural funding included in the 1944 Public Health Service Act, the PHS's National Institute of Health was poised to begin funding a massive new program of biomedical research. In the aftermath of the war, the NIH inherited a number of research programs from the wartime Committee on Medical Research.[86] On July 1, 1946, with little fanfare, Surgeon General Parran redesignated the MCWA program the Communicable Disease Center. Relying on a proven record of disease control and the strong support of Southern state governments and members of Congress, the PHS had constructed a permanent organization that would prove capable of stimulating local-level public health work and coordinating public health efforts across political jurisdictions. Along with implementing the PHS's extended malaria control program, the CDC swiftly emerged as an important training center for public health workers from throughout the

United States.[87] In the years that followed, the CDC trained public health workers for work in Latin America, the Middle East, and Asia and dispatched small groups of scientists and sanitary engineers across the world to assist in antimalaria work.[88]

Thomas Parran chaired the international conference that forged the framework of the new World Health Organization (WHO), and the CDC would work closely with the WHO in the years that followed.[89] Beginning in 1955, the WHO would embark on an ambitious effort to eradicate malaria worldwide. Rather than focusing on measures such as drainage, screening, and the development of local public health capabilities, the eradication program centered around DDT and chloroquine. Though the program made notable headway, the evolution of DDT-resistant mosquitoes, concerns about the environmental impact of DDT, and the emergence of drug-resistant strains of malaria ultimately combined with a lack of international will to bring it to a halt.[90]

Reflecting on these events, Isidore Falk emphasized the interconnections between the growth of federal intervention in public health and the rejection of government-backed insurance. The growth of the PHS's role in American public health between 1935 and the end of World War II, Falk believed, could be attributed "in the first instance" to "the success of the public health programs and beyond that to their acceptance by the public, by representatives of the public in the state legislature, and by the federal Congress. The program initiated by Title VI of the Social Security Act was sound and it was timely."

The quality of the efforts undertaken by the PHS, however, was for Falk only part of the story. "This growth," Falk continued, "also has to be explained in terms of something quite different." There was also, he argued, a "negative-type explanation." The PHS programs included in the Social Security Act, Falk contended, "also won large and continuous support *because* certain other programs did not—namely the program for general medical care for the population." Beginning during the late 1930s and continuing through the Wagner–Murray–Dingell health insurance bills of the 1940s, Falk and his allies had pushed the nation to adopt "a broader, more comprehensive solution to the economic problems of medical care. With each effective blocking of those proposals, the opponents kept constantly taking satisfaction—and seeking strength for their medico-political position—by assuring Congress and the public that every time they spoke up on an important occasion against national health insurance they were *for* something."

Fiercely opposed to insurance, the AMA expressed support for "public health work, and for research in medical care. The more consistently, the more persistently, the drive kept up for health insurance, the more the affirmative support for expanding the public health grants-in-aid and the appropriations for public health and medical research."[91] The AMA's opposition to health insurance, in other words, drove the organization to offer strong support for the growth of a federally backed public health regime.

In August 1946, only a month after MCWA was redesignated the Communicable Disease Center, Congress passed the Hill–Burton Hospital Survey and Construction Act, authorizing more than $1 billion for a new program of federally backed hospital construction to be administered by the PHS.[92] The act was aimed at expanding access to modern hospital facilities for all Americans, particularly those living in underserved communities. Cosponsored by Alabama senator Lister Hill, the act was strongly supported by Southern Democrats. Hill–Burton was also backed by the American Hospital Association and had the support of the AMA.[93] The formula for allocating Hill–Burton money strongly favored poorer states, and beyond this required "that special within-state priority be given to the construction of facilities in rural areas."[94]

Enacted on the basis of the support of the PHS's core Southern constituency, Hill–Burton's language reflected the heightened sensitivities of Southern members of Congress during the postwar period. For many Southern politicians, the implications of federal money and its corollary, federal regulation, for the South's racial status quo were becoming increasingly clear. Since the late 1930s, Southern Democrats had worried aloud that a labor- and Northern-influenced Democratic administration might attempt to use federal money to begin dismantling segregation. Rather than risk any future misunderstanding, Hill–Burton provided explicitly for the construction of "separate but equal" facilities.[95]

Hospital construction under Hill–Burton—a huge undertaking— highlighted the PHS's long-standing entanglement with the South's racial caste system.[96] Following the model of New Orleans's Charity Hospital, built by the federal Public Works Administration during the New Deal, Southern hospitals constructed using Hill–Burton funds typically had internally segregated wards for white and black people. The PHS closely supervised and regulated new construction, often providing blueprints for spatially segregated buildings.[97]

Measured in terms of increased access to facilities, Hill–Burton was a boon for both black and white Southerners. As Karen Kruse Thomas has shown, the program "resulted in the proliferation of modern, well-equipped hospitals that admitted all races of patients but internally segregated them by ward or floor. These multiracial hospitals substantially included blacks in the dramatic postwar expansion, modernization, and geographic redistribution of Southern hospital facilities, which without the federal program would have remained racially separate and grossly inadequate for patients of all races."[98]

These advances were real, but blacks were subjected to pervasive humiliation and discrimination. Where new additions were made to existing hospitals, black patients were relegated to the old facilities. Black physicians were often denied staff privileges at the new hospitals, meaning that they could not treat their patients once they had been admitted.[99] The *Journal of the National Medical Association*—the professional organization of black physicians—deemed the new hospitals "a kind of *de luxe* Jim Crow which is supposed to be more palatable than the customary variety and therefore more acceptable."[100] For the National Medical Association, it was not: "The cruel irony of the fact that the new segregated hospitals are concerned with such a vital human consideration as health should be as stinging a rebuke to the consciences of those who force them [to be segregated], as they are a crushing depressant to those who must accept them."[101] As had often been the case, the PHS was deeply implicated in preserving racial segregation.

While important aspects of the PHS's postwar program were being implemented, it soon became evident that the Wagner–Murray–Dingell bill would not become law. After President Truman's November 1945 speech outlining his support for a new national health program, he went largely silent on the issue.[102] Senate hearings on the Wagner–Murray–Dingell bill, meanwhile, proved a disaster. Senator James Murray chaired the Senate's Committee on Education and Labor. Ohio senator Robert Taft, who announced that he considered the bill to be a dangerous and extreme example of socialism, ostentatiously interrupted Murray's opening statement to the committee on the legislation in April 1946.[103]

Within months, the bill's sponsors decided to abandon it until after the November midterm elections. With the AMA again launching a full-scale assault on the legislation, little enthusiasm among congressional Democrats, and the campaign looming, Wagner, Murray, and Dingell decided that keeping the discussion alive in Congress would only further injure their cause by allowing the AMA to make its case.[104]

In November, the Republicans, who had last controlled Congress during the presidency of Herbert Hoover, won control of both the House and the Senate. Although Surgeon General Parran immediately indicated his commitment to the administration's health program and the Social Security Board continued to push forward with the project, it was obvious that nothing even remotely resembling the Wagner–Murray–Dingell bill would become law during the next session of Congress.[105] As 1946 came to an end, the AMA's House of Delegates passed resolutions condemning Surgeon General Parran and the PHS for supporting the Wagner–Murray–Dingell bill and the president's health program. Such political advocacy by medical professionals employed by the federal government, according to the AMA, was inappropriate and unacceptable.[106]

Employer-Sponsored Health Insurance

With the Wagner–Murray–Dingell bill off the table and a Republican majority in control of Congress, organized labor turned decisively toward collective bargaining as a means of securing health insurance for union members.[107] Labor would remain generally supportive of the idea of national health insurance and would at times offer leadership in the area, but the growth of employer-sponsored health insurance in the years that followed significantly blunted the appeal of a federal program.[108] The passage of the Taft–Hartley Act in 1947 both threatened unions and created strong incentives to focus on collective bargaining as a means of shoring up membership. After the United Mine Workers secured a high-quality health and welfare program under the Taft–Hartley framework through collective bargaining, their leader, John Lewis, explicitly dismissed the idea of national health insurance.[109]

Former assistant treasury secretary Josephine Roche, who had a background in mining and was close with Lewis, was made a trustee of the United Mine Workers' welfare and retirement fund and was designated as its director. Roche recruited Warren Draper, PHS assistant surgeon general and veteran of the rural sanitation program, to design and administer the health fund. Already sixty-five years old when he began working for the union in 1948, Draper remained in this position until 1969, creating an innovative decentralized system that emphasized the importance of preventive medicine.[110]

In the postwar years, enrollment in employer-sponsored health insurance skyrocketed. Commercial insurance companies, which relied on experience rating rather than the community rating model used by Blue Cross and Blue Shield, increasingly came to dominate the field. By 1950, fully

76.6 million Americans had hospital insurance (up from 11.96 million in 1940), and 21.58 million had physicians' insurance (up from 3 million) out of a total population of 152.3 million.[111] The nation had moved decisively toward the private provision of insurance, grounded in the tax-preferred status of employer contributions to premiums for group insurance coverage. Organized medicine had elected to support employer-sponsored health insurance as a means of warding off government-backed insurance, but its growth ultimately had the effect of shifting power toward the purchasers of medical services at the expense of providers.

CHAPTER NINE

HEALTH DIVIDED

Long a central player in debates over federal policy dealing with individual medical services, the PHS was largely sidelined after 1948, when Thomas Parran was ousted from the position of surgeon general after a dispute with Truman's federal security administrator, Oscar Ewing. The already dim prospects for national health insurance, meanwhile, faded further. Although Harry Truman advocated a national health insurance program during the 1948 election and clashed with the AMA over the issue during 1949, the barriers to such a program were high: the Democratic Party was increasingly divided along regional lines, a growing number of Americans received insurance through their employers, and the AMA remained implacably opposed. After Truman's failed 1949 push for insurance, the Social Security Board and other insurance proponents embraced an incremental approach that focused on securing hospital insurance for the elderly. Ultimately, this approach would result in the enactment of Medicare and Medicaid. The PHS, for its part, concentrated on shoring up what were now its core areas of strength: the CDC and the NIH.

The Truman Administration and Thomas Parran

Despite his strong advocacy for President Truman's health program, Thomas Parran had no real relationship with the nation's new chief executive. In August 1947, Truman appointed Indiana Democrat Oscar Ewing to head the Federal Security Agency, which had overseen the PHS since it left the Treasury Department in 1939. An important player in the Democratic Party, Ewing helped persuade President Roosevelt to choose Truman as his running mate in 1944. As FSA chief, Ewing quickly became embroiled in a personal dispute with Parran over a grant application to the NIH.

Dr. Walter Kempner, a German refugee who worked at Duke, had treated Ewing's wife.[1] When Kempner's request for NIH funding was rejected, Ewing decided to appeal directly to Parran. Parran looked into the matter and agreed with the NIH's conclusion that Kempner's work should not be funded. At this point, Ewing turned decisively against the surgeon general.

He began refusing to approve Parran's appointments for various advisory committee positions at the NIH, making it difficult for the organization to function and infuriating Parran. "The situation," Ewing later admitted, "got rather critical. Some of the institutes couldn't function because their advisory committees could not muster quorums." Enraged, Parran confronted Ewing and told him that the appointments had to be approved. Ewing asked, dismissively, "Who is going to make me?"

Parran ultimately relented, but the episode led directly to the end of his tenure as surgeon general. "The whole experience," Ewing explained, "annoyed me so much that when Dr. Parran's term as Surgeon General expired the following May [1948], I did not recommend him for reappointment."[2] In Parran's place, Truman appointed Leonard Scheele, a younger physician who had joined the PHS in the midst of the Great Depression.[3] Dr. Scheele, Ewing recalled, "was just as cooperative as anyone could be."[4]

Parran's ouster marked a crucial turning point for the PHS, causing its leaders to focus on consolidating existing programs such as the CDC and NIH and making clear the limitations on its authority. North Carolina state health officer Carl Reynolds, writing to Parran, expressed dismay. "To my mind," he told Parran, "it proves that [Harry Truman] is a small town, pinhead politician, whose interests lie in what he thinks to be expedient to his political needs,—self-aggrandizement—rather than to the interest and welfare of the people of these United States. The President slipped a cog this time and it is now my fervent hope he will fall in his political quagmire, and I am a Democrat."[5]

Truman and Insurance

Parran's demise meant the end of the PHS's commitment to a comprehensive national health program linking public health and individual medicine. President Truman, however, began to speak out more and more on the issue of health insurance. Facing an election in 1948, Truman campaigned against the "do-nothing" Republican Congress. Among the policies Truman promised to enact if elected to his own term with a Democratic majority was a health insurance program modeled along the lines of that still being pushed by Isidore Falk, Arthur Altmeyer, and the Social Security Administration (formerly the Social Security Board, but renamed and reorganized in 1946).

The Democrats, however, were deeply divided. After Roosevelt's death and the end of World War II, Truman emerged as a restrained but determined advocate of increased civil rights for black Americans.[6] Intraparty tensions over civil rights came to a head at the 1948 Democratic National Convention, held in Philadelphia. After a passionate speech by Minneapolis mayor Hubert Humphrey, the party adopted a pro–civil rights platform that, along with calling for congressional action to ease discrimination, commended President Harry Truman "for his courageous stand on the issue of civil rights."[7] In response, Deep South Democrats, who had hoped someone other than Truman might be nominated, held their own convention in Birmingham and nominated South Carolina governor Strom Thurmond as a "states' rights" Democratic candidate for president.[8] The new breakaway party called itself the States' Rights Democrats. Nine days after Thurmond and his followers bolted from the Democratic convention, Truman issued executive orders mandating the end of race-based discrimination in the armed forces "as rapidly as possible" and instituting fair employment practices in the federal civil service.[9] The process initially moved ahead slowly, but segregation would be ended in military bases throughout the South at the discretion of the president.

Despite the defection of four Deep South states to Thurmond, Truman managed to win a full term of his own in a close election. The Democratic Party, moreover, regained control of Congress after two years of Republican rule. Truman attempted to make good on his campaign promise of national health insurance, although the prospects for success were dim from the beginning. Three major obstacles stood in his way: the AMA, the growth of employer-sponsored health insurance, and the deep divisions within his own political party.

During 1949, the AMA embarked on a massive publicity campaign. Morris Fishbein, long the organization's spokesman on insurance, was removed from his position as *Journal of the American Medical Association* editor in June, a sign of the organization's commitment to more professionalized public relations. Designed by the husband-and-wife firm of Whitaker and Baxter, the new AMA campaign was two-pronged. To begin with, it drew on Cold War fears and the intensely anticommunist atmosphere in Washington, portraying Truman's insurance plan as a dangerous lurch toward totalitarianism. National health insurance, the AMA maintained in a now well-worn formulation, was "one of the final, irrevocable steps toward state socialism." The president's plan, according to the organization, "would regiment doctors and patients alike under a vast bureaucracy of political administrators, clerks, bookkeepers and lay committees."[10]

Second, the AMA argued that the president's plan was designed to address a problem that was no longer a problem. With the growth of employer-sponsored health insurance, the nation's health finance problems were being effectively addressed through voluntary means. Describing private insurance as the "American Way," the AMA maintained that employer-sponsored plans would soon help to cover the entire population. In the same month that Fishbein was removed as editor of the *Journal of the American Medical Association*, the organization endorsed voluntary commercial (rather than just nonprofit and physician-run) health insurance.[11] The AMA's updated approach proved effective, in large part because Americans could see that insurance coverage was in fact becoming more and more common.

While Truman pushed for national health insurance along the lines long favored by the Social Security Administration and confronted a massive publicity campaign from the AMA, members of Congress offered a series of counterproposals. Senator Robert Taft, a fierce critic of the administration's health policy, offered a limited grant-in-aid bill to help states pay for health services for the indigent. Taft had offered a similar bill in 1946, largely for the purpose of having something to contrast the Truman administration's approach with.[12]

Alabama senator Lister Hill, working with Vermont Republican George Aiken, introduced a plan for federal assistance to states to help the indigent purchase nonprofit prepayment insurance plans.[13] Like Hill's earlier hospital construction bill, the new insurance proposal was supported by the American Hospital Association, which helped draft it and viewed it as a means of gaining additional paying patients while warding off national government control. An editorial in the *Journal of the American Medical Association*, meanwhile, asserted that Hill–Aiken was "in accord with the basic principles of freedom of choice of physician and hospital, and absence of interference in the personal relationship between doctor and patient."[14] Had Truman been interested, there are strong reasons to believe that Hill–Aiken could have been enacted.

Meanwhile, a group of Republican lawmakers, led by Vermont's Ralph Flanders and New York's Irving Ives, proposed an innovative plan for subsidizing large-scale enrollment in voluntary health insurance programs. The Flanders–Ives bill, which included among its cosponsors California's Richard Nixon, laid out a plan in which the federal government would set standards that private health insurance plans would have to follow in order to receive funds through a federal–state cooperative program. In contrast to Hill–Aiken and the Taft proposal, there would be no means test for participation in the health insurance plans. Instead, individuals would decide what benefit level they wished to enroll in and pay a capped percentage of their income. Money from the federal government and state governments would then cover the difference between the enrollee's contribution and the actual cost of the plan.[15]

Such an approach, Flanders and Ives believed, would both keep important decisions about medical care out of federal hands and allow for a significant expansion in access to medical services. It also was hoped that by keeping the program open to individuals of all income levels, federally backed plans would be able to retain a high level of quality. In practice, however, Flanders–Ives might have faced significant adverse selection problems. With their own contributions capped, the sickest among the uninsured would likely have been among the first to enroll in the insurance plans, driving up the cost of insurance and requiring the federal government to pick up the slack.

Throughout 1949, the Democratic split over civil rights loomed in the background of Truman's push for insurance. During earlier battles over insurance, Southern Democrats had not played a significant role, in large part because compulsory insurance was understood to be a program aimed at Northern and urban populations. Now, however, the dangers of the president's insurance proposal were obvious from the perspective of many Southern Democrats. As Georgia representative James C. Davis explained, national health insurance might represent a mortal threat to segregation: "Negro doctors would treat white patients. White patients would be interested in Negro hospitals. White doctors would have to treat Negro patients and admit them in their hospitals." According to Davis, certain "persons high in government" intended "to do away with every vestige of segregation in this country if it is possible to do so." As evidence, Davis cited Truman's unilateral desegregation of the armed forces and overt support for civil rights.[16]

Davis's thoughts were echoed by Federal Security Agency chief Oscar Ewing, who was widely loathed by Southern Democrats for his open opposition to segregation. When the president proposed turning the FSA into a Cabinet-level department, Southern Democrats helped to block the move in large part because of Ewing. Ewing's thoughts on the potential implications of national health insurance were clear. "The President's fight for Civil Rights," he contended, "is having much more of an effect than many of us realize. And, with the passage of national health insurance, I believe we shall see, so far as the medical profession is concerned, a steady development in its practical application."[17] Just as Southern Democrats feared,

Ewing argued that federally backed insurance might be used to transform race relations in the region.

It is clear that some form of compromise on the issue of insurance for the indigent might have been reached in 1949. Truman, however, had strong reasons for not taking this approach. To begin with, he was wary of working on the issue with the Southern Democrats who were offering so much opposition to his administration's policies. Politically, a compromise on health insurance for the indigent might have alienated the increasingly important labor movement. It might also have further sapped political support for national health insurance over the long run. A shift toward the Flanders–Ives approach, meanwhile, would have represented a huge leap away from the contributory social insurance approach that Truman favored and that the Social Security Administration believed would prove most effective. Above all else, Truman thought that pushing for national health insurance was the right thing to do. While it is possible to imagine a scenario in which a federal grant-in-aid program resembling Medicaid might have emerged out of the 1949 battle over health insurance, the reality is that a stalemate on insurance was by far the most likely outcome from the moment that Truman began his new term in 1949.

Health Divided

In the years after the 1949 insurance battle, the bifurcated health policy regime that emerged out of the New Deal and World War II became increasingly locked in. As surgeon general, Thomas Parran's successor Leonard Scheele proved a loyal supporter of Truman's health program. The PHS, however, was no longer particularly interested in transforming the American health care system. Instead, the service focused on consolidating its growing strength in the CDC and NIH.

The service itself had changed dramatically over a fairly short period of time. The marine hospitals, once the heart of the PHS's mission, were now a peripheral component of its operations. In the decades that followed, their numbers would dwindle and a series of federal bureaucrats would question the need for their continued existence. The NIH, meanwhile, grew more and more powerful, with its own base of support in Congress and effective control over substantial amounts of research funding.[18] Over time, it became increasingly autonomous.

In Atlanta, the CDC continued to assume control over many of the PHS's most important functions. First under the direction of Raymond Vonderlehr (who had directed the early stages of the Tuskegee study during the 1930s) and then under veteran malariologist Justin Andrews, the CDC carved out new and important avenues of action for itself. In 1951, chief CDC epidemiologist Alexander Langmuir created a new Epidemiological Intelligence Service (EIS). Initially propelled forward by the Korean War and Cold War fears that the Soviet Union or China might deploy biological weapons in an attack on the United States, the EIS would within a few years become among the best known of the CDC's swiftly multiplying operations.[19]

Beginning in 1955, the EIS played a key role in the nation's polio vaccination campaign. It created a special program for monitoring the distribution of the vaccine after the Cutter incident, in which several young children came down with polio after being given a vaccine produced by the Cutter Laboratory, which failed to adequately kill the virus when preparing it.[20] Three years later, when the nation faced a potential flu pandemic, the EIS again oversaw disease surveillance and monitored a large-scale vaccination campaign. In testing the flu vaccine, the CDC remained within the ethical traditions of the PHS: "volunteers" from the federal penitentiary in Atlanta were used in the trials.[21]

The institutional and political world that the PHS had once inhabited had, in many ways, ceased to exist by the 1950s. In 1953, President Eisenhower used his executive authority to reorganize the Federal Security Agency as a Cabinet-level department, henceforth known as the Department of Health, Education, and Welfare (HEW).[22] With the controversial Oscar Ewing gone, the Republican Congress offered no opposition. For the first time, the nation had something approaching a national department of health like that first proposed by Robert Owen more than forty years before. It was an important step, though its immediate significance should not be overstated. For the time being, the department exercised only minimal control over the PHS. During the late 1960s, however, HEW would strip the post of surgeon general of most of its statutory power.

By the end of 1950s, the CDC had emerged as the premier force in coordinating public health activities throughout the nation, distributing grants to state and local health departments, supplying technical information and personnel, and embarking on large-scale epidemiological studies. It continued to be deeply engaged in the efforts of the WHO. Starting in 1955, the CDC assisted in an ultimately unsuccessful campaign to eradicate malaria worldwide.[23] In 1960, the CDC began occupying brand-new facilities in Atlanta on land donated to the PHS by Emory University. The same year, it gained control of the collection of national vital statistics, further cementing its role at the heart of American public health.[24] In 1967, it gained authority over the nation's quarantine activities.[25]

While the federal government asserted a central role in American public health, the proponents of national health insurance began shifting their approach, embracing incremental change as a means of forwarding their cause. In June 1951, Federal Security Agency chief Oscar Ewing announced that the Truman administration would support a program of contributory hospital insurance for people receiving Social Security old-age pensions. Such a plan, Ewing and insurance proponents in the Social Security Administration such as Arthur Altmeyer and Isidore Falk hoped, might pave the way toward a more comprehensive insurance system. The next year, Democrats in Congress introduced legislation providing for sixty days of hospitalization per year for Social Security beneficiaries.[26]

The logic of such an approach was clear. The postwar growth of health insurance coverage in the United States was based largely in employee groups. The elderly, however, were generally not in the workforce and were almost guaranteed to have significant and expensive medical needs. For insurance companies interested in selling profitable policies, the implications were obvious: "the expensive medical needs of the elderly simply made them a bad risk not worth insuring."[27] If insurance proponents could enact legislation covering a sympathetic population that was largely excluded from the existing employer-sponsored system, they could create a pathway toward national health insurance. Hospital insurance, which was viewed as less threatening to the existing practice of medicine than insurance for physicians' services, would be used as an entering wedge. A program could be developed for the elderly, and once proven effective, it could be expanded to the rest of society.[28]

The election of Dwight Eisenhower and the Republican takeover of Congress in 1952, however, ensured that the hospital insurance plan would go nowhere in the short run. With the Republican Party in control in Washington, Isidore Falk, the leading figure pressing for a national health insurance plan since the mid-1930s, decided to leave government service, accepting a position at Yale. Employer-sponsored health insurance, meanwhile, continued to grow. In 1954, a new Internal Revenue Code formalized the tax-exempt status of employer contributions to health insurance premiums, which had been established in 1943 through an administrative ruling. The new code "expanded the scope of this ruling and codified" the earlier ruling, further strengthening the emerging system.[29] From 76.6 million in 1950, the number of Americans with hospital insurance grew to 122.5 million (out of a total population of 180 million) in 1960. The number with physicians' insurance grew from 21.5 million to 83.1 million.[30]

Congress added disability insurance to Social Security in 1956, leading some to believe that hospital insurance for the elderly might be the next step in American social policy. As the issue of the unmet health needs of the elderly drew growing attention during the late 1950s, President Eisenhower offered a proposal intended to incentivize the insurance industry to develop insurance plans capable of covering the elderly.[31] Organized labor, meanwhile, threw its weight behind the old-age hospitalization insurance approach. In 1957, Rhode Island representative Aime Forand introduced legislation that would create a hospital insurance program tied to Social Security. Forand was persuaded to do so by the leaders of the AFL-CIO, who believed that such a program was the best means of providing insurance to retired workers not covered by employer-sponsored health insurance. Though Forand's bill gained little traction, it drew further attention to the large gaps in coverage in the emerging American system of health insurance.[32] Labor's stated belief that such a plan would help to shore up the strength of insurance plans negotiated through collective bargaining, meanwhile, suggested the extent to which the growth of employer-sponsored insurance had reshaped the political debate.

There was no real likelihood that a hospital insurance program tied to Social Security would become law during the Eisenhower administration.[33] The issue was a salient one, however, during the 1960 presidential election. Both Democrat John Kennedy and Republican Richard Nixon offered proposals for dealing with the issue of the elderly uninsured. Kennedy declared himself to be strongly in favor of a hospital insurance plan tied to Social Security, while Nixon endorsed a more limited approach aimed at the indigent elderly.[34] For its part, Congress passed a small-scale grant-in-aid program aimed at expanding access to individual medical services for the elderly, the Kerr–Mills Act, in 1960. Cosponsored by Oklahoma senator Robert Kerr and Senator Wilbur Mills of Arkansas, the program was inoffensive enough to gain broad support. Under Kerr–Mills, states could receive federal assistance for expanding access to health services for the elderly. Indicative of the level of popular interest in the health of the elderly, the program did not prove particularly successful, with only four states participating by 1963.[35] Nonetheless, the precedent it set was important.

As president, Kennedy continued to push for hospital insurance tied to Social Security. Faced with the ongoing strength of the conservative coalition of Southern Democrats and Republicans, the plan stalled. The political dynamics of insurance for the elderly were altered dramatically, however, in the aftermath of Kennedy's assassination and Lyndon Johnson's subsequent landslide victory against Republican Barry Goldwater in the 1964 presidential election. The election brought a new class of liberal Democrats into Congress, meaning that Johnson, unlike Kennedy, could rely on something approaching a liberal majority in the legislative branch. Emphasizing Kennedy's legacy, and using his own vast knowledge of how to push legislation through Congress, Johnson faced a substantially less difficult path forward.[36]

The push for hospital insurance for the elderly had previously been held back by House Ways and Means Committee chairman Wilbur Mills, but Johnson now succeeded in persuading Mills that the Arkansas congressman faced an upswing of support for the Medicare idea. If Mills moved the program forward, he could take full credit for it. Cajoled by Johnson, Mills also endorsed voluntary physicians' insurance for the elderly under Social Security. The idea of a premium-supported program that the elderly could choose to enroll in had been offered as an alternative approach to a mandatory program by the AMA. This alternative was offered in part to undercut the position of liberal proponents of insurance, but it makes clear the extent to which the AMA had become comfortable with the concept of insurance over the preceding two decades. Mills also embraced a program of federal assistance to the states for the creation of health insurance programs for some categories of the indigent. Such an approach had been suggested as an alternative to national health insurance on a number of occasions. Now Mills proposed it as an extension of the existing Kerr–Mills program, to be revamped as Medicaid.[37]

Health politics had been transformed by the emergence of employer-sponsored health insurance, paving the way for a federal approach to expanding access to individual medical services that proved legislatively possible. With strong presidential backing, the support of Wilbur Mills, and a liberal majority in Congress after the 1964 elections, the process of turning Medicare and Medicaid into a reality during 1965 was surprisingly straightforward. In July, President Johnson signed them into law as amendments to the Social Security Act.[38] Medicare Part A created a payroll tax–based national system of hospital insurance for the elderly, while Medicare Part B created a voluntary system of physicians' insurance for the elderly. Medicaid created a federal–state cooperative program for insuring recipients of Aid to Families with Dependent Children, the medically indigent elderly, and other low-income groups. In 1972, Medicare was expanded to include the disabled as well as people with end-stage renal failure.[39]

Medicare's proponents hoped it would lay the groundwork for a national health insurance program, but its impact proved significantly different. Modeled on the existing insurance system, Medicare was designed to avoid alienating the hospitals and physicians who would provide services to Medicare recipients. Under Part A, participating institutions could select "fiscal intermediaries," typically Blue Cross plans, to administer billing and payments. Part B was administered by insurance "carriers," which were mostly Blue Shield plans.[40] This approach helped the federal government ease into its new role as a major payer for health services by relying on the accumulated knowledge and competency of Blue Cross and Blue Shield while also creating a buffer between intervention-wary providers and the federal government.[41]

Grounded in a retrospective payment system, Medicare invited an almost inevitable inflation of medical costs. More seniors could access medical services, while service providers were given a huge amount of leeway in terms of what prices they might charge. As passed in 1965, Medicare allowed hospitals to bill for "reasonable costs." Physicians, meanwhile, could claim their "customary charges."[42] Within a few years, it became evident that the program would prove extremely expensive.[43] Fiscal concerns helped ensure that Medicare would not provide the basis for a national health insurance program; such an expansion, it appeared, would lead to massive and uncontrollable spending. Still, it was not until the 1980s that Congress—faced with ongoing budget deficits—put in place policies for controlling the ever-expanding costs of hospital and physicians' care under Medicare. Legislation in 1983 implemented a prospective payment system that connected payments for hospital care under Part A to a patient's diagnosis through a process known as "diagnosis related groups."[44] A fee schedule grounded in "relative value" was finally put in place for physicians' services in 1989.[45]

Medicaid, meanwhile, emerged as a somewhat patchwork system, with individuals living in different states encountering distinct versions the program as well as differing eligibility standards.[46] Arizona became the last state to sign on to the program in 1982, making it fully nationwide. During the 1980s, Congress enacted guidelines that required states to expand eligibility for the program to new categories of the elderly, children, and pregnant women.[47] Nonetheless, eligibility standards continued to vary across the nation—and remained particularly stringent in the South and West. As a result, a significant portion of the low-income population did not have access to the program.[48]

Together, employer-sponsored health insurance, Medicare, and Medicaid ensured that the majority of Americans had insurance. As a result, the likelihood that the United States would adopt a comprehensive national health insurance system along the lines long favored by the Social Security Administration and liberal Democrats became increasingly small.[49] Challenging a system in which most Americans were covered, particularly those in the middle class, was a politically fraught endeavor. The costs of medical care, however, continued to grow. With fee-for-service payment routed through third-party insurance, the dominant means through which both physicians and hospitals were paid, strong incentives existed toward the provision of more services. The proliferation of medical technology, growing physician specialization, and construction of hospitals after World War II, meanwhile, interacted with fee-for-service and insurance to generate further cost inflation. While other industrialized nations possessed tools for controlling costs through mechanisms such as global budgeting, the United States proved generally incapable of confronting the problem.[50] In the decades that followed, policy makers would confront an entrenched system, with a strong status quo bias, in which health care costs continued to grow. Over time, increasing costs made insurance coverage increasingly more difficult to access.

The Public Health Service

The national health insurance plans of the 1930s and 1940s assumed an important role for the PHS, but the PHS was largely marginalized in the development of federal policies dealing with individual medical services after the ouster of Thomas Parran. The PHS's cautious approach to health insurance had alienated some of the most passionate proponents of insurance, and the reputation of the commissioned corps had gone into decline. Although both the CDC and the NIH continued to grow in prestige, the service's commissioned corps and dwindling number of marine hospitals appeared to many to be vestiges of a bygone era. Increasingly, the CDC and NIH asserted identities that went beyond their status as simply components of the PHS.

Although the administration of Medicare was largely under the auspices of the Social Security Administration, the PHS was involved in a key aspect of its implementation: hospital desegregation. In the years after the Supreme Court's 1954 *Brown v. Board of Education* decision, the service's role in perpetuating the South's racial order, particularly through the Hill–Burton hospital construction program, became increasingly glaring. In 1963, the US court of appeals in Richmond, Virginia, found that Hill–Burton construction involved "extensive state–Federal sharing in the common

plan." As an undertaking of state governments and of the federal government, "separate but equal" hospital construction violated the Fifth and Fourteenth Amendments to the Constitution.[51]

The appellate court's decision was followed by the 1964 Civil Rights Act,
which explicitly prohibited discrimination on the basis of "race, color, or
national origin" in programs receiving federal aid. Together, the court decision and the Civil Rights Act appeared to demand action from the PHS.
The service, however, responded in a manner that was widely regarded
as perfunctory. Though it put in place a new set of regulations outlawing
discriminatory practices by future recipients of Hill–Burton aid, the PHS
appeared at best reluctant to enforce the new rules and took little action
against existing patterns of segregation. Throughout 1964 and 1965, the
NAACP continued to document segregation in Southern hospitals and to
lodge complaints with the Department of Health, Education, and Welfare.[52]

The challenge of desegregating Southern hospitals was exacerbated by
the close relationships of PHS officers with the political leaders of the communities in which they lived and worked, as well as with local medical societies and hospital administrators.[53] "Whatever they believe personally," one
civil rights lawyer noted of the PHS at the time, "they are obviously going
to have to experience a radical change in their thinking if they are going to
administer Title VI. Even if you're a flaming liberal it is hard to tell a guy
you've been playing golf with for eight years that his hospital is going to
have to undergo a revolution."[54] The passage of Medicare, however, marked
the beginning of a new phase of desegregation. In order to become eligible
to receive payments from the federal government for Medicare patients,
hospitals needed to be certified as in compliance with Title VI of the Civil
Rights Act.[55] Despite its poor reputation in the realm of civil rights, the PHS
was the federal agency best positioned to accomplish this, and Surgeon
General William Stewart announced his commitment to the program of
desegregation.

The PHS was generally successful in gaining compliance, but resistance
to desegregation was very real.[56] Medicare payments were slated to begin
on July 1, 1966. As the date approached, a number of Southern hospitals
continued to hold out in the hopes that enforcement of the Civil Rights Act
would not prove harsh. President Johnson, however, took a hard line, warning in a meeting of health professionals in June, "The Federal government
is not going to shy away from its clear responsibility."[57] As the program
took effect, the *Washington Post* reported that "three-fourths of Mississippi's
hospitals" were "denying benefits to the aged. . . . In entire Southern com-

munities—such as Danville, Va., Selma, Ala., and Macon, Ga.—not a single hospital was qualified to accept medicare patients." Mobile, Alabama, "was credited with the 'worst showing' because only 30 of its 3986 hospitals beds were certified for medicare."[58] For Southern hospitals, however, the pressure to accept the money offered by the federal government in the form of Medicare payments quickly proved irresistible. After the initial drama of their failure to comply, the recalcitrant hospitals fell into line fairly rapidly. By October 1966, "only 12 southern hospitals were still not certified."[59] The service had fallen in line with the desegregation effort, but its early reluctance accentuated the feeling of some within the Johnson administration that it was a backward-looking organization, far too sympathetic to the proponents of white supremacy and enmeshed in a racist system that it was unwilling to challenge.[60]

Already by this point HEW secretary John Gardner had decided that it was time to begin reorganizing and streamlining the department, which had been created out of the old Federal Security Agency. During 1966, he began implementing the reorganization, which stripped the PHS and other organizations within HEW of most of their ability to act autonomously. Under the reorganization, "all of the surgeon general's statutory powers" were transferred to the secretary of HEW. Top positions in the service that had once been filled only by career officers could now be filled through the civil service.[61]

For the time being, Surgeon General William Stewart continued to retain operational control over the service. After taking over as secretary of HEW in 1968, however, Wilbur Cohen divested Stewart of almost all authority and shifted control over the PHS to an assistant secretary of HEW.[62] Once a highly autonomous organization under the control of a professional commissioned officer corps with a prominent policy-making role, the PHS was now clearly subordinate to political appointees. Many among the commissioned corps were extremely unhappy about the reorganization, which came close to rendering the surgeon general a figurehead. The last of the marine hospitals, once the lifeblood of the organization, were closed early in the Reagan administration.

The federal government's central role in public health, however, remained. Indeed, the CDC's role in both domestic and international public health programs continued to grow, as did its prestige. In 1968, the CDC played a critical part in the US response to the Hong Kong flu pandemic. With a vaccine on hand, a highly developed ability to monitor vaccination campaigns, and the trust of the public, public health authorities mounted a relatively successful effort against the disease. In 1976, on the advice of the CDC, President Gerald Ford backed an attempt to vaccinate most of the US population against a threatened swine flu epidemic that never materialized. The CDC's ability to persuade the president to support this misguided and ultimately embarrassing endeavor made clear the strength of its reputation.[63] Internationally, the CDC assisted in the WHO's smallpox eradication campaign, which resulted in the declaration that the disease had been eradicated in 1980.[64]

In 1972, the PHS's long-standing "Tuskegee Study of Untreated Syphilis in the Negro Male" was detailed in an Associated Press story. Still in operation more than forty years after its beginning, and decades after penicillin became available, the Tuskegee study was widely understood as shocking in the extent of its indifference to human pain and suffering. The power dynamics involved were similarly disturbing. Under false pretenses, the federal government had used poor black Southerners as subjects in a callous experiment.

The study had implications beyond the men who were denied treatment or the initial public uproar. "Confronted with the experiment's moral bankruptcy," writes James Jones, "many blacks lost faith in the government and no longer believed health officials who spoke on matters of public concern."[65] Unambiguous evidence of federal government experimentation on black subjects fueled a skepticism of public health efforts and biomedical research among many African Americans. When the AIDS epidemic emerged a decade after the Tuskegee revelation, the full extent of the damage done became evident. In many black communities, a belief emerged that AIDS had been introduced by the government with the intention of killing black Americans. The actions of the PHS had a negative impact on black perceptions of health efforts that persists into the present day.[66]

Public Health and Individual Medicine

During the 1930s, a sharp division began to emerge between federal policies dealing with public health and with individual medicine. Strongly supported by Southern Democrats who held key positions in Congress, the PHS carved out an important role in American public health under the auspices of the New Deal. When the military began building new installations and engaging in training maneuvers in the South as the nation mobilized for World War II, the PHS embarked on an expanded effort to protect soldiers, sailors, and airmen against the threat of malaria. Rather than building an emergency effort from scratch, as it had been forced to do during World

War I, the PHS could rely on a strong preexisting set of public health institutions and relationships with state and local authorities. In the aftermath of the war, the PHS's Atlanta-based MCWA program was transformed into the Communicable Disease Center (later renamed the Centers for Disease Control and Prevention). The PHS also achieved major goals in the expansion of funding for biomedical research through the NIH and in the passage of the 1946 Hill–Burton hospital construction act.

While the role of the PHS in American public health grew, wartime federal policies helped to foster a system in which more and more Americans accessed health insurance through employment-based group plans. Although PHS leaders believed that support from President Truman for a comprehensive health plan, including insurance, might lead toward a policy breakthrough and the creation of a federal policy regime encompassing both public health and individual medical services, they were sorely disappointed. In the years that followed, the divided health policy regime that emerged clearly from the war would be further locked in. Sharp regional divisions with the Democratic Party, combined with the growth of employer-sponsored health insurance and effective mobilization by the AMA, helped to guarantee that national health insurance would not be adopted. After the failure of President Truman's push for insurance in 1949, the proponents of national health insurance took a new incremental approach. In time, this approach led to the passage of Medicare and Medicaid. Where a unified federal health policy regime, encompassing both public health and individual medicine, had once appeared a possibility, the United States had instead adopted a set of policies in which approaches to health would be divided.

CONCLUSION

Working to confront the debilitating diseases that plagued the Southern United States during the first decades of the twentieth century, officials from the United States Public Health Service built the foundations of the federal government's modern role in public health. Beginning with the nation's mobilization for World War I, PHS officers assembled a political coalition on the basis of their ability to deliver effective services and to frame these services as necessary for the South's economic development. During the New Deal, the bonds they forged with political leaders and communities provided the basis for an expanded national government role in helping to ensure the health of Americans through population-based efforts. Ultimately, the threat of disease during wartime and solid Southern support led to the emergence of the PHS's Atlanta-based Communicable Disease Center, later renamed the Centers for Disease Control and Prevention.

While the national government established an overt and central position in public health, the United States rejected a comparable or linked national government role in the realm of individual medicine. Divisions among key policy makers over both policy and strategy were central to this outcome, as were interest group alignments, political institutions, and timing. Had federal policy makers pursued compromise with organized medicine in either 1935 or 1938, the United States might have gone down an entirely different path in the realm of health policy. Large-scale government intervention in facilitating access to individual medical services for the indigent, in building infrastructure, and in facilitating access to expensive treatments for lower- and medium-income Americans, under the approach advocated by Thomas Parran, might have preceded the emergence of widespread access to insurance through employer-sponsored plans. As a result, physicians might have found themselves negotiating for higher reimbursement rates or for changes in the developing system rather than arguing that voluntary insurance was succeeding in addressing the nation's health-financing problems. If created, employer-sponsored plans might have served as a supplement to the emerging system. Notably, the approach advocated by Parran and the PHS would have obligated the federal government to help foot the bill for the chronic diseases that helped fuel the growth of health costs in the decades that followed.

The path-dependent nature of policy development strengthened the role of public health institutions during the New Deal and World War II, but the critical juncture of the 1930s and 1940s led to a far different outcome for federal intervention in individual medical services. After a period of fluidity, the emergence of the conservative coalition (and its strengthening after the 1938 midterm elections) combined with mobilization for World War II to foreclose once-plausible policy options. As the PHS continued to expand its role in American public health, federal wage and tax policy helped to fuel the growth of employer-sponsored health insurance.

Over time, the creation of a system intended to integrate public health and individual medicine became increasingly unlikely. As employer-sponsored health insurance grew, constituencies such as organized labor, business, the AMA, and the insurance industry adjusted their expectations and strategies. In the years after Thomas Parran's ouster from the position of surgeon general, the PHS almost completely abandoned the approach to health policy articulated by Parran and men such as Joseph Mountin (who died in 1952). By the mid-1960s, the divided national health policy regime that began to emerge in the 1930s was firmly entrenched.

Continuity and Change in American Health Policy

The bifurcated health policy regime that emerged out of the 1930s and 1940s proved highly resilient. Despite hopes that Medicare might provide the framework for a more universal system, widespread access to insurance through tax-preferred employment-based plans and the ongoing growth of medical costs made building a political coalition in favor of national health insurance proposals difficult. Increasingly, organized labor and the insurance industry emerged as pivotal interest groups in debates over insurance. While successful collective bargaining ensured that union members were generally able to access medical care through employer-sponsored insurance, and Medicare addressed the issue of insurance after retirement, many union leaders continued to hold out hope for a single-payer system based on the Canadian model. Insurers, for their part, had a clear material interest in fighting any government-backed approach that might negatively impact their market position.

By the early 1970s, the ongoing growth of medical costs and gaps in coverage within the nation's health insurance system were major issues of concern for both Democratic and Republican leaders. Democratic senator Edward Kennedy, backed by the United Auto Workers, initiated a new push for a single-payer health insurance system and a guaranteed right to health care. In 1971, President Richard Nixon responded with his own National Health Strategy. Foreshadowing the later failed proposal of President Bill Clinton, the approach adopted in Massachusetts under Governor Mitt Romney in 2006, and the 2010 Patient Protection and Affordable Care Act, the Nixon health strategy relied heavily on a mandate that employers help to pay for employee premiums. It also included a Family Health Insurance Plan, which would have replaced Medicaid with a nationally administered plan for poor families, and a strategy for transforming the incentives driving the growth of health costs through health maintenance organizations (HMOs).[1]

HMOs, the Nixon administration believed, would ultimately shift the health care system away from fee-for-service medicine and toward prepaid group practice. The HMO concept was inspired in part by Kaiser Permanente, which had built an integrated health care delivery system apparently capable of both promoting the health of individuals and controlling costs. Emphasizing preventive medicine and early detection, Kaiser Permanente had (along with the Mayo Clinic and the Ross-Loos Clinic) been viewed as a potential model for improving health outcomes and improving the incentives involved in health care delivery by Thomas Parran after World War II. Under the Nixon health strategy, employers, the Family Health Insurance Plan, and Medicare would be required to offer an HMO option. Where Kaiser operated as a nonprofit, however, the Nixon administration's HMO program embraced for-profit entities as potential providers.[2]

Explaining the importance of HMOs in his national health strategy, Nixon used language strikingly reminiscent of the health reformers who had provoked the concerns of organized medicine beginning during the Progressive Era.[3] His description of the perverse incentives that skewed American medical practice might well have been written by Benjamin Warren and Edgar Sydenstricker fifty-five years before: "The more illnesses [physicians and hospitals] treat—and the more service they render—the more their income rises." While this incentive structure did not mean that physicians did not do their best to treat illness, Nixon argued, "it does mean that there is no economic incentive for them to concentrate on keeping people healthy."[4]

Nixon emphasized the possibility that financing mechanisms could be used to reorient the practice of medicine toward prevention and wellness. Providing a "comprehensive range of medical services in a single organization" for a "fixed contract fee . . . paid in advance by all subscribers," he contended, HMOs would reverse the incentives created by fee-for-service medicine. "Under this arrangement," Nixon explained, "income grows not with the number of days a person is sick but with the number of days he is well." As a result, HMOs "have a strong financial interest in preventing illness, or, failing that, in treating it in its early states, promoting a thorough recovering, and preventing any reoccurrence."[5]

Nixon's declaration of support for health reform was partially motivated by a belief that support for new social policy initiatives might help the Republican Party to gain Democratic votes. He was also persuaded that serious problems confronted the American health system, and he apparently felt no qualms about throwing his weight behind what he believed to be an appropriately market-oriented alternative to the approach being advocated by liberal Democrats such as Edward Kennedy.

Like the AMA's New Deal–era willingness to accept certain forms of government action in the realm of individual medicine, Nixon's position during the early 1970s both offered a path toward expanding access and fell far short of what key figures such as Senator Kennedy would accept. During 1971 and 1972, Kennedy and organized labor resisted Nixon's health strategy, portraying it as a boon to the interests of private insurance companies and remaining committed to a single-payer health plan. In 1973, however, Congress did pass a heavily modified version of the HMO plan.

In retrospect, Kennedy expressed regret that he did not pursue a compromise with the Nixon administration while a deal that might have resulted in legislation was possible. By 1974, Kennedy had decided to break with organized labor and pursue a compromise national health insurance proposal with House Ways and Means Committee chairman Wilbur Mills. The plan, based on a contributory model, would have required copayments and deductibles, an approach that labor leaders opposed.[6] Nixon, meanwhile, expressed a clear willingness to make a deal. The administration's Comprehensive Health Insurance Plan (CHIP), released in 1974 as the Watergate scandal overcame his presidency, included an employer mandate as well as an Assisted Health Insurance Program, which would offer insurance to anyone who did not receive it through their employer or through Medicare.

The Assisted Health Insurance Program would be operated and partially financed by the states, but benefit and eligibility standards would be uniform across the country. Premiums, deductibles, and copayments would be put in place on a sliding scale linked to income, with the poor paying no premiums at all. Individuals, importantly, could not be denied insurance on the basis of preexisting medical conditions. As in Medicare, private insurers would act as fiscal intermediaries for the program. The benefits included in

CHIP were impressive. Under the plan, both employer-sponsored health insurance and the Assisted Health Insurance Program would cover prescription drugs and place limits on the out-of-pocket costs that beneficiaries would confront. Medicare's benefits would be expanded to match those of employer-sponsored insurance and the assisted health program. There was some debate over including an individual mandate to have health insurance, but Nixon and key administration figures such as Health, Education, and Welfare secretary Casper Weinberger viewed the voluntary nature of insurance as critical for both political and ideological reasons.[7]

Ultimately, aides of Nixon and Mills produced a compromise proposal that came far closer to the Nixon CHIP approach than to the single-payer approach that remained the ideal for Kennedy and the labor movement. By this point, however, the Watergate scandal had rendered Nixon's support for a deal worthless. Whatever prospects for health insurance legislation continued to exist after Nixon was forced to resign were further eroded after a bizarre series of public incidents involving an intoxicated Chairman Mills and an exotic dancer known as "Fanne Foxe, the Argentine Firecracker."[8]

The problems of cost and access continued to grow in scope in the decades that followed. After his election in 1992, President Bill Clinton launched a bid to reshape the American health care system and guarantee access to individual health services. Although the initial reception of Clinton's plan was favorable, the decision to attempt to forge a new system that would alter the experience of middle-class Americans who already had insurance proved a significant political miscalculation. With Democrats in Congress divided, fierce opposition from parts of the insurance industry, and mounting popular concern that it would threaten the existing coverage of millions of Americans, the Clinton plan flamed out during 1994.[9] Nonetheless, incremental change remained possible. In 1997, a Republican Congress passed the State Children's Health Insurance Program, a federal–state cooperative program aimed at expanding access to insurance for low-income children, with federal money for the program coming from higher taxes on cigarettes.[10]

In 2003, President George W. Bush signed the Medicare Modernization Act (MMA). The MMA created a new entitlement to prescription drug coverage in Medicare, to be administered by private companies. It also expanded earlier efforts to get private insurance companies involved in offering Medicare plans by creating Medicare Advantage. The program was designed to overcompensate insurance companies for offering coverage to Medicare beneficiaries with the hope of creating a private competitive market. Clearly a boon for seniors, the MMA also offered significant benefits for the pharmaceutical industry (which gained a massive new market and a federal commitment to not negotiating prices) and the insurance industry.[11] Expanding coverage for low-income children and expanding access to benefits for Medicare beneficiaries, SCHIP (later just CHIP) and the MMA also increased the amount of the federal budget committed to funding individual medical services.

The status quo bias of national policies dealing with individual medical services is strong. Where major changes have occurred, they have been designed to leave the employer-sponsored health insurance market undisturbed or to offer clear benefits to major stakeholders, such as the pharmaceutical and insurance industries. These tendencies have been evident in moments where the proponents of change have failed—and also where they have succeeded, as in the passage of the 2010 Patient Protection and Affordable Care Act (ACA, also known as Obamacare). Enacted during a brief window of unified government in the face of fierce opposition, the ACA was both novel in its commitments and conservative in its methods. Under the ACA, the federal government committed itself not just to helping most Americans acquire health insurance but also to facilitating coverage at affordable rates. In key respects, the ACA followed the insurance reform model adopted at the state level in Massachusetts under Governor Mitt Romney in 2006. The ACA's approach also echoed the earlier Nixon proposals.

The ACA sought to fill in the gaps in the existing health insurance system by requiring large employers to offer health insurance, by expanding Medicaid to cover a broader swath of low-income individuals and families, and by creating state-based exchanges to facilitate the purchase of private health insurance for those left out of the employer-sponsored system. State exchanges allowed individuals to access premium subsidies on a sliding scale that was based on household income. The legislation also permitted adult children to stay on their parents' insurance plans until the age of twenty-six. As a means of pooling risk across age and health status, as well as ensuring that individuals do not wait until they are sick to enroll in health insurance, it required almost all Americans to have health insurance or pay a fine.[12]

Bridging the Gap

Adopting the approach to national health policy advocated by Thomas Parran and the PHS during the 1930s and 1940s would have made the

United States something of an outlier among Western nations. Though better integrating population-based efforts and medical services aimed at individuals has been a goal of many nations faced with the growth of chronic disease, public health and individual medicine are typically only loosely connected through primary care providers. In the United States, bridging the gap between public health and individual medicine has proven difficult. Concerns about chronic disease, the incentives created by fee-for-service medicine, and the growth of health care costs have at times fueled calls for a new approach to health policy.

An early attempt to confront chronic disease, and one that represented a potential avenue toward better integrating public health and individual medicine, was the Regional Medical Program, created by Congress in 1965. Sponsored by Alabama senator Lister Hill and Arkansas representative Oren Harris, the legislation that created the program was prompted by a major report on the threats represented by heart disease, cancer, and stroke. The Regional Medical Program attempted to address chronic disease in new ways, including the dissemination of information through medical schools, libraries, and training programs. It also sought to emphasize primary care and prevention, and in some areas, it included programs such as federally funded mobile diagnostic equipment.[13] Despite some real promise, the Regional Medical Program ultimately did not emerge as a meaningful threat to the nation's bifurcated health policy regime. Instead, the program remained heavily oriented toward curative medicine and focused on diffusing knowledge about treatments rather than altering the aspects of lifestyle that contribute to chronic disease.[14]

Both Richard Nixon and Bill Clinton pointed to prepaid health plans as an alternative to fee-for-service medicine that might transform American health care for the better. Such an approach, they believed, would reverse the incentives to provide additional care created by fee-for-service, potentially leading to a new emphasis on preventive medicine and cost control. The ACA similarly included incentives for the creation of accountable care organizations. Although their structures may vary substantially, accountable care organizations are "legal entities that take responsibility for meeting the medical care needs of their patients and are willing to be held accountable—with financial consequences—for doing so." The hope of the accountable care organization program was that such an arrangement would both improve quality and decrease the overall cost, creating savings for payers and generating increased revenues for providers.[15] The ACA also included other initiatives, such as decreased Medicare payments for hospitals deemed to have excess readmissions, intended to create incentives for higher-quality care.[16]

In describing the benefits of the ACA for Americans and for the nation's fiscal health, President Barack Obama often highlighted the inclusion of free preventive services among the ACA's "essential health benefits." These services would save both lives and money, "because it's a lot cheaper to prevent an illness than to treat one."[17] Preventive services and new initiatives aimed at encouraging medical students to pursue careers in primary care are clearly steps in the right direction. Still, the ACA largely followed long-standing trends in accepting the bifurcation of American health policy into separate regimes encompassing public health and individual medicine.

Although firmly entrenched, even the most basic of public health interventions remain controversial. Skepticism of vaccination, based on the false belief that vaccines cause autism, is widespread. Understood as a means of protecting individuals against threats to their health posed by others or by factors such as contaminated water, the concept of public health enjoys broad acceptance. As public health interventions move away from efforts that unambiguously affect the health of populations toward those that appear more personal in nature, the extent of opposition tends to increase. Bans on cigarette smoking in public areas have, after initial resistance, generally gained public acceptance on the grounds that secondhand smoke is dangerous. Proposed interventions such as bans on particular food products or New York City's attempt to ban the sale of large sugary beverages have provoked persistent skepticism. Such regulations, for many, are indicative of a vision of public health that is far too private. Other initiatives, such as requirements that school lunches be healthier, have caused similar reactions.

Highly publicized episodes such as the appearance of Ebola, the Zika virus, or the persistent threat of an influenza pandemic may gain the attention of lawmakers, the media, and the public, but it is rare for such threats to result in meaningful new investments in public health infrastructure. The day-to-day factors that influence the health of Americans, meanwhile, are often seen as outside the scope of appropriate government action. The political realities of public health policy were highlighted by the pushback against the ACA's most significant gesture toward population-based health efforts, the Prevention and Public Health Fund.[18] Almost immediately, the fund came under withering assault from Republicans in Congress. In the widely publicized formulation of Wyoming senator Mike Enzi, it was a "slush fund for jungle gyms." In 2012, the fund, which originally included

$18.75 billion over twelve years, was cut by $6.25 billion as part of a deficit reduction package. During the 2013 fiscal year, the Obama administration diverted around 45 percent of the fund toward setting up and operating the federal government's ACA health exchange Web site, Healthcare.gov.[19]

Perhaps the most serious and enduring challenge to the boundaries between public health and individual medicine in the United States has been the community health center program, which grew out of President Lyndon Johnson's War on Poverty. The program began on a small scale as part of the 1964 Economic Opportunity Act's Community Action, with one center based in a Boston housing project and another in the Mississippi Delta.[20] Expanded under an amendment to the Economic Opportunity Act in 1966, the community health center program continued to grow throughout the 1970s. In ways that were reminiscent of the earlier ideas of men such as Hermann Biggs and Thomas Parran, the centers attempted to bridge the gap between public health and individual medicine.

In addition to providing individual medical services, community health centers adopted a flexible and pragmatic approach, engaging in experiments aimed at improving the overall health of their clients. From the beginning, they recognized and worked to address the environmental and social factors that fueled poor health outcomes.[21] In place since the 1960s, the program has proven highly resilient. Focused on the residents of medically underserved areas—and long derided as "ghetto medicine"—community health centers are unlikely to emerge as a model for better integrating public health and individual medicine. Nonetheless, they point clearly to the many alternative means of delivering health services that exist.

The echoes of the past are omnipresent in contemporary debates over the appropriate role of the national government in American health. In the development of accountable care organizations, and in the ongoing growth of community health centers, we can see glimpses of paths not taken and of a future that is highly fluid. Faced with a population increasingly prone to diseases associated with lifestyle, environment, and longevity, as well as a health care system that has become increasingly sophisticated in its ability to deliver expensive curative treatments, policy makers would do well to recall Thomas Parran's admonition from 1938: "The ideal traffic plan is not that which provides a first aid station at all intersections and stream-lined ambulances to carry away the victims of traffic accidents. Both doctors and drainage are needed to save the inhabitants of a malarious swamp."[22]

NOTES

INTRODUCTION

1. My account follows that of Espinosa, *Epidemic Invasions*. For the definitive account of the disease's impact in the American South, see Humphreys, *Yellow Fever and the South*.

2. "The Fever Quarantine," *New York Times*, November 2, 1897.

3. "Yellow Fever Epidemic: State Troops Called Out to Protect the Railroad Property at Jackson, Miss.," *New York Times*, September, 19, 1897.

4. "An Incendiary Fever Mob," *New York Times*, September 25, 1897.

5. "Yellow Fever Decreasing: A Negro Lynched Near New Orleans for Evading Quarantine," *New York Times*, October 17, 1897.

6. See Duffy, *Sanitarians*; Novak, *People's Welfare*.

7. On the history of the PHS, see particularly Mullan, *Plagues and Politics*.

8. Hacker, *Divided Welfare State*; Gottschalk, *Shadow Welfare State*; Mettler, *Submerged State*.

9. In a 2015 poll that asked respondents about their views of eight federal agencies, the US Centers for Disease Control and Prevention had the highest favorability rating, beating out both NASA and the Department of Defense. See Pew Research Center, "Most View the CDC Favorably; VA's Image Slips," *Pew Research Center*, January 22, 2015, http://www.people-press.org/2015/01/22/most-view-the-cdc-favorably-vas-image-slips/.

10. Scholars such as Paul Starr, Jacob Hacker, Alan Derickson, Daniel M. Fox, Marie Gottschalk, Beatrix Hoffman, and Jill Quadagno have offered nuanced analyses of the role of political institutions, interest groups such as the American Medical Association and organized labor, and political ideology in shaping America's unique health system. See Starr, *Social Transformation* and *Remedy and Reaction*; Hacker, *Divided Welfare State* and "Historical Logic of National Health Insurance"; Derickson, *Health Security for All*; Fox, *Health Policies, Politics*; Gottschalk, *Shadow Welfare State*; Hoffman, *Health Care for Some* and *Wages of Sickness*; Quadagno, *One Nation, Uninsured*. David Blumenthal and James Morone have highlighted the role of the presidency in making health policy, while major works by Theodore Marmor, Jonathan Oberlander, and Laura Katz Olson have examined the Medicare and Medicaid programs that emerged out of earlier failed plans for national health insurance. See Blumenthal and Morone, *Heart of Power*; Marmor, *Politics of Medicare*; Oberlander, *Political Life of Medicare*; Olson, *Politics of Medicaid*.

11. Because previous work on public health has been grounded in the field of history, questions about political context, the role of institutions, and why particular policy outcomes occurred have been far less prominent than they are in the literature on national insurance policy. Nonetheless, several important works have explored themes that overlap with those discussed in this book. Fitzhugh Mullan, Elizabeth Etheridge, and Michael Stobbe have written excellent studies of the United States PHS, the Centers for Disease Control and Prevention, and the Office of the Surgeon General, while

George Rosen and John Duffy have written high-quality general histories of international and American public health. See Mullan, *Plagues and Politics;* Etheridge, *Sentinel for Health;* Stobbe, *Surgeon General's Warning;* Rosen, *History of Public Health;* Duffy, *Sanitarians.* These works have illuminated key aspects of the history of American public health and have informed my research in fundamental ways.

12. Starr, *Social Transformation;* Derickson, *Health Security for All.* Starr devotes an entire chapter to public health in his classic study of American medicine. Focused on policies dealing with individual medicine, Derickson's groundbreaking work is consistently attentive to the work of public health theorists and officials. Both works have substantially influenced my analysis.

13. Richard Bensel defines APD as "the study of the processes through which political institutions have been reproduced or changed in the United States." APD, Bensel writes, "involves the longitudinal investigation of such institutions, including explanations of their origin, the conditions sustaining their existence (i.e., reproducibility), and the reasons for their demise." Bensel, "Tension," 104–105.

14. Orren and Skowronek, *Search for American Political Development.*

15. In important ways, my approach follows the polity-centered approach of Theda Skocpol and the bureaucracy-focused approach of Daniel Carpenter. See Skocpol, *Protecting Soldiers and Mothers;* Carpenter, *Reputation and Power* and *Forging of Bureaucratic Autonomy.* On the policy-making and coalition-building roles of elites, see Grossmann, *Artists of the Possible.*

16. Bensel, *Sectionalism and American Political Development;* Sanders, *Roots of Reform.*

17. See Katznelson, Geiger, and Kryder, "Limiting Liberalism"; Lieberman, "Race, Institutions" and *Shifting the Color Line;* Quadagno, *Color of Welfare.*

18. For the classic analysis of the role of Southern Democrats in national government in guaranteeing white supremacy and local autonomy, see Key, *Southern Politics.* See also Katznelson, Geiger, and Kryder, "Limiting Liberalism."

19. On the role of Southern Democrats in making the New Deal, see particularly Katznelson, *Fear Itself.*

20. While potentially misleading, the antistatist reputation of early twentieth-century Southern elites is well known. C. Vann Woodward traced the origins of the white South's late nineteenth-century aversion to government action to the reaction against federal intervention during Reconstruction. Intense dissatisfaction with Republican policies after the Civil War "became reaction against governmental interference of any kind." "The distrust and suspicion of legislative action and political power that accompanies any laissez-faire philosophy," Woodward argued, "was more deep-seated in the South than elsewhere. Laissez faire became almost a test of Southern patriotism." Woodward, *Origins of the New South,* 65.

21. For important discussions of the role of nonstate actors in providing social services, see particularly Dillon, "Middlemen in the Chinese Welfare State"; Cammett, "Partisan Activism"; Thachil, *Elite Parties.*

22. As Carol Nackenoff and Julie Novkov have argued, fully understanding state formation often requires looking outside of the state. Political activities and activists are "not just conditioned by institutions, structures, and previous social policies," they

also forge alliances that are "instrumental in the creation of new public powers and administrative capacities." See Nackenoff and Novkov, "Statebuilding in the Progressive Era," 4. On social movements and American political development, see Francis, *Civil Rights*, 14.

23. On this category of argument, see Troesken, *Water, Race, and Disease*. In the case of typhoid, as Troesken shows, effectively combating typhoid required that cities not discriminate on the basis of race in providing access to sewers and clean drinking water. Indeed, Troesken finds that "blacks benefited more than whites, in terms of disease reduction, from investments in water and sewer lines and water purification systems" during this period. See *Water, Race, and Disease*, 204. Evan Lieberman, meanwhile, finds in an important comparative study that government responses to the AIDS pandemic have been heavily influenced by the extent and character of ethnic divisions within societies. In nations with strong "internal boundaries dividing societies into substantial and recognizable *ethnic* groups," discussions of the disease and the risk of infection from it "are infused with ideas about ethnic difference." As groups within a society attempt to assign blame and "avoid the group shame associated with a stigmatized problem, the effect is a dampening of potential support for AIDS policies, leading to weaker and slower responses." See Lieberman, *Boundaries of Contagion*, 3. See also Doyle, *New Cities, New Men*, 280–281. Doyle argues that the "democracy of disease" (280–281) in urban areas caused white reformers to favor public health measures for black Southerners.

24. Pierson, *Politics in Time*, 21.

25. The great exception to this is Derickson, *Health Security for All*.

26. See Parran, "Public Responsibility."

27. Terris, "Hermann Biggs' Contribution," 389–390.

28. See Hacker, *Divided Welfare State*.

29. For the definitive account of organized labor's role in the development of health insurance in the United States, see Gottschalk, *Shadow Welfare State*.

CHAPTER ONE. HEALTH AT HOME, HEALTH ABROAD

1. Quoted in Gostin, *Public Health Law*, 94. On the role of federalism in shaping American political development, see particularly Robertson, *Federalism*.

2. A number of scholars have detailed the ways in which war, trade, and international relations have impacted the development of domestic policy in the United States and in other nations. See, e.g., Katznelson and Shefter, *Shaped by War and Trade*; Saldin, *War, the American State, and Politics*; Bensel, *Yankee Leviathan*.

3. Ettling's *Germ of Laziness* is the classic account of the fight against hookworm in the United States. Important discussions may also be found in Link, *Paradox of Southern Progressivism*; Elman, McGuire, and Wittman, "Extending Public Health."

4. Rosenberg, "Social Class and Medical Care," 35.

5. Ibid., 40–41.

6. Rosen, *History of Public Health*; Duffy, *Sanitarians*, 193–194. On the reception of the germ theory in the United States, see Tomes, "American Attitudes."

7. Schmeckebier, *Public Health Service*, 8–9.

8. Harrison, *Contagion*, 119; Humphreys, *Yellow Fever and the South*.

9. Warner, "Local Control," 413.

10. See ibid.

11. Schmeckebier, *Public Health Service,* 11.

12. Ibid., 15.

13. Ibid., 16.

14. Ibid., 20.

15. Ibid., 23.

16. Ibid., 19; *Annual Report of the Surgeon General of the Public Health Service of the United States (1915),* 127; "Government Plans Control: Will Take Over Quarantine Station, Says Report," *New York Times,* February 15, 1921.

17. Baumgartner and Jones, *Agendas and Instability.*

18. For an important analysis of the impact that strains on state and local resources may have on the development of American federalism, see Callen, *Railroad and American Political Development.*

19. Lodge, *War with Spain,* iv.

20. Espinosa, *Epidemic Invasions,* 32–33.

21. Ibid., 33.

22. LePrince and Orenstein, *Mosquito Control in Panama,* 237–238.

23. Ibid., 243.

24. Ibid., 5. See also "The Bite of a Tiny Mosquito in East Texas Was the Beginning of a Great Health Crusade," *East Texas,* February 1931, 10, 22–23, clipping in Colonel Joseph A. LePrince, US Public Health Officer, Collection, Memphis Public Library and Information Center, Box I, Life and Work of LePrince, Folder 1—Biographical Information: Newspaper Articles.

25. LePrince and Orenstein, *Mosquito Control in Panama,* 4.

26. Trask, "Malaria."

27. Ashford and Gutierez Igaravidez, *Uncinariasis (Hookworm Disease),* 24.

28. Ibid., 25.

29. Ibid.

30. Ibid., 28.

31. Ibid., 35.

32. Ettling, *Germ of Laziness,* 27–28; Stiles, "Early History," 289.

33. Whether Ashford or Stiles deserved credit for the discovery of hookworm in the new world remained an ongoing point of contention. See "Hookworm Discoverer: Army Officials Declare Maj. B. K. Ashford Found It First," *Washington Post,* October 31, 1909.

34. Sullivan, *Our Times,* 311; Dock and Bass, *Hookworm Disease,* 29.

35. Ettling, *Germ of Laziness,* 32; Stiles, *Significance of the Recent American Cases,* 211; Bjorkman, "Cure for Two Million Sick," 11609; Sullivan, *Our Times,* 311.

36. The new species was also known by another name given to it by Stiles, *Uncinaria americanus.*

37. For an excellent account and analysis of the plague outbreak in the Bay area, see Risse, *Plague, Fear, and Politics.*

38. Furman, *Profile,* 229–231.

39. Stobbe, *Surgeon General's Warning,* 39.

40. Ibid., 42; "Campaign against Plague-Infected Squirrels in California."

41. Parascandola, "Public Health Service," 110.

42. Schmeckebier, *Public Health Service*, 26.

43. Parascandola, "Public Health Service," 110.

44. Stiles, "Early History," 296.

45. Stiles, *Report upon the Prevalence*, 97.

46. Stiles, "Hook-worm Disease in the South."

47. Burke, *Reminiscences of Georgia*, 205–206.

48. Claytor, "Treatment of Uncinariasis," 308.

49. Stiles, "Significance of the Recently Recognized Hookworm Disease," 443.

50. Stiles, "Early History," 296; Sullivan, *Our Times*, 316.

51. The newspaper was the *Denver Republican*. See "Hunting Down the Lazy Germ: Scientists Trying to Remove All Excuses for That Tired Feeling," *Washington Post*, October 25, 1903. See also "Fight with Lazy Bug: Ridding the South of the Hookworm Scourge," *Washington Post*, July 20, 1903. On the press's reaction to Stiles's findings, see Ettling, *Germ of Laziness*, 35–38.

52. For a discussion of the relationship between hookworm disease and ideas about "poor whites," see Wray, *Not Quite White*.

53. "Crusade to Transform the South's 'Poor Whites' into Industrious Citizens," *Washington Post*, September 27, 1908.

54. Carter, "Vampire of the South," 618.

55. Stiles, "Industrial Conditions," 595, 98; "Crusade to Transform the South's 'Poor Whites' into Industrious Citizens," *Washington Post*, September 27, 1908; Wray, *Not Quite White*, 124; Ettling, *Germ of Laziness*, 173.

56. Stiles, "Medical Influence of the Negro," 24.

57. "Crusade to Transform the South's 'Poor Whites' into Industrious Citizens," *Washington Post*, September 27, 1908. See also Stiles, "Hookworm Disease," 1085–1086. See also Carter, "Vampire of the South," 629–631.

58. "Hookworm Evil Real: Dr. Stiles Tells Scientists of Its Spread in the South," *Washington Post*, December 29, 1909.

59. Stiles, "Medical Influence of the Negro," 28. See also Carter, "Vampire of the South," in which Carter, relying on Stiles's work, advised the readers of *McClure's* that "the one real hope of curing the white man lies in curing the black man" (631).

60. Stiles, "Medical Influence of the Negro," 28. A similar argument was being made during this period about typhoid. See Troesken, *Water, Race, and Disease*.

61. *Annual Report of the Surgeon General of the Public Health and Marine Hospital Service of the United States (1908)*, 54.

62. "Rockefeller Gift to Kill 'Hookworm,'" *New York Times*, October 29, 1909

63. Starr, *Social Transformation*, 150, 52–53.

64. Duffy, *Sanitarians*, 207.

65. See Fox, "Abraham Flexner's Unpublished Report."

66. Sealander, *Private Wealth and Public Life*, 47; Carpenter, *Forging of Bureaucratic Autonomy*, 231; Sanders, *Roots of Reform*, 322; *General Education Board*, 25; United States Department of Agriculture, *Status and Results*, 5.

67. United States Department of Agriculture, *Status and Results*, 6.

68. Sealander, *Private Wealth and Public Life*, 48; Sanders, *Roots of Reform*, 323–324.

69. See Sealander, *Private Wealth and Public Life*, 53.

70. Stiles, "Early History," 303.

71. "Insulted by Hookworm Gift," *Washington Post*, November 2, 1909.

72. Ettling, *Germ of Laziness*, 132–133.

73. The eleven states were those of the former Confederacy, with the exception of Florida, and the border state of Kentucky.

74. An excellent and detailed description of one hookworm campaign may be found in Washburn, *Hookworm Campaign*.

75. See Rockefeller Sanitary Commission for the Eradication of Hookworm Disease, *Fifth Annual Report* (1915), 13.

76. Lumsden, Roberts, and Stiles, "Preliminary Note."

77. State Board of Health of South Carolina, *Thirty-Third Annual Report*, 24.

78. Contemporary studies of the "American" hookworm (*Necator americanus*) have suggested that the disease's prevalence tends to be higher among teenagers and adults than among young children. As a result, it is possible to use the RSC's surveys of children aged six to eighteen as a proxy for the entire population of a county. See Crompton, "Public Health Importance of Hookworm Disease," S41. Surveys were compiled from Rockefeller Sanitary Commission for the Eradication of Hookworm Disease, second through fifth annual reports (1911–1915). The missing infection rates for counties that were not surveyed have been derived from neighboring counties with similar characteristics through the use of State Economic Area groups, following the SEA descriptions in Ruggles et al., *Integrated Public Use Microdata Series*. County population data was accessed through the Minnesota Population Center, *National Historical Geographic Information System: Version 2.0*, http://www.nhgis.org.

79. See Ferrell and Mead, *History of County Health Organizations*.

CHAPTER TWO. PUBLIC HEALTH AND HEALTH INSURANCE

1. See Owen, "Conservation of Life and Health."

2. Committee on Public Health and National Quarantine, United States Senate, *Proposed Department of Public Health*, 6.

3. See Schmeckebier, *Public Health Service*, 35.

4. Ibid., 32.

5. Committee on Public Health and National Quarantine, United States Senate, *Proposed Department of Public Health*, 6.

6. "Scientists Favor US Health Bureau: Many Organizations Join in Indorsing the Bill Introduced by Senator Owen," *New York Times*, April 18, 1910.

7. See Waserman, "Quest for a National Health Department."

8. Ibid., 366.

9. Ibid., 358.

10. Taft, "Sanitation and Health of the South," 334–335.

11. For the classic account of American-led public health intervention in the Philippines, see Anderson, *Colonial Pathologies*.

12. Taft, "Sanitation and Health of the South," 334–335.

13. "Might Prolong Life: Senator Owen Urges Federal Health Department Bill," *Washington Post*, March 25, 1910.

14. Ibid.

15. *National Public Health*, 107.

16. Committee on Public Health and National Quarantine, United States Senate, *Proposed Department of Public Health*, 108–109.

17. In a statement typical of those made by industry representatives, Hiram Messenger of the Traveler's Insurance Company explained that "while we have certain laws for registration of births and deaths and the causes of deaths in all the States, there is a great lack of uniformity, and there is a great lack of proper enforcement of those laws." Here, he contended, "is right where the United States Government ought to come in." Committee on Public Health and National Quarantine, United States Senate, *Proposed Department of Public Health*, 31.

18. Ibid., 17.

19. Hamilton, "Cost of Caring."

20. Fisher, *Memorial*, 68.

21. Waserman, "Quest for a National Health Department," 372–373.

22. Fisher, *Memorial*, 66–67.

23. "Defines Opposition to Owen Bill," *New York Times*, June 18, 1910.

24. Waserman, "Quest for a National Health Department," 375.

25. On Wyman's proposals for expanding the Public Health and Marine Hospital Service, see *Annual Report of the Surgeon General of the Public Health and Marine Hospital Service of the United States (1911)*, 283.

26. Quoted in Furman, *Profile*, 281.

27. Ibid., 286.

28. Tobey, *National Government*, 102; *Annual Report of the Surgeon General of the Public Health Service of the United States (1912)*, 9.

29. See "Campaign against Plague-Infected Squirrels in California."

30. Furman, *Profile*, 288; *Annual Report of the Surgeon General of the Public Health Service of the United States (1912)*, 317, 30.

31. Schmeckebier, *Public Health Service*, 40.

32. See Ezdorf, "Demonstrations of Malaria Control."

33. *Annual Report of the Surgeon General of the Public Health Service of the United States (1917)*, 20; Rockefeller Foundation International Health Board, *Third Annual Report*, 20.

34. *Annual Report of the Surgeon General of the Public Health Service of the United States (1912)*, 36.

35. Etheridge, *Butterfly Caste*, 4; Searcy, "Epidemic of Acute Pellagra," 37.

36. Roe, *Plague of Corn*, 30; *Transactions of the Seventh Annual Conference*, 67; Etheridge, *Butterfly Caste*, 4.

37. Hegyi, Schwartz, and Hegyi, "Pellagra," 2.

38. Ibid., 3.

39. *Transactions of National Conference on Pellagra*, 13; Lavinder, "Theory of the Parasitic Origin."

40. Goldberger, "Cause and Prevention of Pellagra," 25; Lavinder, "Pellagra." See also in the *New York Times* the following: "More Causes of Pellagra," October 9, 1909; "The Cause of Pellagra," June 19, 1910, "Put Pellagra Cases in South at 50,000: First Study of Commission in One County Shows that Disease Is Not Decreasing," December 3, 1912.

41. Goldberger, "Etiology of Pellagra," 21.

42. Goldberger, Waring, and Willets, "Prevention of Pellagra," 33.

43. Ibid., 37.

44. For a discussion of this issue, see Marks, "Epidemiologists Explain Pellagra."

45. Goldberger and Wheeler, "Experimental Production of Pellagra," 67.

46. Ibid., 67–68.

47. "The 'meat,'" writes Robert Higgs of the "Three Ms" diet, "hardly deserved its name, consisting almost entirely of fat." Higgs, *Competition and Coercion*, 105. See Goldberger, "Cause and Prevention of Pellagra," 25.

48. Goldberger and Wheeler, "Experimental Production of Pellagra," 73.

49. Ibid., 75.

50. See Goldberger, Wheeler, and Sydenstricker, "Study of the Relation of Family Income," 64. See also Vance, *Human Geography*, 438.

51. Rodgers, *Atlantic Crossings*, 223–224.

52. Starr, *Social Transformation*, 239.

53. Roosevelt, "Confession of Faith," 134–135.

54. "Declaration of the Principles of the Progressive Party," 317.

55. Derickson, *Health Security for All*, 8–9.

56. See especially Fishback and Kantor, *Prelude to the Welfare State*.

57. Starr, *Social Transformation*, 236. See also Hoffman, *Wages of Sickness*, 27.

58. Rubinow, "Standards of Sickness Insurance," 251.

59. John B. Andrews, "Progress toward Health Insurance," 2, in *No. 123 Reprints of Reports and Addresses of the National Conference of Social Work, 1917 Meeting at Pittsburgh* (1917), Research Files, Social Security, Box 209, Edwin Witte Papers, Manuscript Library, Wisconsin Historical Society, Madison (hereafter Witte Papers).

60. Ibid.

61. Thomasson, "From Sickness to Health," 235–236.

62. Ibid., 235.

63. Hoffman, *Wages of Sickness*, 28; Lubove, *Struggle for Social Security*, 64–65, 71–72.

64. I. S. Falk, interview by Peter A. Corning, 1968, Columbia Center for Oral History Archives, Butler Library, Columbia University, New York, NY; King, "Edgar Sydenstricker." Sydenstricker's sister, Pearl Buck, would later win the Nobel Prize for literature.

65. Warren and Sydenstricker, *Health Insurance*, 53.

66. Ibid., 58.

67. Ibid., 68.

68. Ibid.

69. Rubinow, "Review: *Health Insurance* by B. S. Warren and Edgar Sydenstricker," 936, 937; Frankel, "Some Fundamental Considerations," 598.

70. Warren and Sydenstricker, "Health Insurance," 777.

71. Ibid., 783.

72. Ibid.

73. Blue, "Some of the Larger Problems," 1901.

74. Lubove, *Struggle for Social Security;* Fishback and Kantor, *Prelude to the Welfare State.*

75. Lubove, *Struggle for Social Security,* 85.

76. Quoted in ibid., 85.

77. Hamovitch, "History," 284.

78. "Health Insurance Endorsed by Workers," reprint of letter to San Francisco *Bulletin,* March 2, 1918, from Daniel C. Murphy, president of the California Federation of Labor; New York State Federation of Labor, "Health Insurance: Official Endorsement of the New York State Federation of Labor, with Report of Its Committee on Health" (1918). Both are in Research Files, Social Security, Box 209, Witte Papers.

79. Hoffman, *Wages of Sickness,* 69.

80. Andrews, "Progress toward Health Insurance," 6, in Research Files, Social Security, Box 209, Witte Papers.

81. Hoffman, *Wages of Sickness,* 84.

82. Quoted in Lubove, *Struggle for Social Security,* 77.

83. Quoted in, and follows, ibid.

84. Hoffman, *Wages of Sickness,* 79.

85. Ibid., 84.

86. Ibid., 69.

87. Numbers, *Almost Persuaded,* 105.

88. Cooper, *Woodrow Wilson,* 374.

89. On the symbolic use of antistatism by elites or interest groups to further particular interests, see Quadagno and Street, "Ideology and Public Policy."

90. Lubove, *Struggle for Social Security,* 83. Hoffman, *Wages of Sickness,* 56. The insurance industry and Christian Scientists, it was charged, were quietly leading the opposition to insurance. See, e.g., "Health Insurance Endorsed by Workers," reprint of letter to the San Francisco *Bulletin,* March 2, 1918, from Daniel C. Murphy, President of the California Federation of Labor, in Research Files, Social Security, Box 209, Witte Papers.

91. Lubove, *Struggle for Social Security,* 84–89.

CHAPTER THREE. WAR AND ITS AFTERMATH

1. Warren and Bolduan, "War Activities," 1253–1254.

2. Tindall, *Emergence of the New South,* 54.

3. Warren and Bolduan, "War Activities," 1247–1248. The South is defined here as the eleven former states of the Confederacy plus Kentucky and Oklahoma. The extracantonment zone around Washington, DC, included parts of Virginia and is counted as Southern.

4. For a summary of PHS work in all extracantonment zones, see *Annual Report of the Surgeon General of the Public Health Service of the United States (1918),* 103–160, and *(1919),* 86–106. See also Blue, "Conserving the Nation's Man Power." Watkins, "Extra-cantonment Zone Sanitation," 2153.

5. See, e.g., "Report of Inspection of Extra Cantonment Sanitary Activities, Camp Shelby, Hattiesburg, Miss., December 5, 1917," Box 416, Records of the Public Health Service, Central File, 1897–1923, National Archives, College Park, MD (hereafter National Archives).

6. On the significance of Yakima from Lumsden's perspective, see Ferrell and Mead, *History of County Health Organizations*, 2–4.

7. Counties were surveyed in Alabama (2), Georgia (1), Illinois (1), Indiana (1), Iowa (1), Kansas (1), Maryland (2), Mississippi (1), Missouri (1), North Carolina (1), South Carolina (1), Tennessee (1), and West Virginia (1). See Lumsden, *Rural Sanitation*.

8. See [*Sundry Civil Bill for 1919*], 248. Thomas Parran Jr., "Reminiscences of Thomas Parran," interviews conducted by Harlan Phillips, July 16 and 18, 1962, Columbia Center for Oral History Archives, Butler Library, Columbia University, New York, NY.

9. Parran, "Reminiscences." See also, e.g., Grubbs, *By Order of the Surgeon General*, 287.

10. Parran, "Reminiscences."

11. See *Annual Report of the Surgeon General of the Public Health Service of the United States (1918)*, 103–160, and *(1919)*, 86–106. Watkins, "Extra-cantonment Zone Sanitation," 2155.

12. *Annual Report of the Surgeon General of the Public Health Service of the United States (1919)*, 103.

13. Schmeckebier, *Public Health Service*, 48.

14. Trask, "Malaria," 3447.

15. Ibid., 3445–3446.

16. Biographical information is from Griffitts, "Henry Rose Carter." Griffitts, who knew Carter, reports that Carter (born in 1852) was shot in the leg during the Civil War after grabbing a gun and becoming briefly involved in an engagement with Union troops.

17. The "right hand" quotation is from the introduction, by the Department of Agriculture's L. O. Howard, of LePrince's book. See LePrince and Orenstein, *Mosquito Control in Panama*. On LePrince's wide-ranging career, which spanned antimalaria work from the aftermath of the Spanish-American War through the Tennessee Valley Authority, see "LePrince, Malaria Fighter."

18. LePrince, "Mosquito Control about Cantonments and Shipyards," 552.

19. Ibid., 553.

20. LePrince, "Aftermath of Malaria Control," 414–415.

21. Warren and Bolduan, "War Activities," 1248–1249. A description of the PHS's wartime antimalaria work may be found in LePrince, "Mosquito Control about Cantonments and Shipyards."

22. Warren and Bolduan, "War Activities," 1251.

23. Crosby, *America's Forgotten Pandemic*, 56. Crosby's is the definitive account of the Spanish flu epidemic.

24. For a detailed account of the PHS response to the flu, see *Annual Report of the Surgeon General of the Public Health Service of the United States (1919)*.

25. Hatchett, Mecher, and Lipsitch, "Public Health Interventions," 7582.

26. Schmeckebier, *Public Health Service*, 50–51; Pierce, "Public Health Service Program," 1057.

27. On the PHS's postwar plans, see Warren, "Coordination and Expansion" and "Unified Health Service."

28. Warren, "Coordination and Expansion," 2773.

29. Ibid.

30. Ibid.

31. Warren, "Unified Health Service," 380–381.

32. Ibid., 381.

33. Ibid.

34. Ibid., 379.

35. Fox, "Abraham Flexner's Unpublished Report."

36. Warren, "Unified Health Service," 383.

37. "Malaria: A Serious Health Problem of Nation-wide Concern," 545.

38. *Rural Sanitation* [Hearings], 8.

39. Oscar Dowling, president of Louisiana State Board of Health, to Surgeon General Rupert Blue, January 21, 1919. See also, e.g., W. H. Kellog, Secretary of the California State Board of Health, to Rupert Blue, January 24, 1919; S. J. Crumbine, Secretary of the Kansas State Board of Health, to Rupert Blue, January 24, 1919. All in Records of the Public Health Service (RG 90), Central File, 1897–1923, January 1918–January 1919, Box 219, National Archives.

40. "Program for each state health officer for assisting in the enactment of bill providing for rural health work," Included with form letter to state health officials from W. S. Rankin, January 21, 1919, Box 219, Records of the Public Health Service (RG 90), Central File, 1897–1923, 2240 (January 1918–January 1919), National Archives.

41. Sanders, *Roots of Reform*, 392. Lever's attitude toward federal power and money is neatly summarized in a statement quoted by Sanders: "When there is a great general good to be accomplished by legislation, I am not so squeamish about the Constitution."

42. "Statement" included with form letter to state health officials from W. S. Rankin, January 21, 1919, Box 219, Records of the Public Health Service (RG 90), Central File, 1897–1923, 2240 (January 1918–January 1919), National Archives.

43. *Rural Sanitation* [Hearings], 31.

44. Ibid.

45. See, e.g., M. V. Ziegler, Medical Officer in Charge, to the Surgeon General, April 16, 1919, Box 219, Records of the Public Health Service (RG 90), Central File, 1897–1923, January 1918–January 1919, National Archives; L. L. Lumsden to Surgeon General, April 19, 1919, Box 219, Records of the Public Health Service (RG 90), Central File, 1897–1923, January 1918–January 1919, National Archives.

46. *Transactions of the Seventeenth Annual Conference*, 16, 23. "The other way to get immediate action on a reasonably adequate scale," Lumsden told the assembled health officers, "is to get enacted or appropriated the item for rural sanitation contained in the sundry civil bill" (16).

47. Ibid., 16.

48. Ettling, *Germ of Laziness*, 136. After heading one of the nation's leading state departments of health in Ohio, Freeman went on to become a professor of public health at Johns Hopkins. In 1935, he offered congressional testimony in favor of the inclusion of federal grants-in-aid to states for public health work in the Social Security Act.

49. *Transactions of the Seventeenth Annual Conference*, 18–19.

50. "Resignation of Herbert Quick from Federal Farm Loan Board—Representative Lever Named as Successor," collected in *Commercial and Financial Chronicle*, July 19, 1919, 109:224; *Official Congressional Directory*, iii. Lever was appointed to the position on July 17 and officially resigned from Congress on August 1.

51. See Warren, "Coordination and Expansion."

52. See [*Appropriations for Sundry Civil Expenses*], 25–26.

53. *Annual Report of the Surgeon General of the Public Health Service of the United States (1919)*, 52; Lumsden, "Cooperative Rural Health Work" (1920), 2334.

54. Lumsden, "Cooperative Rural Health Work" (1920), 2334.

55. Lumsden, "Rural Hygiene," 2524.

56. Warren, "Coordination and Expansion," 2768.

57. See Lumsden, "Cooperative Rural Health Work" (1920).

CHAPTER FOUR. "SOME VERY DANGEROUS PRECEDENTS"

1. Stobbe, *Surgeon General's Warning*, 52–53.

2. Warren, "Coordination and Expansion," 2762.

3. As Surgeon General Hugh Cumming would later recall, "I had to organize as best we could out of nothing . . . the hospitalization of the ex-service men after the World War. President Harding saw fit to make them separate, much to my relief, I might say, and set up a different organization." See *Economic Security Act* [Committee on Ways and Means], 329.

4. Stobbe, *Surgeon General's Warning*, 57.

5. See "Orders Relief for Pellagra Victims: Harding Asks Public Health Service for Full Report on Cotton Belt Conditions," *New York Times*, July 26, 1921. Harding was alerted to the increase in pellagra by reading a *New York Times* article. See also "Asks Famine Inquiry: Harding Calls for Health Service and Red Cross to Aid South," *Washington Post*, July 26, 1921.

6. "South Resents Federal Alarm over Pellagra: Cotton Belt Authorities Declare There Is No Occasion for Government Aid," *New York Times*, July 27, 1921. See also "Surprise in Washington: No Reason Seen to Withdraw Statements on the Situation," *New York Times*, July 27, 1921; "Pellagra Reports Rouse Ire of South: State Officials Deny that Disease Will Spread to 100,000 in Cotton Belt," *Washington Post*, July 27, 1921.

7. "South Resents Federal Alarm over Pellagra: Cotton Belt Authorities Declare There Is No Occasion for Government Aid," *New York Times*, July 27, 1921; Vance, *Human Geography*, 438–439.

8. "Wants Refutation of Pellagra Scare: Byrnes Asks Harding to Go On with Investigation and to Punish Federal Officials," *New York Times*, July 31, 1921.

9. On the politics of Sheppard–Towner, see particularly Skocpol, *Protecting Soldiers and Mothers*; Moehling and Thomasson, "Political Economy of Saving Mothers and Babies."

10. Smillie, *Public Health*, 468. Quoted in Furman, *Profile*, 279. Smillie's description of Wyman's response came from Milton Rosenau, who played an important early role in the service's Hygienic Laboratory.

11. From 1912 until the creation of the Department of Labor in 1913, the bureau was a part of the Department of Commerce. See Tobey, *National Government*, 233.

12. Furman, *Profile*, 350; Skocpol, *Protecting Soldiers and Mothers*, 517.

13. See Fox, *Health Policies, Politics*, 38.

14. Schmeckebier, *Public Health Service*, 85.

15. Mullan, *Plagues and Politics*, 85.

16. Tobey, *National Government*, 136.

17. See *Annual Report of the Surgeon General of the Public Health Service of the United States (1920)*, 20; Rockefeller Foundation International Health Board, *Seventh Annual Report*, 15–16; LePrince, "Co-operative Antimalaria Campaigns."

18. Lumsden, "Cooperative Rural Health Work" (1920), 2334.

19. On Lumsden's thoughts during this period, see his "Rural Hygiene."

20. Parran, "Cooperative County Health Work," 983–984.

21. *Transactions of the Seventeenth Annual Conference*, 26–27.

22. Lumsden, "Cooperative Rural Health Work" (1920), 2335, and "Cooperative Rural Health Work" (1921), 2481.

23. In most counties, the health officer was a physician. In some counties, however, the health officer was not a physician but rather a trained sanitarian.

24. Lumsden, "Cooperative Rural Health Work" (1920), 2335.

25. W. K. Sharp (Office of Field Investigations, Rural Sanitation) to Surgeon General, July 10, 1919, Records of the Public Health Service, Central File, 1897–1923m 2240 (February–May 1919), Box 220. Lumsden describes the use of franking by "field agents" in a 1926 memo to the surgeon general written after the objection of an Alabama postmaster to field agent J. A. Hill's furnishing of "penalty envelopes or labels to private physicians for the purpose of enabling the latter to transmit in the mails free of postage" bacteriological specimens. See J. H. Hill to L. L. Lumsden, June 21, 1926, L. L. Lumsden to Surgeon General via W. F. Draper, June 26, 1926, Records of the Public Health Service, General Subject File, 1924–1935, State Boards of Health, Alabama 0620-2323, Box 377, NC-34, E-10, NWCH, HM 1999, National Archives.

26. Lumsden, "Cooperative Rural Health Work" (1920).

27. See Lumsden, "Cooperative Rural Health Work" (1930), 2618.

28. Lumsden, "Cooperative Rural Health Work" (1927). The Cape Cod project, wrote Lumsden, "is of especial interest in that it furnishes a test of the applicability of the general plan of cooperative rural health work to the conditions of local government by town units obtaining in Massachusetts and other New England States." See Lumsden, "Cooperative Rural Health Work" (1922), 2362.

29. On the International Health Board, see Farley, *To Cast Out Disease*.

30. Ferrell and Mead, *History of County Health Organizations*.

31. Lumsden, "Cooperative Rural Health Work" (1930), 2619–2620.

32. See Starr, *Social Transformation*, 182–183; Sardell, *US Experiment in Social Medicine*, 25–26.

33. On the activities of the program, see, e.g., Lumsden, "Cooperative Rural Health Work" for 1920 and 1930.

34. Lumsden, "Public Health and Private Practice," 38.

35. Ibid., 42–43.

36. Winslow, "Untilled Fields," 6.

37. Ibid., 10.

38. Starr, *Social Transformation*, 180.

39. Terris, "Hermann Biggs' Contribution," 388.

40. Ibid., 390; Starr, *Social Transformation*, 195.

41. Terris, "Hermann Biggs' Contribution," 389–390.

42. Ibid., 395, 96; "To Extend Health Work," *New York Times*, March 26, 1920; Green, "Social Responsibilities"; MacKenzie, "Legislative Campaign," 146.

43. In an article detailing the need for the Biggs plan, his director of laboratories and research criticized insurance as at best an ineffective and often-abused safeguard against financial loss. See Terris, "Hermann Biggs' Contribution," 396; Wadsworth, "Development of the State Department of Health," 55.

44. Lumsden, "Public Health and Private Practice," 43.

45. Furman, *Profile*, 370; Mullan, *Plagues and Politics*, 95, 99.

46. Barry, *Rising Tide*, 285.

47. One function of these camps was to ensure that local black laborers would not leave for work elsewhere. Writes James Cobb: "The national guardsmen charged with camp security appeared to have the dual mission of keeping refugees in and others—particularly labor agents—out." Cobb, *Most Southern Place on Earth*, 123. See also, e.g., Dulles, *American Red Cross*, 272.

48. Townsend, "Full-Time County Health Program," 1200–1201.

49. J. A. LePrince, "Suggested Plan for Sanitary Control at Flood Area Plantations and Farm Tenant Homes," Records of the Public Health Service, General Subject File, 1924–1935, Closed Stations: Virginia, Richmond Malaria Investigation—Richmond Relief Station, Box 354, NC-34, E-10, NWCH, HM 1999, National Archives.

50. LePrince's recommendation was based on a recent study of how to effectively screen tenant shacks by the service's C. P. Coogle. See *Annual Report of the Surgeon General of the Public Health Service of the United States (1927)*, 39. See also Coogle, "Methods and Costs of Screening," L. L. Williams, Medical Officer in Charge, Office of Malaria Investigations, to Dr. Felix J. Underwood, Mississippi State Health Officer, May 27, 1929, Records of the Public Health Service, General Subject File, 1924–1935, State Boards of Health, Mississippi, Box 416, National Archives.

51. Townsend, "Full-Time County Health Program," 1200–1201.

52. Ibid. See also Deklein, "Recent Health Observations," 148.

53. DeKruif, *Fight for Life*, 11.

54. DeKruif, *Hunger Fighters*, 365–366. Goldberger's initial experiments with brewer's yeast were conducted on dogs. Inspired by an article by two Yale professors and an encounter with a foxhound owner in Georgia who had lost a dog after feeding it nothing but cornbread in order to "thin her down for the hunt," Goldberger established that "black tongue" was the canine version of pellagra. Experimenting with dogs allowed Goldberger quite a bit more leeway than experimenting with humans. Notably, in his first canine experiment, Goldberger fed dogs the diet that he had given the prisoners at Rankin Prison Farm. As Paul DeKruif wrote in 1928 in *Hunger Fighters*, "It killed them" (364).

55. Townsend, "Full-Time County Health Program," 1206; Deklein, "Recent Health Observations," 150.

56. Goldberger and Sydenstricker, "Pellagra in the Mississippi Flood Area."

57. Ibid., 276–277.

58. DeKruif, *Fight for Life*, 16–17.

59. Goldberger and Sydenstricker, "Pellagra in the Mississippi Flood Area," 290.

60. Ibid., 279.

61. "Goldberger, who, because of the desperate tricks he turned with the lives of other men and with his own," DeKruif wrote, "you might take for a Messiah, had no Messianic delusions." DeKruif, *Hunger Fighters*, 362.

62. DeKruif, *Fight for Life*, 16–17.

63. Furman, *Profile*, 364.

64. Lumsden, "Cooperative Rural Health Work" (1927), 2594–2595.

65. Townsend, "Full-Time County Health Program," 1202.

66. Ibid.

67. Ibid., 1202–1203. See also Rockefeller Foundation, *Annual Report for 1927*, 145; O'Neill, "Relief Measures," 159.

68. Townsend, "Full-Time County Health Program," 1203.

69. *First Deficiency Appropriation Bill, 1928*, 631; *Flood Control*, 3074; Ferrell and Mead, *History of County Health Organizations*, 5.

70. Lumsden, "Cooperative Rural Health Work" (1928), 3154.

71. Townsend, "Full-Time County Health Program," 1207.

72. *Second Deficiency Appropriation Bill, 1928*, 466.

73. Ibid., 469.

74. Ibid., 469.

75. Eisenhower, *United States Department of Agriculture*, 1.

76. Furman, *Profile*, 369–70.

77. Leslie Lumsden to Hugh Cumming, August 10, 1931, Box 325, Records of the Public Health Service (RG 90), General Subject File, 1924–1935, Closed Stations: Louisiana, National Archives.

78. Furman, *Profile*, 370. See C. E. Waller to L. L. Lumsden, March 9, 1932, Records of the Public Health Service, General Subject File, 1924–1935, State Boards of Health, Box 440, National Archives.

79. *Emergency Appropriation for Cooperation with State Health Departments in Rural Sanitation, etc.*; "Statement of Dr. A. T. McCormack," 2. The apparent contrast between Hoover's role during 1927 as secretary of commerce and his administration's restrained approach to the 1930–1931 drought crisis was often referenced by the proponents of a more vigorous federal response. See "Robinson Pleads for Drought Area," *New York Times*, January 8, 1931.

80. *Emergency Appropriation for Cooperation with State Health Departments in Rural Sanitation, etc.*, 6.

81. Ibid., 16.

82. Ibid.; "Letter from James M. Smith to Dr. C. W. Garrison, dated December 28, 1930," 165. In addition to being submitted and reprinted along with the other letters

from local public health officials, Smith's letter was read aloud by C. W. Garrison during his testimony.

83. As signed, the appropriations bill was the outcome of a conference committee. There were no roll-call votes on the public health provisions of the bill.

84. Ferrell and Mead, *History of County Health Organizations*, 5.

85. *Annual Report of the Surgeon General of the Public Health Service of the United States (1931)*, 87–88.

86. *Demonstration Work in Rural Sanitation*, 808.

87. Ferrell and Mead, *History of County Health Organizations*.

CHAPTER FIVE. ECONOMIC SECURITY

1. The most significant exception is Kooijman, *Pursuit of National Health*, 68. Kooijman offers a thoroughly researched and impressive account of the push for national health insurance in the United States.

2. King, "Edgar Sydenstricker," 412.

3. Starr, *Social Transformation*, 260.

4. Cunningham and Cunningham, *The Blues*, 5; Thomasson, "From Sickness to Health," 237.

5. Ibid., 237.

6. Starr, *Social Transformation*, 296.

7. On the evaluation of insurance, see Thomasson, "From Sickness to Health" and "Importance of Group Coverage."

8. See Committee on the Costs of Medical Care, *Medical Care for the American People*, 118. On the importance of using the financing of care to transform the practice of medicine, see Falk, "Reminiscences" (1968).

9. Committee on the Costs of Medical Care, *Medical Care for the American People*, 201.

10. Committee on the Costs of Medical Care, "Editorial and Abstract Summary," 1953.

11. Ibid., 9.

12. Ibid., 1951.

13. Falk, "Reminiscences" (1968).

14. Kennedy, *Freedom from Fear*, 144; Schlesinger, *Coming of the New Deal*, 339.

15. Schlesinger, *Coming of the New Deal*, 326.

16. See ibid., 20–21.

17. "Peek Stresses Aim of Farm Relief Act," *Wall Street Journal*, May 17, 1933.

18. For the classic work on the AAA and the NRA, see Finegold and Skocpol, *State and Party*.

19. *A. L. A. Schechter Corp v. United States*, 295 US 495 (1935).

20. Falk, "Reminiscences" (1968).

21. Jones, *Bad Blood*.

22. Furman, *Profile*, 393.

23. Falk, "Reminiscences" (1968).

24. Parran, "New Health Program for New York State" and "Public Medical Care in New York State."

25. See Thomas Parran Jr. to W. S. Leathers, January 9, 1935, 90/F-14, Box 2, Thomas Parran Jr. Papers, University of Pittsburgh Archives Service Center, Pittsburgh (hereafter Parran Papers). That Parran would likely be appointed surgeon general was mentioned in the national press as early as 1934. See "Hears Dr. Cumming Is Likely to Resign," *New York Times*, November 19, 1934.

26. See Schlesinger, *Coming of the New Deal*, 20–21; Kennedy, *Freedom from Fear*, 171.

27. Furman, *Profile*, 382; Mullan, *Plagues and Politics*, 99.

28. *Annual Report of the Surgeon General of the Public Health Service of the United States (1934)*, 58.

29. Furman, *Profile*, 383.

30. *Annual Report of the Surgeon General of the Public Health Service of the United States (1934)*, 60; Kennedy, *Freedom from Fear*, 176.

31. *Annual Report of the Surgeon General of the Public Health Service of the United States (1934)*, 59. The 64,000 worker estimate is from Williams, "Civil Works Administration Emergency Relief," 59.

32. Williams, "Civil Works Administration Emergency Relief," 13.

33. Ibid., 12. Hugh Cumming to Harry Hopkins, July 3, 1934, Box 440, Records of the Public Health Service (RG 90), General Subject File, 1924–1935, State Boards of Health, Tennessee—Cities and Counties, Texas, National Archives.

34. Brown, *Public Relief*, 256.

35. Ibid., 256.

36. Wilbur J. Cohen, "Chronological Summary of Activities of the Committee on Economic Security and Developments in Social Security Legislation," in Box 65, Witte Papers; Schlesinger, *Coming of the New Deal*, 304.

37. On the organization of the CES, see Witte, *Development of the Social Security Act*.

38. Sydenstricker, CES executive director Edwin Witte later recalled, "was the person everyone agreed best qualified to make this study." Witte, *Development of the Social Security Act*, 174.

39. "Administration Studies Social Insurance"; Kooijman, *Pursuit of National Health*, 54.

40. Witte, *Development of the Social Security Act*, 174–175.

41. Thomas Parran to Edgar Sydenstricker, September 22, 1934, Box 20, Parran Papers.

42. Ibid.

43. Ibid.

44. Ibid. Derickson cites this exchange in his crucial study of health insurance in the United States. See Derickson, *Health Security for All*, 66.

45. Sydenstricker to Parran, September 24, 1934, 90/F-14, Box 20; Michael M. Davis to Thomas Parran, October 15, 1934, Box 21; and Michael M. Davis to Edwin Witte, October 9, 1934, Box 21, all in the Parran Papers. Falk, "Reminiscences" (1968). For an outline of Sydenstricker's views during this period, see Sydenstricker, "Health in the New Deal."

46. Michael M. Davis to Edwin Witte, October 9, 1934, Box 67, Witte Papers.

47. Ibid.

48. Edgar Sydenstricker to Thomas Parran, November 7, 1934, Box 21, Parran Papers.

49. "Reports of the Committee on Economic Security: Committee Activities," CES meeting, October 1, 1934, Box 65, Witte Papers.

50. "Medical Advisory Committee," in Committee on Economic Security, Technical Board, Medical Advisory Board, Box 2, Records of the Social Security Administration (RG 47), National Archives.

51. Witte, *Development of the Social Security Act*, 177.

52. Hirshfield, *Lost Reform*, 49; Kooijman, *Pursuit of National Health*, 58.

53. Witte, *Development of the Social Security Act*, 179.

54. Kooijman, *Pursuit of National Health*, 58.

55. Witte, *Development of the Social Security Act*, 178–179.

56. Edgar Sydenstricker to Frances Perkins, November 19, 1934, Box 20, Parran Papers.

57. Hirshfield, *Lost Reform*, 61–62.

58. Edgar Sydenstricker to Frances Perkins, November 19, 1934, Box 20, Parran Papers.

59. Ibid.

60. Isidore Sydney Falk, "Reminiscences of Isidore Sydney Falk: Oral History, 1963," conducted by Harlan Phillips, Columbia University Center for Oral History, New York, NY.

61. On Southern Democrats and the New Deal, see particularly Katznelson, *Fear Itself*.

62. Falk, "Reminiscences" (1963).

63. Arthur Altmeyer, "Interview #2 with Arthur Altmeyer," conducted by Peter A. Corning, Washington, DC, 1966.

64. *Report to the President of the Committee on Economic Security*, 41.

65. Ibid., 40.

66. Ibid., 42.

67. See particularly Kooijman, *Pursuit of National Health*, 63.

68. Witte, *Development of the Social Security Act*, 182.

69. Altmeyer, "Interview #2."

70. See Kooijman, *Pursuit of National Health*, 67–68.

71. Ibid.

72. See Falk, "Reminiscences" (1963, 1968). Sydenstricker's thinking on the subject is detailed in Sydenstricker, "Group Medicine or Health Insurance." Sydenstricker had endorsed this view as early as 1917.

73. The most significant exception is Kooijman, *Pursuit of National Health*, 68. Even Kooijman, however, does not discuss the details and implications of Parran's plan.

74. Committee on Economic Security Medical Advisory Board, minutes of meetings, Tuesday afternoon session, January 29, 1935.

75. Ibid.

76. Altmeyer, "Interview #2."

77. Committee on Economic Security Medical Advisory Board, minutes of meetings, Tuesday afternoon session, January 29, 1935.

78. See DeWitt, "Decision to Exclude."

79. For accounts that suggest that Southern congressmen were at the center of the exclusion, see Lieberman, "Race, Institutions"; Katznelson, *Fear Itself*.

80. For a crucial discussion of the exclusion issue, see DeWitt, "Decision to Exclude." On the broader context, see Berkowitz, *America's Welfare State*, 25.

81. On the Biggs plan and its relationship to insurance as well as later proposals, see particularly Terris, "Hermann Biggs' Contribution"; Parran, "Public Responsibility."

82. Committee on Economic Security Medical Advisory Board, minutes of meetings, Tuesday afternoon session, January 29, 1935.

83. Ibid.

84. Ibid.

85. See Parran, "Public Responsibility," 542.

86. Parran outlined his views clearly in a speech delivered in May 1935. See ibid.

87. Committee on Economic Security Medical Advisory Board, minutes of meetings, Tuesday afternoon session, January 29, 1935.

88. Ibid.

89. Ibid.

90. Ibid.

91. Ibid.

92. Committee on Economic Security Medical Advisory Board, minutes of meetings, Wednesday evening session, January 30, 1935.

93. Hirshfield, *Lost Reform*, 55–56.

94. Witte, *Development of the Social Security Act*, 171.

95. See Carpenter, *Forging of Bureaucratic Autonomy* and *Reputation and Power*.

96. Witte, *Development of the Social Security Act*, 171.

97. Ibid., 171–172.

98. Robyn Muncy has written the definitive biography of Roche. See Muncy, *Relentless Reformer*.

99. "Hears Dr. Cumming is Likely to Resign," *New York Times*, November 19, 1934.

100. *Economic Security Act* [Committee on Finance], 408.

101. *Economic Security Act* [Committee on Ways and Means], 312.

102. Ibid., 315. Later in the hearing, Vinson told Waller that he did "not see any logical connection between the marine hospital appropriation and the Public Health Service appropriation" (321).

103. Ibid., 316.

104. Falk, "Reminiscences" (1963).

105. Witte, *Development of the Social Security Act*, 173.

106. Ibid., 173.

CHAPTER SIX. "THE RELIGION OF MANKIND'S FUTURE"

1. Rockefeller Foundation, International Health Division, *Annual Report, 1935*, https://assets.rockefellerfoundation.org/app/uploads/20150530122123/Annual-Report-1935.pdf.

2. Furman, *Profile*, 395.

3. Ibid., 97.

4. Thomas Parran Jr., interview by Harlan Phillips, July 16 and 18, 1962, Columbia Center for Oral History Archives, Butler Library, Columbia University, New York, NY.

5. Furman, *Profile,* 400.

6. For a definitive account of the Tuskegee Study, see Jones, *Bad Blood.*

7. Thomas, *Deluxe Jim Crow,* 65.

8. Agee, *Cotton Tenants,* 193.

9. Ibid., 196.

10. Ibid., 199.

11. Ibid., 210–211.

12. The states included in this calculation are those of the former Confederacy, plus Kentucky (where malaria was a problem along the Mississippi River), Oklahoma (where malaria was a problem in the eastern part of the state), and Missouri (absent in most of the state, malaria was a significant issue in the southeastern boot-heel area).

13. Rates were calculated from the Census Bureau's annual mortality statistics. Reports for individual years may be found online at http://www.cdc.gov/nchs/products/vsus/vsus_1890_1938.htm and http://www.cdc.gov/nchs/products/vsus/vsus_1939_1964.htm.

14. Humphreys, "How Four Once Common Diseases Were Eliminated," 1737.

15. Humphreys, *Malaria,* 112.

16. Gregory, *Southern Diaspora,* 28–32.

17. See Wright, *Old South, New South,* 235; Schulman, *From Cotton Belt to Sunbelt,* 31.

18. For a detailed analysis of the decline of malaria at the county level in Alabama, see Sledge and Mohler, "Eliminating Malaria." In an important study, Carl Kitchens has found a similar impact for Works Progress Administration programs aimed at malaria in Georgia. See Kitchens, "Effects of the Works Progress Administration's Antimalaria Programs."

19. Williams, "Civil Works Administration Emergency Relief," 11–14.

20. Sledge and Mohler, "Eliminating Malaria."

21. Ibid.

22. Williams, "Report of the Subcommittee on Malaria Prevention Activities," 818.

23. Andrews and Grant, "Experience in the United States," 69–74.

24. Faust, "Malaria Mortality," 4, 8–9.

25. DeKruif, *Fight for Life,* 25.

26. Ibid., 25–26.

27. Ibid., 27.

28. Out of 1,858 schoolchildren surveyed by the Rockefeller Sanitary Commission in Sunflower County, only twenty-seven, or 1.45 percent, were found to be infected. The commission's records show that a total of twenty-eight people were treated for the disease. See Rockefeller Sanitary Commission for the Eradication of Hookworm Disease, *Fifth Annual Report* (1915), 70, 72.

29. Sunflower County had an average malaria mortality rate of 109 per 100,000,000 population in 1919–1921, indicating a particularly severe malaria problem. See Maxcy, "Distribution of Malaria," 1129.

30. Ferrell and Mead, *History of County Health Organizations,* 272. The county's health budget ranged from an initial point of $6,250 in 1927 to a high of $25,500 in 1931.

31. DeKruif, *Fight for Life*, 27–28.

32. Stiles, "Early History," 305.

33. Stiles, "Decrease of Hookworm," 1765.

34. Upton, "Incidence and Severity," 925.

35. *Annual Report of the Surgeon General of the Public Health Service of the United States (1937)*, 33–34.

36. See Hollings and Victor, *Making Government Work*, 136.

37. Kennedy, *Freedom from Fear*, 330–331. See also, e.g., "Death Blow to AAA Presages Like Fate for Other New Deal Measures," *Washington Post*, January 12, 1936; "Roosevelt Puts Court on Trial before Nation," *New York Times*, January 10, 1937.

38. "President's Message," *New York Times*, February 6, 1937.

39. "Party Lines Are Split as Democrats Attack Plan," *Washington Post*, February 7, 1937.

40. Polsby, *How Congress Evolves*, 10.

41. Kennedy, *Freedom from Fear*, 332–333; Polsby, *How Congress Evolves*, 7–8.

42. Kelly, Harbison, and Belz, *American Constitution*, 484; Kennedy, *Freedom from Fear*, 334–336.

43. Moore, "Senator Josiah W. Bailey," 25.

44. Grantham, *The South in Modern America*, 129–130; Kennedy, *Freedom from Fear*, 340; Moore, "Senator Josiah W. Bailey"; "Senators Give Coalition Plea Wide Publicity," *Washington Post*, January 19, 1938.

45. Katznelson, *Fear Itself*, 170; Mickey, *Paths out of Dixie*, 137.

46. National Emergency Council, *Report on Economic Conditions of the South*, 1.

47. Ibid., 29–30.

48. Ibid., 32.

49. Katznelson, *Fear Itself*, 170.

50. "Roosevelt Asks Defeat of George and Talmadge as Foes of Liberalism," *New York Times*, August 12, 1938; "President Says 'Friend' Doesn't 'Speak Same Language,'" *Washington Post*, August 12, 1938.

51. "President Appeals to South Carolina," *New York Times*, August 12, 1938.

52. Quoted in "Negro Issue Raised in South at 'Purge,'" *New York Times*, August 23, 1938. See also "'White Supremacy' Issue Revived in the South," *New York Times*, August 28, 1938.

53. "Enemies of the New Deal in South Now United," *Washington Post*, September 18, 1938.

CHAPTER SEVEN. AN INTEGRATED APPROACH

1. Falk, "Reminiscences" (1968).

2. "Statement by the President," August 15, 1935, Box 3, Arthur J. Altmeyer Papers, Wisconsin Historical Society, Madison (hereafter Altmeyer Papers).

3. On Roche, see Muncy, *Relentless Reformer*.

4. Arthur Altmeyer to Franklin Roosevelt, June 17, 1937, Box 2, Altmeyer Papers.

5. On the Social Security Board, see esp. Altmeyer, *Formative Years of Social Security*.

6. Waller, "Social Security Act," 1193.

7. Falk, "Proposals for National Health Insurance," 168–169; Kooijman, *Pursuit of National Health*, 89.

8. "Memorandum on Relationship between the US Public Health Service and the Children's Bureau," July 20, 1935, Box 3, Altmeyer Papers.

9. Parran, "Career in Public Health."

10. See Viseltear, "Emergence of the Medical Care Section."

11. Falk, "Reminiscences" (1968).

12. Weisz, "Epidemiology and Health Care Reform."

13. "National Health Conference, July 18–19–20, 1938," held at the Mayflower Hotel, Washington, DC, Box 3, Altmeyer Papers; "A National Health Program: A Summary," press release intended for morning newspapers, July 19, 1938, 90/F-14, Box 39, Parran Papers. The president was given the report on February 14.

14. Josephine Roche to Franklin Roosevelt, October 13, 1938, Box 2; National Health Conference, July 18–19–20, 1938, called by the Interdepartmental Committee to Coordinate Health and Welfare Activities, Mayflower Hotel, Washington, DC, Box 3, both in Altmeyer Papers.

15. Although "presidentially sponsored," the conference was clearly the idea of the Interdepartmental Committee. Arthur Altmeyer drafted the presidential letter asking Josephine Roche to call the National Health Conference. See Memorandum to Mr. Rudolph Forster, from Arthur Altmeyer, on the report of the Technical Committee on Medical Care, March 8, 1938, Box 3, Altmeyer Papers.

16. Altmeyer, "National Health Conference and the Future of Public Health"; Muncy, *Relentless Reformer,* 190–191; Falk, "Reminiscences" (1968).

17. "National Health Conference, July 18–19–20, 1938," Mayflower Hotel, Washington, DC, Box 3, Altmeyer Papers.

18. "Speech Delivered to the National Health Conference, Monday Morning, July 18, by Dr. Thomas Parran, Surgeon General of the US Public Health Service," 90/F-14, Box 39, Parran Papers.

19. Ibid.

20. Ibid.

21. Ibid.

22. Ibid.

23. "National Health Conference, July 18–19–20, 1938," 51, Mayflower Hotel, Washington, DC, Box 3, Altmeyer Papers.

24. Draper, "National Health Program," 46.

25. On this point, see Altmeyer, "National Health Conference and the Future of Public Health," 5; Parran, "Health of the Nation," 1378; Hugh O'Connor, "New Deal Mapping Health Insurance," *New York Times,* October 26, 1938.

26. "National Health Conference, July 18–19–20, 1938," 11, Mayflower Hotel, Washington, DC, Box 3, Altmeyer Papers.

27. Draper, "National Health Program," 46.

28. For the definitive account of the FSA's health work, see Grey, *New Deal Medicine.*

29. Ibid., 43.

30. Ibid., 56. See also Mott and Roemer, *Rural Health and Medical Care.* On migratory farm workers, see their "Federal Program."

31. Draper, "National Health Program," 46.

32. Fox, *Health Policies, Politics*, 88–89; Viseltear, "Emergence of the Medical Care Section," 989. Thomas Parran was among those who signed the group's statement of principles.

33. Altmeyer, *Formative Years of Social Security*, 96; Arthur Altmeyer, "Interview #3 with Arthur Altmeyer," conducted by Peter A. Corning, Washington, DC, 1966.

34. Altmeyer, *Formative Years of Social Security*, 96.

35. Arthur Altmeyer, interview by Peter A. Corning, 1966, https://www.ssa.gov/history/ajaoral3.html. The organization had already suggested that it would be open to disability insurance. See Arthur Altmeyer to Franklin Roosevelt, June 17, 1937, Box 2, Altmeyer Papers.

36. Falk, "Reminiscences" (1968).

37. Ibid.

38. Altmeyer, *Formative Years of Social Security*, 96.

39. See "Proceedings of the Special Session."

40. For Daniel Hirschfield, the rationale behind the AMA's posture was obvious. These endorsements, he writes, "were no doubt the result of a decision first to isolate compulsory health insurance and then to eliminate it from serious consideration by the administration." See Hirshfield, *Lost Reform*, 126, 2.

41. Fishbein, "American Medicine," 502.

42. "Proceedings of the Special Session" (1938).

43. "Professional Associations on the Proposed National Health Program," 694.

44. Kentucky state health commissioner A. T. McCormack apparently believed that the AMA would be inclined to support the PHS-backed approach, suggesting at the meeting that Title VI of the Social Security Act be amended to allow for the distribution of funds for public medical services through state health departments. In December 1938, he wrote to Surgeon General Parran about the recent meeting of the Southern Medical Association and also about an important development in his state. With the support of then-AMA president Irvin Abell, a firm opponent of government-backed insurance, McCormack had persuaded the Kentucky State Medical Association to pass a resolution "that a Bureau of Medical Service be created in the State Department of Health *immediately*." See A. T. McCormack to Thomas Parran, December 6, 1938, Box 3, Parran Papers.

45. Schickler and Caughey, "Public Opinion," 163.

46. Hirshfield, *Lost Reform*, 116–117, 138.

47. Kooijman, *Pursuit of National Health*, 95.

48. See Altmeyer, *Formative Years of Social Security*, 115. For a contemporary assessment of the bill and its antecedents, see Maslow, "Background of the Wagner National Health Bill."

49. According to Arthur Altmeyer, Roosevelt did not express private support for the bill either. Altmeyer, "Interview #2."

50. See Thomas Parran to Paul DeKruif, February 28, 1939, Box 1, Parran Papers.

51. Michael M. Davis to Thomas Parran, March 24, 1939, Box 1, Parran Papers.

52. Ibid.

53. Ibid.

54. Altmeyer, *Formative Years of Social Security*, 116. The AMA publically signaled its plans for fighting the bill. See William Laurence, "Doctors Map Fight on New Health Bill," *New York Times*, May 16, 1938.

55. Quoted in "Federal Officials Back Health Bill," *New York Times*, June 3, 1939.

56. Huthmacher, *Senator Robert F. Wagner*, 266.

57. Ibid.

CHAPTER EIGHT. DIVERGENT PATHS

1. Thomas Parran to W. B. Grayson, State Board of Health, Arkansas, October 24, 1940, Box 766; and A. B. McCreary, Florida Department of Health, to Joseph Mountin, October 14, 1940, Box 795, both in Records of the Public Health Service (RG 90), General Classified Records, Group X—National Defense, 1940–1946, National Archives.

2. R. A. Vonderlehr to the Surgeon General, Memorandum, December 7, 1940, Box 722; and Thomas Parran to Honorable Andrew J. May, US House of Representatives, March 11, 1941, Box 722, both in Records of the Public Health Service (RG 90), General Classified Records, Group X—National Defense, 1940–1946, National Archives. On venereal disease and World War II, see particularly Lord, *Condom Nation*, 71–92.

3. On the early stages of the antimosquito program, see M. V. Ziegler to I. C. Riggin, July 23, 1941, and "Orientation Course for Public Health Personnel: Mosquito Control Course," July 15–31, 1941, both in Box 738, Records of the Public Health Service (RG 90), General Classified Records, Group X—National Defense, 1940–1946, National Archives.

4. On Mountin, see Parran, "Career in Public Health."

5. Furman, *Profile*, 418.

6. Lord, *Condom Nation*, 90. On inductions, see, e.g., R. A. Vonderlehr to H. J. Childress, Upshur County Health Officer, Gilmer, TX, November 5, 1942, Box 722, Records of the Public Health Service (RG 90), General Classified Records, Group X—National Defense, 1940–1946, National Archives.

7. Thomas Parran to Honorable Andrew J. May, US House of Representatives, March 11, 1941, in Box 722, Records of the Public Health Service (RG 90), General Classified Records, Group X—National Defense, 1940–1946, National Archives.

8. Lord, *Condom Nation*, 91; Pearce, "Rapid Treatment Centers."

9. Thomas Parran to Honorable Andrew J. May, US House of Representatives, March 11, 1941, Box 722, Records of the Public Health Service (RG 90), General Classified Records, Group X—National Defense, 1940–1946, National Archives.

10. Memorandum on States Relations Field Offices, November 25, 1942; Malaria Control in Defense Areas, *Breakdown of Functions*, undated, early 1942; on the importance of shifting all malaria control work to MCWA, see C. L. Williams to Joseph Mountin, April 2, 1942, all in Box 416, Records of the Public Health Service (RG 90), Group VI: Government Establishments, National Archives.

11. Tetzlaff, "Operation," 557. See also *Malaria Control in War Areas, 1942–43*, 34.

12. Sullivan and Wiley, "Sanitation Activities," 618.

13. Andrews and Grant, "Experience in the United States," 68.

14. Ibid., 69.

15. Tetzlaff, "Operation," 557.

16. Sledge and Mohler, "Eliminating Malaria."

17. Andrews and Grant, "Experience in the United States," 61–62.

18. Ibid., 69.

19. Ibid.

20. Ibid., 66.

21. *Malaria Control in War Areas, 1942–43*, 52; *Malaria Control in War Areas, 1943–44*, 18–21.

22. *Malaria Control in War Areas, 1942–43*, 51, 55–64; *Malaria Control in War Areas, 1943–44*, 22–27. For a comprehensive account of MCWA activities, see Etheridge, *Sentinel for Health*, "War and the Mosquito," 1–17.

23. *Malaria Control in War Areas, 1943–44*, 9, 47–53.

24. Altmeyer, "Interview #2." Wolman, "Beveridge Report."

25. Rodgers, *Atlantic Crossings*, 496.

26. Perkins, *The Roosevelt I Knew*, 283.

27. The report was not particularly well received at the time, and Congress soon stopped funding the National Resources Planning Board. See Poen, *Harry S. Truman*, 37; Merriam, "National Resources Planning Board."

28. "Congress Gets Security Bill Adapting Beveridge Plan," *New York Times*, June 4, 1943.

29. Kooijman, *Pursuit of National Health*, 97; Rorty, "Health under the Social Security Tent."

30. See Altmeyer, *Formative Years of Social Security*, 146; Altmeyer, "Interview #2."

31. Altmeyer, "Interview #2." Rose Ehrlich and Michael M. Davis, "Four National Health Bills Compared," October 1, 1943, Research Files, Social Security, Box 210, Witte Papers.

32. Arthur Altmeyer to Thomas Parran, January 4, 1943, Box 26, Wilbur J. Cohen Papers, Wisconsin Historical Society, Madison (hereafter Cohen Papers)

33. Rose Ehrlich and Michael M. Davis, "Four National Health Bills Compared," October 1, 1943, Research Files, Social Security, Box 210, Witte Papers.

34. See C.-E. A. Winslow to Robert Wagner, October 13, 1944, Box 26, Cohen Papers.

35. See "Wagner–Murray–Dingell Bill."

36. Kooijman, *Pursuit of National Health*, 100–101. Marjorie Shearon, a PHS employee and former Social Security Board staffer who harbored paranoid and possibly anti-Semitic beliefs about the power of the Social Security Board's Isidore Falk, wrote an analysis of the Wagner–Murray–Dingell bill that found that its risks outweighed any potential rewards. Falk, she believed, had designed the bill with the intention of expanding the power of the Social Security Board at the expense of the PHS. As the titular head of a program actually operated by the Social Security Board, the surgeon general could easily be scapegoated were the program to go wrong. Although Shearon was correct that the plan as designed was at best administratively problematic, a point noted by a number of other people, the Social Security Board certainly did not design the program with the intention of placing blame for its failings with the PHS. Later, after clashing with Parran and PHS statistician George St. John Perrott, Shearon would

become an advisor to opponents of national health insurance. On Shearon and Falk, see Derickson, "House of Falk."

37. "Wagner–Murray–Dingell Bill for Social Security," 600.

38. Viseltear, "Emergence of the Medical Care Section." The APHA, Surgeon General Parran later noted, "was not a strong factor in initiating or pushing legislation through Congress." See Thomas Parran Jr., interview by Harlan Phillips.

39. "Wagner–Murray Bill," 1275.

40. Daniel Fox terms the focus on creating networks of hospitals, connected to research universities, "hierarchical regionalism." "In the United States, as in Great Britain," writes Fox, "almost everyone concerned with every aspect of health policy assumed that is was necessary to establish and improve regional hierarchies of hospitals and doctors." Fox, *Health Policies, Politics*, 163.

41. "Public Health of Tomorrow," address given at Postwar Planning Session of the American Hospital Association in Buffalo, NY, September 16, 1943, Box 44, Parran Papers.

42. Ibid.

43. Mountin, "Evolving Pattern," 1403.

44. Ibid., 1406–1407.

45. Ibid., 1403.

46. See Snyder, "Passage and Significance."

47. Ibid.

48. Mullan, *Plagues and Politics*, 122.

49. Furman, *Profile*, 430.

50. For a thorough discussion of the evolution and politics of extramural funding through the NIH, see Fox, "Politics of the NIH Extramural Program." See also Parran, "Reminiscences."

51. Fox, "Politics of the NIH Extramural Program."

52. Starr, *Social Transformation*, 342–343; Stobbe, *Surgeon General's Warning*, 93.

53. Falk, "Reminiscences" (1968).

54. Etheridge, *Sentinel for Health*, 16–17.

55. See Parran, *Health of the Nation*. "US Health Service Combats Malaria," *New York Times*, April 1, 1944.

56. See Masterson, *Malaria Project*; Patterson, *Mosquito Crusades*.

57. *Malaria Control in War Areas, 1943–44*, 28.

58. See Masterson, *Malaria Project*, 33, 40.

59. *Malaria Control in War Areas, 1943–44*, 29.

60. On prison medical experiments, see Hornblum, "They Were Cheap and Available," 1437.

61. "Malaria Remedy Tested in Prison," *New York Times*, July 23, 1944; Coatney, "Reminiscences," 8. Later the Atlanta experiments would be continued at the penitentiary in Seagoville, TX.

62. See Reverby, "Normal Exposure."

63. Williams, "Extended Malaria Control," 464.

64. Andrews and Grant, "Experience in the United States," 102.

65. Ibid., 105.

66. Ibid., 102–103.

67. On the use of DDT during the 1940s, see Humphreys, "Kicking a Dying Dog." On the elimination of malaria, see Sledge and Mohler, "Eliminating Malaria."

68. Hoffman, *Health Care for Some*, 48; "Corporal Kelly and His Son"; "More Federal Aid for Babies Urged," *New York Times*, October 25, 1944.

69. Mullan, *Plagues and Politics*, 120.

70. Mott and Roemer, "Federal Program."

71. Health Insurance Association of America, *Source Book*.

72. See Thomasson, "Importance of Group Coverage."

73. Health Insurance Association of America, *Source Book*.

74. An analysis of this speech and its context may be found in Sunstein, *Second Bill of Rights*, 9–16.

75. Poen, *Harry S. Truman*, 48–50.

76. Davis, *Medical Care for Tomorrow*, 280.

77. Falk, "Reminiscences" (1968).

78. Poen, *Harry S. Truman*, 81.

79. "Rural Health—Today and Tomorrow," speech given at the Georgia Conference on Social Welfare, Atlanta, September 13, 1945, Box 47, Parran Papers.

80. "Report on S. 1606," Thomas Parran to Watson B. Miller, Administrator, Federal Security Agency, December 7, 1945, Box 27, Cohen Papers.

81. "A National Health Program—American Style," speech given at the US Conference of Mayors, December 12, 1945, New York City, Box 47, Parran Papers. Parran discusses the FSA as a precedent in "Rural Health—Today and Tomorrow," delivered to the Georgia Conference on Social Welfare, Atlanta, September 13, 1945, Box 47, Parran Papers.

82. Falk, "Reminiscences" (1968). "The fact that the Social Security Board was a separate agency from the Public Health Service," Falk explained in describing the politics of Parran's position beginning with the 1938 National Health Conference, "didn't spare him altogether the criticisms that were anti-federal that were emerging."

83. Poen, *Harry S. Truman*, 104.

84. "Medical Centers of the Future," William and Charles Mayo Memorial Lecture, Dartmouth College, Hanover, NH, December 16, 1945, Box 47, Parran Papers.

85. Ibid.

86. Fox, "Politics of the NIH Extramural Program."

87. Etheridge, *Sentinel for Health*, 24; Tisdale, "National Program for Training," 1362; Boyd, Stubbs, and Weinstein, "Tropical Disease Education Program." Workers were trained both in Atlanta and at the CDC's auxiliary training facility in Columbus, GA.

88. See Tisdale, "National Program for Training," 1368; Etheridge, *Sentinel for Health*, 24. See, e.g., Ziony, "Malaria Control in Iran." On the role of the United States in providing assistance in matters of health to other nations, see "International Technical Assistance in Public Health."

89. Snyder, "New York," 632.

90. Nájera, González-Silva, and Alonso, "Some Lessons."

91. Falk, "Reminiscences" (1963).

92. "Truman Signs Bill for Billion US–State Hospital Program," *Washington Post*, August 14, 1946; "Hospital Measure Sent to President," *New York Times*, August 1, 1946; *Annual Report of the Federal Security Agency*, 417.

93. "Hill–Burton Hospital Construction Bill."

94. Clark et al., "Impact of Hill–Burton," 553–554, 48.

95. For important discussions of Hill–Burton's "separate but equal" provision and its impact, see Thomas, *Deluxe Jim Crow*; Cornely, "Segregation and Discrimination"; Quadagno, *One Nation, Uninsured*, 77–93.

96. See Thomas, *Deluxe Jim Crow*. My discussion largely follows Thomas's important analysis.

97. Ibid., 71.

98. Ibid., 205.

99. See, e.g., "End of Segregation in All Hospitals Urged," *Baltimore Afro-American*, July 25, 1953; "Hospital Discrimination Must End!"

100. "Crushing Irony of De Luxe Jim Crow," 386. See Thomas, *Deluxe Jim Crow*, 174.

101. See "Hospital Discrimination Must End!"

102. Poen, *Harry S. Truman*, 68.

103. Ibid., 88.

104. *New York Times*, July 10, 1946, 25: "HOLD HEALTH BILL DEAD FOR SESSION Sponsors Decide Measure Is Too Controversial to Get to the Voting Stage Now. HEARINGS ALMOST ENDED. Program for Insurance and Adding to Social Security Goes Over to January. Bill Must Start Anew Provisions of the Measure."

105. Derickson, *Health Security for All*, 102.

106. Stobbe, *Surgeon General's Warning*, 84; "Doctors Censure Surgeon General," *New York Times*, December 12, 1946, 31.

107. Hacker, *Divided Welfare State*, 232.

108. For the definitive study of labor and the development of health insurance in the United States, see Gottschalk, *Shadow Welfare State*.

109. Hacker, *Divided Welfare State*, 233.

110. See Krajcinovic, *From Company Doctors to Managed Care*, 54; Goldstein, "Obituary: Warren Fales Draper."

111. Health Insurance Association of America, *Source Book*.

CHAPTER NINE. HEALTH DIVIDED

1. My account follows that of Stobbe, *Surgeon General's Warning*, 85. On Kempner's "rice diet," see Kempner, "Some Effects of the Rice Diet."

2. J. R. Fuchs, "Oral History Interview with Oscar R. Ewing," May 1, 1969, Harry S. Truman Library and Museum, Independence, MO, 203, http://www.trumanlibrary .org.

3. Stobbe, *Surgeon General's Warning*, 92.

4. Fuchs, "Oral History," 208.

5. Carl V. Reynolds to Thomas Parran, February 14, 1948, Box 130, Parran Papers.

6. "Guardians for Civil Rights Proposed by Truman Board," *New York Times*, October 30, 1947. See Mickey, *Paths out of Dixie*, 140.

7. "Platform Adopted by Democratic Convention at Philadelphia," *Washington Post*, July 15, 1948; "South Beaten on Race Issue as Rights Plank Is Widened," *New York Times*, July 15, 1948.

8. "Southerners Name Thurmond to Lead Anti-Truman Fight," *New York Times*, July 18, 1948. See also "Dixie Rebels Nominate Thurmond and Wright," *Washington Post*, July 18, 1948; Key, *Southern Politics*, 334–335.

9. "Presses for Rights: President Acts Despite Split in His Party over the Chief Issue," *New York Times*, July 27, 1948; "Truman Orders Equal Rights in US Jobs, Armed Services," *Washington Post*, July 27, 1948.

10. "AMA Statement on Truman Health Plan," *New York Times*, April 25, 1949.

11. Poen, *Harry S. Truman*, 151.

12. Falk, "Reminiscences" (1968).

13. "Senator Warns Hospital Session," *New York Times*, September 27, 1949. See also "Truman to Submit a Health Program Costing Billions," *New York Times*, March 31, 1949.

14. "Hill Bill for Extension of Medical Care." For a positive description of the bill components, published in the same issue of the *Journal of the American Medical Association*, see "Federal Voluntary Health Insurance Bill."

15. John Morris, "GOP Independents to File Bill For Private Health Aid to All: GOP Group to File New Bill," *New York Times*, May 31, 1949.

16. "Rep. Davis Fears Racism in Socialized Medicine," *Atlanta Daily World*, November 20, 1949.

17. Ewing, "President's Health Program," 433. The incoming president of the American Medical Association, for his part, sent a written statement to the national convention of the National Medical Association, the professional organization of black physicians, asserting that the group should not support Truman's plan on the assumption that it would lead to desegregation: "The highest law of the land, the Constitution of the United States, expressly outlaws prejudice on account of race, creed or color. This in itself proves that legislation is not sufficient to eliminate the blots of bigotry and prejudice. No, gentlemen, compulsory health insurance must be evaluated solely on the basis of its ability to deliver what it promises." See "Fight Health Plan, AMA Asks Negroes," *New York Times*, August 10, 1949. On Southern opposition to Ewing, see "23 Democrats Join GOP Bloc of 37 in Rejection Despite White House Appeal," *Washington Post*, August 17, 1949.

18. Fox, "Politics of the NIH Extramural Program."

19. Langmuir and Andrews, "Biological Warfare Defense."

20. Etheridge, *Sentinel for Health*, 74; Stobbe, *Surgeon General's Warning*, 103.

21. Etheridge, *Sentinel for Health*, 84–85.

22. Stobbe, *Surgeon General's Warning*, 99.

23. Nájera, González-Silva, and Alonso, "Some Lessons."

24. Etheridge, *Sentinel for Health*, 115. On the CDC's new facilities, see "Highlights from the 1959 Report."

25. Mullan, *Plagues and Politics*, 162.

26. Marmor, *Politics of Medicare*, 10–11. See also Altmeyer, "Interview #2." "Aid for Pensioners Urged in Congress," *New York Times*, April 11, 1952. Hacker, *Divided Welfare State*, 235.

27. Oberlander, *Political Life of Medicare*, 23.

28. On the political strategy behind Medicare, see particularly Marmor, *Politics of Medicare;* Oberlander, *Political Life of Medicare.*

29. Thomasson, "From Sickness to Health," 241.

30. Health Insurance Association of America, *Source Book*, 12.

31. Kooijman, *Pursuit of National Health*, 134.

32. *Pursuit of National Health*, 137–138; Oberlander, *Political Life of Medicare*, 26; Starr, *Social Transformation*, 368.

33. Marmor, *Politics of Medicare*, 23.

34. Oberlander, *Political Life of Medicare*, 28; John D. Morris, "Nixon to Support Eisenhower Plan for Care of Aged," *New York Times*, May 7, 1960.

35. Marmor, *Politics of Medicare*, 29.

36. Blumenthal and Morone, *Heart of Power*, 178, 85.

37. See ibid., 188–189.

38. Ibid., 195.

39. Oberlander, *Political Life of Medicare*, 40–41.

40. Cunningham and Cunningham, *The Blues*, 147.

41. See Starr, *Social Transformation*, 375.

42. Marmor, *Politics of Medicare*, 97.

43. Oberlander, *Political Life of Medicare*, 47.

44. Ibid., 120.

45. Ibid., 128.

46. Hanson, "Medicaid and the Politics of Redistribution."

47. Olson, *Politics of Medicaid*, 55.

48. For an overview of the political history of Medicaid, see ibid.

49. On this point, see particularly Starr, *Remedy and Reaction;* Hacker, *Divided Welfare State.*

50. See Jacobs, *Health of Nations* and "Politics of America's Supply State."

51. "Bias in Hospitals Barred by Court: Color Line under Hill–Burton Act Held Unconstitutional," *New York Times*, November 2, 1963; "Hospitals on Federal Aid Ruled Open to Negroes," *Washington Post*, November 2, 1963; "Constitutional Law."

52. See Langer, "Hospital Discrimination."

53. Quadagno, *One Nation, Uninsured*, 84.

54. Quoted, without attribution, in Langer, "Hospital Discrimination," 1356.

55. See Quadagno, *One Nation, Uninsured*, 86–93, and "Promoting Civil Rights."

56. Informed by undersecretary of HEW Wilbur Cohen that a medical facility in his district was not in compliance with the Civil Rights Act, South Carolina representative L. Mendel Rivers replied that he had received Cohen's letter "concerning the compliance of my State of South Carolina with your Civil Rights Act." Sarcastically expressing delight that Cohen did not believe his constituents sought to disobey the laws of the United States, Rivers asserted that the law was being followed and that HEW should not threaten to hold back funding. "I presume and assume that the motives of my people will not be impugned in the future and that your representatives will discontinue harassing my people and denying my State its just proportion of monies to which it is entitled under the Law of the Land." See Rivers to Cohen, May 5, 1966, Box 88, Cohen Papers.

57. Langer, "Hospital Integration."

58. "Segregation Mars Start of Medicare," *Washington Post*, July 1, 1966.

59. Quadagno, "Promoting Civil Rights," 84.

60. Quoted in Stobbe, *Surgeon General's Warning*, 135. My account follows that of Stobbe.

61. Ibid., 136.

62. Ibid., 137.

63. The classic analysis of the decision-making process that led to the swine flu immunization program may be found in Neustadt and Fineberg, *The Epidemic that Never Was*. See also Dehner, *Influenza*, 128–144; Boffey, "Anatomy of a Decision," 640.

64. Henderson, "Eradication."

65. Jones, *Bad Blood*, 220.

66. Hip-hop artist Kanye West, for instance, referenced the AIDS conspiracy theory in his 2005 hit single, "Heard 'Em Say": "Before you go ask me to get a job today / Can I least get a raise on the minimum wage? / And I know the government administer AIDS." West's delivery of this line is knowing and slightly sarcastic.

CONCLUSION

1. On Nixon's health plans, see esp. Blumenthal and Morone, *Heart of Power;* Wainess, "Ways and Means."

2. Starr, *Social Transformation,* 397.

3. Ibid., 396.

4. Richard Nixon, "Special Message to the Congress Proposing a National Health Strategy," *American Presidency Project,* February 18, 1971, http://www.presidency.ucsb .edu/ws/?pid=3311.

5. Ibid.

6. Blumenthal and Morone, *Heart of Power,* 143.

7. Wainess, "Ways and Means," 315.

8. Blumenthal and Morone, *Heart of Power,* 245.

9. Skocpol, *Boomerang;* Hacker, *Road to Nowhere.*

10. Oberlander and Lyons, "Beyond Incrementalism?"

11. Berenson, "Medicare Disadvantaged"; Oberlander, "Through the Looking Glass."

12. For important discussions of the structure of the ACA, see Jonathan Oberlander and Theodore R. Marmor, "The Health Bill Explained at Last," *New York Review of Books,* August 19, 2010; Davidson, *New Era in US Health Care;* Starr, *Remedy and Reaction.*

13. Fox, *Power and Illness,* 68.

14. Ibid., 69; Starr, *Social Transformation,* 370.

15. Davidson, *New Era in US Health Care,* 85–86.

16. Kocher and Adashi, "Hospital Readmissions."

17. Barack Obama, "Remarks by the President on Preventive Care, February 10, 2012," *White House, Office of the Press Secretary,* February 10, 2012, http://www.white house.gov/the-press-office/2012/02/10/remarks-president-preventive-care.

18. Shaw et al., "Patient Protection and Affordable Care Act."

19. Sarah Kliff, "The Incredible Shrinking Prevention Fund," *Washington Post,* April 19, 2013.

20. For a comprehensive discussion, see Sardell, *US Experiment in Social Medicine.*

21. Ibid. Mickey, "Dr. StrangeRove."

22. "Speech Delivered to the National Health Conference, Monday Morning, July 18, by Dr. Thomas Parran, Surgeon General of the US Public Health Service," 90/F-14, Box 39, Parran Papers.

BIBLIOGRAPHY

"The Administration Studies Social Insurance." *Journal of the American Medical Association* 103, no. 8 (1934): 609–610.

Agee, James. *Cotton Tenants: Three Families.* Brooklyn: Melville House, 2013.

Altmeyer, Arthur J. *The Formative Years of Social Security.* Madison: University of Wisconsin Press, 1966.

———. "The National Health Conference and the Future of Public Health." *American Journal of Public Health* 29, no. 1 (1939): 1–10.

Anderson, Warwick. *Colonial Pathologies: American Tropical Medicine, Race, and Hygiene in the Philippines.* Durham, NC: Duke University Press, 2006.

Andrews, Justin, and Jean Grant. "Experience in the United States." In *Preventive Medicine in World War II*, vol. 6, *Communicable Diseases: Malaria*, 61–112. Washington, DC: Office of the Surgeon General, Department of the Army, 1963.

Annual Report of the Federal Security Agency, Section Three, United States Public Health Service, for the Fiscal Year 1947. Washington, DC: US Government Printing Office, 1947.

Annual Report of the Surgeon General of the Public Health and Marine Hospital Service of the United States. Fiscal years 1908 and 1911. Washington, DC: US Government Printing Office, 1909–1911.

Annual Report of the Surgeon General of the Public Health Service of the United States. Fiscal years 1912, 1915, 1917–1920, 1927, 1931, 1934, and 1937. Washington, DC: US Government Printing Office, 1913–1937.

[*Appropriations for Sundry Civil Expenses*]. Hearings before the Subcommittee on Appropriations, United States Senate, Sixty-Sixth Congress, First Session, on HR 6176, a Bill Making Appropriations for Sundry Civil Expenses of the Government for the Fiscal Year Ending June 30, 1920 and for Other Purposes. Washington, DC: US Government Printing Office, 1919.

Ashford, Bailey K., and Pedro Gutierrez Igaravidez. *Uncinariasis (Hookworm Disease) in Porto Rico.* Senate Document No. 808. Washington, DC: US Government Printing Office, 1911.

Barry, John M. *Rising Tide: The Great Mississippi Flood of 1927 and How It Changed America.* New York: Simon & Schuster, 1997.

Baumgartner, Frank R., and Bryan D. Jones. *Agendas and Instability in American Politics.* 2nd ed. Chicago: University of Chicago Press, 2009.

Bensel, Richard. *Sectionalism and American Political Development, 1880–1980.* Madison: University of Wisconsin Press, 1984.

———. "The Tension between American Political Development as a Research Community and as a Disciplinary Subfield." *Studies in American Political Development* 17 (2003): 103–106.

———. *Yankee Leviathan: The Origins of Central State Authority in America, 1859–1877.* New York: Cambridge University Press, 1990.

Berenson, Robert. "Medicare Disadvantaged and the Search for the Elusive 'Level

Playing Field.'" *Health Affairs (Milwood)* (2004, Suppl. Web Exclusives): W4-572–W4-585.

Berkowitz, Edward D. *America's Welfare State: From Roosevelt to Reagan.* Baltimore, MD: Johns Hopkins University Press, 1991.

Bjorkman, Frances Maule. "The Cure for Two Million Sick: The Discovery of the Hookworm Disease by Dr. C. W. Stiles—Its Cure Will Restore a Whole Class of People to Health and Industrial Efficiency." *World's Work* 18, no. 1 (1909): 11608–11612.

Blue, Rupert. "Conserving the Nation's Man Power: Disease Weakens Armies, Cripples Industry, Reduces Production. How the Government Is Sanitating the Civil Zones around Cantonment Areas. A Nation-wide Campaign for Health." *National Geographic* 32 (1917): 254–278.

———. "Some of the Larger Problems of the Medical Profession." *Journal of the American Medical Association* 66, no. 25 (1916): 1899–1902.

Blumenthal, David, and James Morone. *The Heart of Power.* Berkeley: University of California Press, 2010.

Boffey, Philip M. "Anatomy of a Decision: How the Nation Declared War on Swine Flu." *Science* 192, no. 4240 (1976): 636–641.

Boyd, William S., Trawick H. Stubbs, and Paul P. Weinstein. "The Tropical Disease Education Program of the United States Public Health Service." *Public Health Reports* 61, no. 20 (1946): 707–711.

Brown, Josephine Chapin. *Public Relief, 1929–1939.* New York: Henry Holt, 1940.

Burke, Emily P. *Reminiscences of Georgia.* Oberlin, OH: James M. Fitch, 1850.

Callen, Zachary. *Railroad and American Political Development.* Lawrence: University Press of Kansas, 2016.

Cammett, Melani Claire. "Partisan Activism and Access to Welfare in Lebanon." *Studies in Comparative International Development* 46 (2011): 70–97.

"Campaign against Plague-Infected Squirrels in California." *Public Health Reports* 26, no. 16 (1911): 544–548.

Carpenter, Daniel P. *The Forging of Bureaucratic Autonomy: Reputations, Networks, and Policy Innovation in Executive Agencies, 1862–1928.* Princeton, NJ: Princeton University Press, 2001.

———. *Reputation and Power: Organizational Image and Pharmaceutical Regulation at the FDA.* Princeton, NJ: Princeton University Press, 2010.

Carter, Marion Hamilton. "The Vampire of the South." *McClure's Magazine* 33, no. 6 (1909): 617–631.

Clark, Lawrence J., Marilyn J. Field, Theodore L. Koontz, and Virginia L. Koontz. "The Impact of Hill–Burton: An Analysis of Hospital Bed and Physician Distribution in the United States, 1950–1970." *Medical Care* 18, no. 5 (1980): 532–550.

Claytor, Thomas A. "The Treatment of Uncinariasis." *Journal of the American Medical Association* 41, no. 5 (1903): 308–313.

Coatney, G. Robert. "Reminiscences: My Forty-Year Romance with Malaria." *Transactions of the Nebraska Academy of Sciences and Affiliated Societies* 13 (1985): 5–11.

Cobb, James C. *The Most Southern Place on Earth: The Mississippi Delta and the Roots of Regional Identity.* New York: Oxford University Press, 1992.

The Commercial and Financial Chronicle, a Weekly Newspaper Representing the Industrial Interests of the United States. Vol. 109. New York: William B. Dana, 1919.

Committee on Public Health and National Quarantine, United States Senate. *Proposed Department of Public Health.* Hearings before the United States Senate Committee on Public Health and National Quarantine, Sixty-First Congress, Second Session. Washington, DC: US Government Printing Office, 1910.

Committee on the Costs of Medical Care. "Editorial and Abstract Summary." *Journal of the American Medical Association* 99, no. 23 (1932): 1950–1952, 1954–1958.

———. *Medical Care for the American People: The Final Report of the Committee on the Costs of Medical Care.* Chicago: University of Chicago Press, 1932.

"Constitutional Law: Discrimination by Private Hospitals Participating in Hill–Burton Program Held to Be Violation of Fifth and Fourteenth Amendments." *Duke Law Journal* 1964, no. 4 (1964): 908–914.

Coogle, C. P. "Methods and Costs of Screening Farm Tenant Homes in Mississippi: Post Flood Malaria Control." *Southern Medical Journal* (1928): 738–747.

Cooper, Jr., John Milton. *Woodrow Wilson: A Biography.* New York: Knopf, 2009.

Cornely, P. B. "Segregation and Discrimination in Medical Care in the United States." *American Journal of Public Health* 46 (1956): 1074–1081.

"Corporal Kelly and His Son." *American Journal of Nursing* 44, no. 4 (1944): 366–370.

Crompton, D. W. T. "The Public Health Importance of Hookworm Disease." *Parasitology* 121 (2000): S39–S50.

Crosby, Alfred W. *America's Forgotten Pandemic: The Influenza of 1918.* 2nd ed. New York: Cambridge University Press, 2003.

"The Crushing Irony of De Luxe Jim Crow." *Journal of the National Medical Association* 44, no. 5 (1952): 386–387.

Cunningham, Robert, III, and Robert Cunningham Jr. *The Blues: A History of the Blue Cross and Blue Shield System.* DeKalb: Northern Illinois University Press, 1997.

Davidson, Stephen M. *A New Era in US Health Care: Critical Next Steps under the Affordable Care Act.* Stanford, CA: Stanford University Press, 2013.

Davis, Michael M. *Medical Care for Tomorrow.* New York: Harper & Brothers, 1955.

"Declaration of the Principles of the Progressive Party." In *Progressive Principles: Selections from Addresses Made During the Presidential Campaign of 1912,* edited by Elmer H. Youngman, 314–330. London: Effingham Wilson, 1913.

Dehner, George. *Influenza: A Century of Science and Public Health Response.* Pittsburgh, PA: University of Pittsburgh Press, 2012.

Deklein, William. "Recent Health Observations in the Mississippi Flood Area." *American Journal of Public Health* 18, no. 2 (1928): 145–151.

DeKruif, Paul. *The Fight for Life.* New York: Harcourt, Brace, 1938.

———. *Hunger Fighters.* New York: Harcourt, Brace, 1928.

Demonstration Work in Rural Sanitation. Hearings before the Committee on Agriculture and Forestry, United States Senate, Seventy-Second Congress, First Session, on S. 1234, a Bill to Authorize an Emergency Appropriation for Special Study of and Demonstration Work in Rural Sanitation. Washington, DC: US Government Printing Office, 1932.

Derickson, Alan. *Health Security for All: Dreams of Universal Health Care in America.* Baltimore, MD: Johns Hopkins University Press, 2005.

———. "The House of Falk: The Paranoid Style in American Health Politics." *American Journal of Public Health* 87, no. 11 (1997): 1836–1843.

DeWitt, Larry. "The Decision to Exclude Agricultural and Domestic Workers from the 1935 Social Security Act." *Social Security Bulletin* 70, no. 4 (2010): 49–68.

Dillon, Nara. "Middlemen in the Chinese Welfare State: The Role of Philanthropists in Refugee Relief in Wartime Shanghai." *Studies in Comparative International Development* 46 (2011): 22–45.

Dock, George, and Charles C. Bass. *Hookworm Disease: Etiology, Pathology, Diagnosis, Prognosis, Prophylaxis, and Treatment.* St. Louis, MO: C. V. Mosby, 1910.

Doyle, Don H. *New Cities, New Men, New South: Atlanta, Nashville, Charleston, Mobile, 1860–1910.* Chapel Hill: University of North Carolina Press, 1990.

Draper, Warren F. "A National Health Program." *New England Journal of Medicine* 220, no. 2 (1939): 43–47.

Duffy, John. *The Sanitarians: A History of American Public Health.* Urbana: University of Illinois Press, 1990.

Dulles, Foster Rhea. *The American Red Cross: A History.* New York: Harper & Brothers, 1953.

Economic Security Act [Committee on Finance]. Hearings before the Committee on Finance, United States Senate, Seventy-Fourth Congress, First Session, on S. 1130, a Bill to Alleviate the Hazards of Old Age, Unemployment, Illness, and Dependency, to Establish a Social Insurance Board in the Department of Labor, to Raise Revenue, and for Other Purposes. Washington, DC: US Government Printing Office, 1935.

Economic Security Act [Committee on Ways and Means]. Hearings before the Committee on Ways and Means, House of Representatives, Seventy-Fourth Congress, First Session, on HR 4120, a Bill to Alleviate the Hazards of Old Age, Unemployment, Illness, and Dependency, to Establish a Social Insurance Board in the Department of Labor, to Raise Revenue, and for Other Purposes. Washington, DC: US Government Printing Office, 1935.

Eisenhower, Milton E., ed. *United States Department of Agriculture, Yearbook of Agriculture 1931.* Washington, DC: US Government Printing Office, 1931.

Elman, Cheryl, Robert McGuire, and Barbara Wittman. "Extending Public Health: The Rockefeller Sanitary Commission and Hookworm in the American South." *American Journal of Public Health* 104, no. 1 (2014): 47–58.

Emergency Appropriation for Cooperation with State Health Departments in Rural Sanitation, etc. Hearing before the Committee on Agriculture and Forestry, United States Senate, Seventy-First Congress, Third Session, on S. 5440, a Bill to Authorize an Emergency Appropriation for Special Study of, and Demonstration Work in, Rural Sanitation. Washington, DC: US Government Printing Office, 1931.

Espinosa, Mariola. *Epidemic Invasions: Yellow Fever and the Limits of Cuban Independence, 1878–1930.* Chicago: University of Chicago Press, 2009.

Etheridge, Elizabeth W. *The Butterfly Caste: A Social History of Pellagra in the South.* Westport, CT: Greenwood, 1972.

———. *Sentinel for Health: A History of the Centers for Disease Control.* Berkeley: University of California Press, 1992.

Ettling, John. *The Germ of Laziness*. Cambridge, MA: Harvard University Press, 1981.

Ewing, Oscar R. "The President's Health Program and the Negro." *Journal of Negro Education* 18, no. 3 (1949): 436–443.

Ezdorf, R. H. von. "Demonstrations of Malaria Control." *Public Health Reports* 31, no. 10 (1916): 614–629.

Falk, I. S. "Proposals for National Health Insurance in the USA: Origins and Evolution, and Some Perceptions for the Future." *Milbank Memorial Fund Quarterly* 55, no. 2 (1977): 161–191.

Farley, John. *To Cast Out Disease*. New York: Oxford University Press, 2004.

Faust, E. C. "Malaria Mortality in the Southern United States for the Year 1937." In *Malaria and Its Control: Some Papers Read at the 21st Meeting of the National Malaria Committee, Oklahoma City, Okla., Nov. 15–18, 1938*. Tallahassee, FL: National Malaria Committee, 1939.

"Federal Voluntary Health Insurance Bill: A Condensation Prepared by the Bureau of Legal Medicine and Legislation, American Medical Association, April 1, 1949." *Journal of the American Medical Association* 139, no. 15 (1949): 1007–1008.

Ferrell, John, and Pauline Mead. *History of County Health Organizations in the United States, 1908–33*. Public Health Bulletin No. 222. Washington, DC: US Government Printing Office, 1936.

Finegold, Kenneth, and Theda Skocpol. *State and Party in America's New Deal*. Madison: University of Wisconsin Press, 1995.

First Deficiency Appropriation Bill, 1928. Hearing before the Subcommittee of House Committee on Appropriations in Charge of Deficiency Appropriations, Seventieth Congress, First Session. Washington, DC: US Government Printing Office, 1927.

Fishback, Price, and Shawn Kantor. *A Prelude to the Welfare State: The Origins of Workers' Compensation*. Chicago: University of Chicago Press, 2000.

Fishbein, Morris. "American Medicine and the National Health Program." Speech given December 13, 1938. *New England Journal of Medicine* 220, no. 12 (1939): 495–504.

Fisher, Irving. *Memorial Relating to the Conservation of Human Life*. Washington, DC: US Government Printing Office, 1912.

Flood Control. Hearings before the Committee on Flood Control, House of Representatives, Seventieth Congress, First Session, on the Control of the Destructive Flood Waters of the United States. Washington, DC: US Government Printing Office, 1928.

Fox, Daniel. "Abraham Flexner's Unpublished Report: Foundations and Medical Education, 1909–1928." *Bulletin of the History of Medicine* 54, no. 4 1980): 475–496.

———. *Health Policies, Politics: The British and American Experience, 1911–1965*. Princeton, NJ: Princeton University Press, 1986.

———. "The Politics of the NIH Extramural Program, 1937–1950." *Journal of the History of Medicine* 42, no. 4 (1987): 447–466.

———. *Power and Illness: The Failure of American Health Policy*. Berkeley: University of California Press, 1993.

Francis, Megan Ming. *Civil Rights and the Making of the Modern American State*. New York: Cambridge University Press, 2014.

Frankel, Lee. "Some Fundamental Considerations in Health Insurance." In *Proceedings of the Conference on Social Insurance, Called by the Industrial Accident Boards and Commissions, Washington, DC, December 5 to 9, 1916*, 598–605. Washington, DC: US Government Printing Office, 1917.

Furman, Bess. *A Profile of the United States Public Health Service, 1798–1948*. Washington, DC: US Department of Health, Education, and Welfare, National Institutes of Health, National Library of Medicine, 1973.

The General Education Board: An Account of Its Activities, 1902–1914. 3rd ed. New York: General Education Board, 1916.

Goldberger, Joseph. "The Cause and Prevention of Pellagra." In Terris, *Goldberger on Pellagra*.

———. "The Etiology of Pellagra: The Significance of Certain Epidemiological Observations with Respect Thereto." In Terris, *Goldberger on Pellagra*.

Goldberger, Joseph, and Edgar Sydenstricker. "Pellagra in the Mississippi Flood Area: Report of an Inquiry Relating to the Prevalence of Pellagra in the Area Affected by the Overflow of the Mississippi and Its Tributaries in Tennessee, Arkansas, Mississippi, and Louisiana in the Spring of 1927." In Terris, *Goldberger on Pellagra*.

Goldberger, Joseph, C. H. Waring, and David G. Willets. "The Prevention of Pellagra: A Test of Diet among Institutional Inmates." In Terris, *Goldberger on Pellagra*.

Goldberger, Joseph, and G. A. Wheeler. "The Experimental Production of Pellagra in Human Subjects by Means of Diet." In Terris, *Goldberger on Pellagra*, 64–94.

Goldberger, Joseph, G. A. Wheeler, and Edgar Sydenstricker. "A Study of the Relation of Family Income and Other Economic Factors to Pellagra Incidence in Seven Cotton-Mill Villages of South Carolina in 1916." In Terris, *Goldberger on Pellagra*, 225–267.

Goldstein, David. "Obituary: Warren Fales Draper, MD, 1883–1970." *Archives of Environmental Health: An International Journal* 21, no. 2 (1970): 230.

Gostin, Lawrence O. *Public Health Law: Power, Duty, Restraint*. 2nd ed. Berkeley: University of California Press, 2008.

Gottschalk, Marie. *The Shadow Welfare State: Labor, Business, and the Politics of Health Care in the United States*. Ithaca, NY: ILR Press/Cornell University Press, 2000.

Grantham, Dewey W. *The South in Modern America: A Region at Odds*. Edited by Henry Steele Commager and Richard B. Morris. New York: HarperCollins, 1994.

Green, Frederick. "The Social Responsibilities of Modern Medicine." *Journal of the American Medical Association* 76, no. 22 (1921): 1477–1483.

Gregory, James N. *The Southern Diaspora: How the Great Migration of Black and White Southerners Transformed America*. Chapel Hill: University of North Carolina Press, 2005.

Grey, Michael R. *New Deal Medicine: The Rural Health Programs of the Farm Security Administration*. Baltimore, MD: Johns Hopkins University Press, 1999.

Griffitts, T. H. D. "Henry Rose Carter: The Scientist and the Man." *Southern Medical Journal* 32, no. 8 (1939): 841–848.

Grossmann, Matt. *Artists of the Possible: Governing Networks and American Policy Change since 1945*. New York: Oxford University Press, 2014.

Grubbs, Samuel B. *By Order of the Surgeon General*. Greenfield, IN: William Mitchell, 1943.

Hacker, Jacob S. *The Divided Welfare State: The Battle over Public and Private Social Benefits in the United States*. New York: Cambridge University Press, 2002.

———. "The Historical Logic of National Health Insurance: Structure and Sequence in the Development of British, Canadian, and US Medical Policy." *Studies in American Political Development* 12 (1998): 57–130.

———. *The Road to Nowhere: The Genesis of President Clinton's Plan for Health Security*. Princeton, NJ: Princeton University Press, 1997.

Hamilton, Diane. "The Cost of Caring: The Metropolitan Life Insurance Company's Visiting Nurse Service, 1909–1953." *Bulletin of the History of Medicine* 63 (1989): 414–434.

Hamovitch, Maurice. "History of the Movement for Compulsory Health Insurance in the United States." *Social Service Review* 27, no. 3 (1953): 281–299.

Hanson, Russell L. "Medicaid and the Politics of Redistribution." *American Journal of Political Science* 28, no. 2 (1984): 313–339.

Harrison, Mark. *Contagion: How Commerce Has Spread Disease*. New Haven, CT: Yale University Press, 2012.

Hatchett, Richard J., Carter E. Mecher, and Marc Lipsitch. "Public Health Interventions and Epidemic Intensity during the 1919 Influenza Pandemic." *Proceedings of the National Academy of Sciences of the United States of America* 104, no. 18 (2007): 7582–7587.

Health Insurance Association of America. *Source Book of Health Insurance Data, 1984–1985*. Washington, DC: Health Insurance Association of America.

Hegyi, Juraj, Robert A. Schwartz, and Vladimir Hegyi. "Pellagra: Dermatitis, Dementia, and Diarrhea." *International Journal of Dermatology* 43 (2004): 1–5.

Henderson, Donald. "Eradication: Lessons from the Past." *Bulletin of the World Health Organization* 76 (1998): 7–21.

Higgs, Robert. *Competition and Coercion: Blacks in the American Economy, 1865–1914*. New York: Cambridge University Press, 1977.

"Highlights from the 1959 Report of the Communicable Disease Center." *Public Health Reports (1896–1970)* 75, no. 12 (1960): 1171–1172.

"The Hill Bill for Extension of Medical Care." *Journal of the American Medical Association* 139, no. 15 (1949): 1005.

"The Hill–Burton Hospital Construction Bill." *Journal of the American Medical Association* 129, no. 12 (1945): 804.

Hirshfield, Daniel S. *The Lost Reform: The Campaign for Compulsory Health Insurance in the United States from 1932 to 1943*. Cambridge, MA: Harvard University Press, 1970.

Hoffman, Beatrix. *Health Care for Some: Rights and Rationing in the United States since 1930*. Chicago: University of Chicago Press, 2012.

———. *The Wages of Sickness: The Politics of Health Insurance in Progressive America*. Chapel Hill: University of North Carolina Press, 2001.

Hollings, Ernest, and Kirk Victor. *Making Government Work*. Columbia: University of South Carolina Press, 2008.

Hornblum, Allen M. "They Were Cheap and Available: Prisoners as Research Subjects in Twentieth Century America." *BMJ* 315 (1997): 1437–1441.

"Hospital Discrimination Must End!" *Journal of the National Medical Association* 45, no. 4 (1953): 284–286.

Humphreys, Margaret. "How Four Once Common Diseases Were Eliminated from the American South." *Health Affairs (Milwood)* 28, no. 6 (2009): 1734–1744.

———. "Kicking a Dying Dog: DDT and the Demise of Malaria in the American South." *Isis* 87, no. 1 (1996): 1–17.

———. *Malaria: Poverty, Race, and Public Health in the United States.* Baltimore, MD: Johns Hopkins University Press, 2001.

———. *Yellow Fever and the South.* Baltimore, MD: Johns Hopkins University Press, 1992.

Huthmacher, Joseph. *Senator Robert F. Wagner and the Rise of Urban Liberalism.* New York: Atheneum, 1968.

"International Technical Assistance in Public Health." *Public Health Reports* 67, no. 4 (1952): 333–357.

Jacobs, Larry. *The Health of Nations: Public Opinion and the Making of Health Policy in the US and Britain.* Ithaca, NY: Cornell University Press, 1993.

———. "Politics of America's Supply State: Health Reform and Technology." *Health Affairs (Milwood)* 14, no. 2 (1995): 143–157.

Jones, James H. *Bad Blood: The Tuskegee Syphilis Experiment.* New York: Free Press, 1993.

Katznelson, Ira. *Fear Itself: The New Deal and the Origins of Our Time.* New York: Liveright, 2013.

Katznelson, Ira, Kim Geiger, and Daniel Kryder. "Limiting Liberalism: The Southern Veto in Congress, 1933–1950." *Political Science Quarterly* 108, no. 2 (1993): 283–306.

Katznelson, Ira, and Martin Shefter, eds. *Shaped by War and Trade: International Influences on American Political Development.* Princeton, NJ: Princeton University Press, 2002.

Kelly, Alfred, Winfred Harbison, and Herman Belz. *The American Constitution: Its Origins and Development.* 7th ed. Vol. 2. New York: Norton, 1991.

Kempner, Walter. "Some Effects of the Rice Diet Treatment of Kidney Disease and Hypertension." *Bulletin of the New York Academy of Medicine* 22, no. 7 (1946): 358–370.

Kennedy, David M. *Freedom from Fear: The American People in Depression and War, 1929–1945.* New York: Oxford University Press, 1999.

Key, V. O. *Southern Politics in State and Nation.* 1949. New ed., Knoxville: University of Tennessee Press, 1984.

King, Willford I. "Edgar Sydenstricker." *Journal of the American Statistical Association* 31, no. 194 (1936): 411–414.

Kitchens, Carl. "The Effects of the Works Progress Administration's Anti-malaria Programs in Georgia, 1932–1947." *Explorations in Economic History* 50, no. 4 (2013): 567–581.

Kocher, Robert, and Eli Adashi. "Hospital Readmissions and the Affordable Care Act: Paying for Coordinated Quality Care." *Journal of the American Medical Association* 306, no. 16 (2011): 1794–1795.

Kooijman, Jaap. . . . *And the Pursuit of National Health*. Amsterdam: Rodopi, 1999.

Krajcinovic, Ivana. *From Company Doctors to Managed Care: The United Mine Workers' Noble Experiment*. Ithaca, NY: ILR Press/Cornell University Press, 1997.

Langer, Elinor. "Hospital Discrimination: HEW Criticized by Civil Rights Groups." *Science* 149, no. 3690 (1965): 1355–1357.

———. "Hospital Integration: Equality versus Availability." *Science* 152, no. 3730 (1966): 1727.

Langmuir, Alexander, and Justin Andrews. "Biological Warfare Defense: The Epidemic Intelligence Service of the Communicable Disease Center." *American Journal of Public Health* 42 (1952): 235–238.

Lavinder, C. H. "Pellagra: Brief Comments on Our Present Knowledge of the Disease." *Public Health Reports* 28, no. 47 (1913): 2461–2463.

———. "The Theory of the Parasitic Origin of Pellagra." *Public Health Reports* 25, no. 22 (1910): 735–737.

LePrince, J. A. "The Aftermath of Malaria Control in Extra-cantonment Areas." *Southern Medical Journal* 13, no. 6 (1920): 413–416.

———. "Co-operative Antimalaria Campaigns in the United States in 1920." *Southern Medical Journal* 14, no. 4 (1921): 297–306.

———. "Mosquito Control about Cantonments and Shipyards." *Public Health Reports* 34, no. 12 (1919): 547–553.

LePrince, Joseph A., and A. J. Orenstein. *Mosquito Control in Panama: The Eradication of Malaria and Yellow Fever in Cuba and Panama*. New York: G. P. Putnam's Sons, 1916.

"LePrince, Malaria Fighter." *Public Health Reports* 71, no. 8 (1956): 756–758.

Lieberman, Evan. *Boundaries of Contagion: How Ethnic Politics Have Shaped Government Responses to Aids*. Princeton, NJ: Princeton University Press, 2009.

Lieberman, Robert. "Race, Institutions, and the Administration of Social Policy." *Social Science History* 19, no. 4 (1995): 514–515.

———. *Shifting the Color Line: Race and the American Welfare State*. Cambridge, MA: Harvard University Press, 2001.

Link, William A. *The Paradox of Southern Progressivism, 1880–1930*. Chapel Hill: University of North Carolina Press, 1992.

Lodge, Henry Cabot. *The War with Spain*. New York: Harper & Brothers, 1899.

Lord, Alexandra M. *Condom Nation: The US Government's Sex Education Campaign from World War I to the Internet*. Baltimore, MD: Johns Hopkins University Press, 2010.

Lubove, Roy. *The Struggle for Social Security, 1900–1935*. Cambridge, MA: Harvard University Press, 1968.

Lumsden, L. L. "Cooperative Rural Health Work of the Public Health Service . . . ," fiscal years 1920–1922, 1927–1930. *Public Health Reports*, 1920–1922, 1927–1930.

———. "Public Health and Private Practice." In *Transactions of the Section on Preventive Medicine and Public Health of the American Medical Association at the Seventy-Second Annual Session, Held at Boston, Mass., June 6 to 10, 1921*. Chicago: American Medical Association Press, 1921.

———. "Rural Hygiene." Lecture delivered May 22, 1919, New York City. *Public Health Reports* 34, no. 45 (1919): 2518–2538.

———. *Rural Sanitation: A Report on Special Studies Made in 15 Counties in 1914, 1915, 1916*. Public Health Bulletin No. 94. Washington, DC: US Government Printing Office, 1918.

Lumsden, L. L., Norman Roberts, and Charles Wardell Stiles. "Preliminary Note on a Simple and Inexpensive Apparatus for Use in Safe Disposal of Night Soil." *Public Health Reports* 25, no. 45 (1910): 1619–1623.

MacKenzie, Frederick. "The Legislative Campaign in New York for the 'Welfare Bills.'" *American Labor Legislation Review* 10 (1920): 136–149.

"Malaria: A Serious Health Problem of Nation-wide Concern." *Public Health Reports* 34, no. 12 (1919): 543–546.

Malaria Control in War Areas, 1942–43, and *Malaria Control in War Areas, 1943–44*. Atlanta, GA: US Public Health Service, 1943, 1944.

Marks, Harry M. "Epidemiologists Explain Pellagra: Gender, Race, and Political Economy in the Work of Edgar Sydenstricker." *Journal of the History of Medicine* 58 (2003): 34–55.

Marmor, Theodore. *The Politics of Medicare*. 2nd ed. Hawthorne, NY: Aldine de Gruyter, 2000.

Maslow, Harold. "The Background of the Wagner National Health Bill." *Law and Contemporary Problems* 6 (1939): 606–618.

Masterson, Karen. *The Malaria Project: The US Government's Secret Mission to Find a Miracle Cure*. New York: New American Library, 2014.

Maxcy, Kenneth F. "The Distribution of Malaria in the United States as Indicated by Mortality Reports." *Public Health Reports* 38, no. 21 (1923): 1125–1138.

Merriam, Charles. "The National Resources Planning Board: A Chapter in American Planning Experience." *American Political Science Review* 38, no. 6 (1944): 1075–1088.

Mettler, Suzanne. *The Submerged State: How Invisible Government Policies Undermine American Democracy*. Chicago: University of Chicago Press, 2011.

Mickey, Robert. "Dr. StrangeRove; or, How Conservatives Learned to Stop Worrying and Love Community Health Centers." In *The Health Care "Safety Net" in a Post-reform World*, edited by Mark Hall and Sara Rosenbaum, 21–66. New Brunswick, NJ: Rutgers University Press, 2012.

———. *Paths out of Dixie: The Democratization of Authoritarian Enclaves in America's Deep South, 1944–1972*. Princeton, NJ: Princeton University Press, 2015.

Moehling, Carolyn, and Melissa Thomasson. "The Political Economy of Saving Mothers and Babies: The Politics of State Participation in the Sheppard–Towner Program." *Journal of Economic History* 72, no. 1 (2012): 75–103.

Moore, John Robert. "Senator Josiah W. Bailey and the 'Conservative Manifesto' of 1937." *Journal of Southern History* 31, no. 1 (1965): 21–39.

Mott, F. D., and M. I. Roemer. "A Federal Program of Public Health and Medical Services for Migratory Farm Workers." *Public Health Reports* 60, no. 9 (1945): 229–249.

———. *Rural Health and Medical Care*. New York: McGraw-Hill, 1948.

Mountin, Joseph. "The Evolving Pattern of Tomorrow's Health." *American Journal of Public Health* 33 (1943): 1401–1407.

Mullan, Fitzhugh. *Plagues and Politics: The Story of the United States Public Health Service*. New York: Basic Books, 1989.

Muncy, Robyn. *Relentless Reformer: Josephine Roche and Progressivism in Twentieth-Century America.* Princeton, NJ: Princeton University Press, 2015.

Nackenoff, Carol, and Julie Novkov. "Statebuilding in the Progressive Era: A Continuing Dilemma in American Political Development." In *Statebuilding from the Margins: Between Reconstruction and the New Deal,* edited by Carol Nackenoff and Julie Novkov, 1–31. Philadelphia: University of Pennsylvania Press, 2014.

Nájera, Jose, Matiana González-Silva, and Pedro Alonso. "Some Lessons from the Future from the Global Malaria Eradication Programme (1955–1969)." *PLoS Medicine* 8, no. 1 (2011): e1000412.

National Emergency Council. *Report on Economic Conditions of the South.* Washington, DC: US Government Printing Office, 1938.

National Public Health. Papers, Opinions, Letters, etc., Relative to the National Public Health, in the Consideration of Senate Bill (S. 6049), "a Bill Establishing a Department of Public Health, and for Other Purposes." 61st Congress, 2nd Session, Senate Document 637. Washington, DC: US Government Printing Office, 1910.

Neustadt, Richard, and Harvey Fineberg. *The Epidemic that Never Was: Policy-making and the Swine Flu Affair.* New York: Vintage Books, 1983.

Novak, William J. *The People's Welfare: Law and Regulation in Nineteenth-Century America.* Chapel Hill: University of North Carolina Press, 1996.

Numbers, Ronald L. *Almost Persuaded: American Physicians and Compulsory Health Insurance, 1912–1920.* Baltimore, MD: Johns Hopkins University Press, 1978.

Oberlander, Jonathan. *The Political Life of Medicare.* Chicago: University of Chicago Press, 2003.

———. "Through the Looking Glass: The Politics of the Medicare Prescription Drug, Improvement, and Modernization Act." *Journal of Health Politics, Policy, and Law* 32, no. 2 (2007): 187–219.

Oberlander, Jonathan, and Barbara Lyons. "Beyond Incrementalism? SCHIP and the Politics of Health Reform." *Health Affairs (Milwood)* 28 (2009): w399–w410.

Official Congressional Directory, for the Use of the United States Congress, 66th Congress, 2nd Session, Beginning December 1, 1919. Washington, DC: Government Printing Office, 1920.

Olson, Laura Katz. *The Politics of Medicaid.* New York: Columbia University Press, 2010.

O'Neill, J. H. "Relief Measures During and Following the Mississippi Valley Flood." *American Journal of Public Health* 18, no. 2 (1928): 154–160.

Orren, Karen, and Stephen Skowronek. *The Search for American Political Development.* New York: Cambridge University Press, 2004.

Owen, Robert L. "The Conservation of Life and Health." *Life and Health* 25, no. 6 (1910): 325.

Parascandola, John. "The Public Health Service and the Control of Biologics." *Public Health Reports* 110, no. 6 (1995): 110–111.

Parran, Thomas, Jr. "A Career in Public Health." *Public Health Reports* 67, no. 10 (1952): 930–943.

———. "Cooperative County Health Work." *Public Health Reports* (1925): 983–992.

———. "The Health of the Nation." *American Journal of Public Health* 28 (1938): 1375–1380.

————. *The Health of the Nation: Report of the Surgeon General of the US Public Health Service, Federal Security Agency, before the Subcommittee of the Committee on Appropriations, House of Representatives, Seventy-Eighth Congress, Second Session*. Washington, DC: US Government Printing Office, 1944.

————. "A New Health Program for New York State." *Journal of the American Medical Association* 97, no. 11 (1931): 763–766.

————. "Public Medical Care in New York State." *Journal of the American Medical Association* 101, no. 5 (1933): 342–345.

————. "Public Responsibility for Public and Personal Health: The Biggs Health Center Plan of 1920 in Retrospect." *Bulletin of the New York Academy of Medicine* 11, no. 9 (1935): 533–548.

Patterson, Gordon. *The Mosquito Crusades: A History of the American Anti-mosquito Movement from the Reed Commission to the First Earth Day*. New Brunswick, NJ: Rutgers University Press, 2009.

Pearce, Donna. "Rapid Treatment Centers: For Venereal Disease Control." *American Journal of Nursing* 43, no. 7 (1943): 658–660.

Perkins, Frances. *The Roosevelt I Knew*. New York: Viking, 1946.

Pierce, C. C. "Public Health Service Program for Nation-wide Control of Venereal Disease." *Public Health Reports* 34, no. 20 (1919): 1056–1062.

Pierson, Paul. *Politics in Time: History, Institutions, and Social Analysis*. Princeton, NJ: Princeton University Press, 2004.

Poen, Monte. *Harry S. Truman versus the Medical Lobby: The Genesis of Medicare*. Columbia: University of Missouri Press, 1979.

Polsby, Nelson W. *How Congress Evolves: Social Bases of Institutional Change*. New York: Oxford University Press, 2004.

"Proceedings of the Special Session: Minutes of the Special Session of the House of Delegates of the American Medical Association, Held at Chicago, September 16–17, 1938." *Journal of the American Medical Association* 111, no. 13 (1938): 1191–1217.

"Professional Associations on the Proposed National Health Program." *Social Service Review* 12, no. 4 (1938): 693–697.

Quadagno, Jill. *The Color of Welfare: How Racism Undermined the War on Poverty*. New York: Oxford University Press, 1994.

————. *One Nation, Uninsured: Why the US Has No National Health Insurance*. New York: Oxford University Press, 2005.

————. "Promoting Civil Rights through the Welfare State: How Medicare Integrated Southern Hospitals." *Social Problems* 47, no. 1 (2000): 68–89.

Quadagno, Jill, and Debra Street. "Ideology and Public Policy: Antistatism in American Welfare State Transformation." *Journal of Policy History* 17, no. 1 (2005): 52–71.

Report to the President of the Committee on Economic Security. Washington, DC: US Government Printing Office, 1935.

Reverby, Susan. "'Normal Exposure' and Inoculation Syphilis: A PHS 'Tuskegee' Doctor in Guatemala, 1946–1948." *Journal of Policy History* 23, no. 1 (2011): 6–28.

Risse, Guenter B. *Plague, Fear, and Politics in San Francisco's Chinatown*. Baltimore, MD: Johns Hopkins University Press, 2012.

Robertson, David Brian. *Federalism and the Making of America*. New York: Routledge, 2012.

Rockefeller Foundation. *Annual Report for 1927*. New York: Rockefeller Foundation, 1927.

Rockefeller Foundation International Health Board. *Third Annual Report, January 1, 1916–December 31, 1916*, and *Seventh Annual Report, January 1, 1920–December 31, 1920*. New York: Rockefeller Foundation, 1917, 1921.

Rockefeller Sanitary Commission for the Eradication of Hookworm Disease. Second to fifth annual reports. Washington, DC: Rockefeller Sanitary Commission for the Eradication of Hookworm Disease, 1911–1915.

Rodgers, Daniel T. *Atlantic Crossings: Social Politics in a Progressive Age*. Cambridge, MA: Belknap Press, 1998.

Roe, Daphne A. *A Plague of Corn: The Social History of Pellagra*. Ithaca, NY: Cornell University Press, 1973.

Roosevelt, Theodore. "A Confession of Faith: Address before the National Convention of the Progressive Party in Chicago, August 6, 1912." In *Progressive Principles: Selections from Addresses Made During the Presidential Campaign of 1912*, edited by Elmer H. Youngman, 115–173. London: Effingham Wilson, 1913.

Rorty, James. "Health under the Social Security Tent." *Antioch Review* 3, no. 4 (1943): 498–511.

Rosen, George. *A History of Public Health*. Baltimore, MD: Johns Hopkins University Press, 1993.

Rosenberg, Charles E. "Social Class and Medical Care in Nineteenth-Century America: The Rise and Fall of the Dispensary." *Journal of the History of Medicine* 29, no. 1 (1974): 32–54.

Rubinow, I. M. "Review: *Health Insurance* by B. S. Warren and Edgar Sydenstricker." *American Economic Review* 6, no. 4 (1916): 936–939.

———. "Standards of Sickness Insurance: I." *Journal of Political Economy* 23, no. 3 (1915): 221–251.

Ruggles, Steven, J. Trent Alexander, Katie Genadek, Ronald Goeken, Matthew B. Schroeder, and Matthew Sobek. *Integrated Public Use Microdata Series: Version 5.0*. Machine-readable database. Minneapolis: University of Minnesota, 2010.

Rural Sanitation. Hearings before the Committee on Agriculture of the House of Representatives, Sixty-Fifth Congress, Third Session, February 17, 1919. Washington, DC: US Government Printing Office, 1919.

Saldin, Robert P. *War, the American State, and Politics since 1898*. New York: Cambridge University Press, 2011.

Sanders, Elizabeth. *Roots of Reform: Farmers, Workers, and the American State, 1877–1917*. Chicago: University of Chicago Press, 1999.

Sardell, Alice. *The US Experiment in Social Medicine: The Community Health Center Program, 1965–1986*. Pittsburgh, PA: University of Pittsburgh Press, 1988.

Schickler, Eric, and Devin Caughey. "Public Opinion, Organized Labor, and the Limits of New Deal Liberalism, 1936–1945." *Studies in American Political Development* 25 (2011): 162–189.

Schlesinger, Arthur, Jr. *The Coming of the New Deal*. Boston: Mariner, 2003.

Schmeckebier, Laurence F. *The Public Health Service: Its History, Activities and Organization*. Baltimore, MD: Johns Hopkins University Press, 1923.

Schulman, Bruce J. *From Cotton Belt to Sunbelt: Federal Policy, Economic Development, and the Transformation of the South, 1938–1980*. New York: Oxford University Press, 1991.

Sealander, Judith. *Private Wealth and Public Life: Foundation Philanthropy and the Reshaping of American Social Policy from the Progressive Era to the New Deal*. Baltimore, MD: Johns Hopkins University Press, 1997.

Searcy, George H. "An Epidemic of Acute Pellagra." *Journal of the American Medical Association* 49, no. 1 (1907): 37–38.

Second Deficiency Appropriation Bill, 1928. Hearing before the Subcommittee of House Committee on Appropriations in Charge of Deficiency Appropriations, Seventh Congress, First Session. Washington, DC: US Government Printing Office, 1928.

Shaw, Frederic, Chisara Asomugha, Patrick Conway, and Andrew Rein. "The Patient Protection and Affordable Care Act: Opportunities for Prevention and Public Health." *Lancet* 384, no. 9937 (2014): 75–82.

Skocpol, Theda. *Boomerang: Health Reform and the Turn against Government*. New York: Norton, 1997.

———. *Protecting Soldiers and Mothers: The Political Origins of Social Policy in the United States*. Cambridge, MA: Belknap Press, 1992.

Sledge, Daniel, and George Mohler. "Eliminating Malaria in the American South." *American Journal of Public Health* (2013).

Smillie, Wilson G. *Public Health: Its Promise for the Future*. 1955. Reprint, New York: Arno Press, 1976.

Snyder, Lynne Page. "New York, the Nation, the World: The Career of Surgeon General Thomas J. Parran Jr., MD (1892–1968)." *Public Health Reports* 110 (1995): 630–632.

———. "Passage and Significance of the 1944 Public Health Service Act." *Public Health Reports* 109, no. 6 (1994): 721–724.

Starr, Paul. *Remedy and Reaction: The Peculiar American Struggle over Health Care Reform*. New Haven, CT: Yale University Press, 2011.

———. *The Social Transformation of American Medicine*. New York: Basic Books, 1982.

State Board of Health of South Carolina. *Thirty-Third Annual Report of the State Board of Health of South Carolina, for the Fiscal Year 1912*. Columbia, SC: Gonzales and Bryan, 1913.

Stiles, Charles Wardell. "Decrease of Hookworm in the United States." *Public Health Reports* 45, no. 31 (1930): 1763–1781.

———. "Early History, in Part Esoteric, of the Hookworm (Uncinariasis) Campaign in Our Southern United States." *Journal of Parasitology* 25, no. 4 (1939): 283–308.

———. "Hookworm Disease in Its Relation to the Negro." *Public Health Reports* 24, no. 31 (1909): 1083–1089.

———. "Hook-worm Disease in the South—Frequency of Infection by the Parasite (*Uncinaria americana*) in Rural Districts." *Public Health Reports* 17, no. 43 (1902): 2433–2434.

———. "The Industrial Conditions of the Tenant Class (White and Black) as Influenced by the Medical Conditions." In *The South in the Building of the Nation*, 594–601. Richmond, VA: Southern Historical Publication Society, 1909.

———. "The Medical Influence of the Negro in Connection with Anemia in the White, Address Given to the North Carolina Board of Health and State Medical Society, June 17, 1908." In *Biennial Report of the North Carolina Board of Health, 1907–1908*, 22–28. Raleigh, NC: E. M. Uzzell, 1909.

———. *Report upon the Prevalence and Geographic Distribution of Hookworm Diseases (Uncinariasis or Ancylostomiasis) in the United States*. Washington, DC: US Government Printing Office, 1903.

———. *The Significance of the Recent American Cases of Hookworm Disease (Uncinariasis, or Ancylostomiasis) in Man*. Washington, DC: US Government Printing Office, 1902.

———. "The Significance of the Recently Recognized Hookworm Disease for the Texas Practitioner." In *Transactions of the State Medical Association of Texas, Thirty-Fifth Annual Session, Held at San Antonio, Texas, April 28th, 29th, 30th and May 1st, 1903*, 353–445. Austin, TX: Von Boeckman-Jones, 1903.

Stobbe, Mike. *Surgeon General's Warning: How Politics Crippled the Nation's Doctor*. Berkeley: University of California Press, 2014.

Sullivan, E. C., and J. S. Wiley. "Sanitation Activities in the Southeastern States in Connection with National Defense." *Public Health Reports* 57, no. 17 (1942): 617–625.

Sullivan, Mark. *Our Times: The United States 1900–1925*. Vol. 3. New York: Charles Scribner's Sons, 1930.

[*Sundry Civil Bill for 1919*]. Hearings before Subcommittee of House Committee on Appropriations in Charge of Sundry Civil Bill for 1919. Washington, DC: US Government Printing Office, 1918.

Sunstein, Cass. *The Second Bill of Rights: FDR's Unfinished Revolution and Why We Need It More than Ever*. Basic Books, 2004.

Sydenstricker, Edgar. "Group Medicine or Health Insurance: Which Comes First?" *American Labor Legislation Review* 24, no. 2 (1934): 79–86.

———. "Health in the New Deal." *Annals of the American Academy of Political and Social Science* 176 (1934): 131–137.

Taft, William Howard. "Sanitation and Health of the South: Remarks at the Georgia–Carolina Fair, Augusta, Georgia, November 8, 1909." In *The Collected Works of William Howard Taft*, edited by David H. Burton, 333–337. Athens: Ohio University Press, 2002.

Terris, Milton. "Hermann Biggs' Contribution to the Modern Concept of the Health Center." *Bulletin of the History of Medicine* 20, no. 3 (1946): 387–412.

———, ed. *Goldberger on Pellagra*. Baton Rouge: Louisiana State University Press, 1964.

Tetzlaff, Frank. "Operation of the United States Public Health Service Malaria Control Program." *Public Health Reports* 63, no. 18 (1948): 557–563.

Thachil, Tariq. *Elite Parties, Poor Voters: How Social Services Win Votes in India*. New York: Cambridge University Press, 2014.

Thomas, Karen Kruse. *Deluxe Jim Crow: Civil Rights and American Health Policy, 1935–1954*. Athens: University of Georgia Press, 2011.

Thomasson, Melissa A. "From Sickness to Health: The Twentieth-Century Development of US Health Insurance." *Explorations in Economic History* 39, no. 3 (2002): 233–252.

———. "The Importance of Group Coverage: How Tax Policy Shaped US Health Insurance." *American Economic Review* 93, no. 4 (2003): 1373-'84.

Tindall, George B. *The Emergence of the New South, 1913–1945.* Baton Rouge: Louisiana State University Press, 1967.

Tisdale, Ellis S. "A National Program for Training Public Health Personnel." *Public Health Reports* 66, no. 42 (1951): 1361–1368.

Tobey, James A. *The National Government and Public Health.* Baltimore, MD: Johns Hopkins University Press, 1926.

Tomes, Nancy J. "American Attitudes towards the Germ Theory of Disease: Phyllis Allen Richmond Revisited." *Journal of the History of Medicine* 52 (1997): 17–50.

Townsend, J. G. "The Full-Time County Health Program Developed in the Mississippi Valley Following the Flood." *Public Health Reports* 43, no. 20 (1928): 1199–1207.

Transactions of National Conference on Pellagra: Held under the Auspices of the State Board of Health of South Carolina at the State Hospital for the Insane, October 29th, 1908. Columbia, SC: State Co. Printers, 1909.

Transactions of the Seventeenth Annual Conference of State and Territorial Health Officers with the United States Public Health Service, Held at Washington, DC, June 4 and 5, 1919. Washington, DC: US Government Printing Office, 1920.

Transactions of the Seventh Annual Conference of State and Territorial Health Officers with the United States Public Health and Marine-Hospital Service, Held June 2, 1909, in Washington, DC. Washington, DC: US Government Printing Office, 1910.

Trask, John W. "Malaria: A Public Health and Economic Problem in the United States." *Public Health Reports* 31, no. 51 (1916): 3445–3452.

Troesken, Werner. *Water, Race, and Disease.* Cambridge, MA: MIT Press, 2004.

Upton, R. G. "Incidence and Severity of Hookworm Infestation in East Texas." *American Journal of Public Health* 26 (1936): 924–926.

United States Department of Agriculture. *Status and Results of Extension Work in the Southern States, 1903–1921.* Circular 248. Washington, DC: US Government Printing Office, 1922.

Vance, Rupert B. *Human Geography of the South: A Study in Regional Resources and Human Adequacy.* 2nd ed. Chapel Hill: University of North Carolina Press, 1932.

Viseltear, Arthur. "Emergence of the Medical Care Section of the American Public Health Association, 1926–1948." *American Journal of Public Health* 63, no. 11 (1973): 986–1007.

Wadsworth, Augustus B. "The Development of the State Department of Health in Relation to Health Insurance and Industrial Hygiene." *American Journal of Public Health* 10, no. 1 (1920): 53–59.

"The Wagner–Murray Bill." *American Journal of Public Health* 33, no. 10 (1943): 1274–1276.

"The Wagner–Murray–Dingell Bill." *American Journal of Nursing* 44, no. 4 (1944): 326–331.

"Wagner–Murray–Dingell Bill for Social Security." *Journal of the American Medical Association* 122, no. 9 (1943): 600–601.

Wainess, F. J. "The Ways and Means of National Health Care Reform, 1974 and Beyond." *Journal of Health Politics, Policy and Law* 24, no. 2 (1999): 305–333.

Waller, C. E. "The Social Security Act in Its Relation to Public Health." *American Journal of Public Health* 25, no. 11 (1935): 1186–1194.

Warner, Margaret. "Local Control versus National Interest: The Debate over Southern Public Health, 1878–1884." *Journal of Southern History* 50, no. 3 (1984): 407–428.

Warren, B. S. "Coordination and Expansion of Federal Health Activities." *Public Health Reports* 34, no. 49 (1919): 2761–2779.

———. "A Unified Health Service." *Public Health Reports* 34, no. 9 (1919): 377–385.

Warren, Benjamin S., and Charles F. Bolduan. "War Activities of the United States Public Health Service." *Public Health Reports* 34, no. 23 (1919): 1243–1267.

Warren, B. S., and Edgar Sydenstricker. *Health Insurance: Its Relation to the Public Health.* Public Health Bulletin 76. Washington, DC: US Government Printing Office, 1916.

———. "Health Insurance, the Medical Profession, and the Public Health: Including the Results of a Study of Sickness Expectancy." *Public Health Reports* 34, no. 16 (1919): 775–789.

Waserman, Manfred. "The Quest for a National Health Department in the Progressive Era." *Bulletin of the History of Medicine* 49, no. 3 (1975): 353–380.

Washburn, Benjamin Earle. *The Hookworm Campaign in Alamance County, North Carolina.* Raleigh, NC: E. M. Uzzell, 1914.

Watkins, J. A. "Extra-cantonment Zone Sanitation, Camp Shelby, near Hattiesburg, Miss." *Public Health Reports* 32, no. 51 (1917): 2149–2164.

Weisz, George. "Epidemiology and Health Care Reform: The National Health Survey of 1935–1936." *American Journal of Public Health* 101, no. 3 (2011): 438–447.

Williams, Louis L. "Civil Works Administration Emergency Relief Administration Malaria Control Program in the South." *American Journal of Public Health* 25, no. 1 (1935): 11–14.

———. "The Extended Malaria Control Program." *Public Health Reports* 60, no. 17 (1945): 464–469.

———. "Report of the Subcommittee on Malaria Prevention Activities, 1937." *Southern Medical Journal* 31 (1938): 818–819.

Winslow, C. E.-A. "The Untilled Fields of Public Health." Canadian Red Cross Society, 1920.

Witte, Edwin E. *The Development of the Social Security Act: A Memorandum on the History of the Committee on Economic Security and Drafting and Legislative History of the Social Security Act.* Madison: University of Wisconsin Press, 1962.

Wolman, Leo. "The Beveridge Report." *Political Science Quarterly* 58, no. 1 (1943): 1–10.

Woodward, C. Vann. *Origins of the New South, 1877–1913.* Baton Rouge: Louisiana State University Press/Littlefield Fund for Southern History of the University of Texas, 2005.

Wray, Matt. *Not Quite White: White Trash and the Boundaries of Whiteness.* Durham, NC: Duke University Press, 2006.

Wright, Gavin. *Old South, New South: Revolutions in the Southern Economy since the Civil War.* Baton Rouge: Louisiana State University Press, 1996.

Ziony, Miriam. "Malaria Control in Iran." *Public Health Reports* 65, no. 11 (1950): 351–367.

INDEX

AALL (American Association for Labor Legislation), 8–9, 46–50, 52–56
ACA (2010 Patient Protection and Affordable Care Act), 3
  incentives for higher-quality care and, 201–202
  Nixon health strategy and, 197
  passage of, 200
  public health funds diverted to Healthcare.gov, 203
accountable care organizations, 201, 203
AFL (American Federation of Labor)
  on Forand bill, 187
  on National Board of Health, 39
  on Progressive-Era health insurance proposal, 52–53
Agee, James, 126–127
Agricultural Adjustment Act, 102–103, 128–129, 132, 135
Altmeyer, Arthur
  CES and, 106, 112–113
  on health insurance during the 1940s, 162, 180
  on hospital insurance for the elderly, 186
  National Health Program and, 141, 143, 145, 149–151, 153
AMA (American Medical Association), 8–12, 25, 64, 96, 196, 198
  Blue's presidential address to, 51–52
  on CCMC majority report, 99–102
  CES and, 106, 108–110, 112–113, 119
  Cumming's wish to become president of, 93
  federal public health efforts and, 5, 98, 111, 120, 157, 174–175
  FERA and, 105
  hospital construction and, 167, 175
  Medicare and, 188
  on National Board of Health, 34, 38–40, 56

  on National Health Program, 141, 149–154
  on 1939 Wagner bill, 155–156
  Parran plan and, 114–119
  on Progressive-Era plans for insurance, 53–55, 56
  resistance to health centers, 86
  on Sheppard–Towner Act, 78
  on Wagner–Murray–Dingell bills, 163–164, 172, 174–177, 179, 181–182, 194
American Association for Labor Legislation. *See* AALL (American Association for Labor Legislation)
American Federation of Labor. *See* AFL (American Federation of Labor)
American Journal of Public Health, editorial on 1943 Wagner–Murray–Dingell bill, 164
American Medical Association. *See* AMA (American Medical Association)
American Public Health Association. *See* APHA (American Public Health Association)
APHA (American Public Health Association), 69, 71, 143, 144, 164
Ashford, Bailey K., 21–22, 38

Bailey, Josiah
  on court-packing plan, 136
  on New Deal, 138–139
  on rural sanitation program, 95
Barkley, Alben, on rural sanitation program, 93, 95
Beveridge, Sir William, 161–162
Bierring, Walter, 109, 118–119
Biggs, Hermann
  community health centers, impact on, 203
  health centers plan, 10, 85–86

national health program and, 11–12, 125–126, 137, 141, 154, 187, 196
cotton
    Agricultural Adjustment Act and, 102, 128–129
    mills, 45, 63, 137
    pellagra and, 45, 77, 88, 89, 132
court-packing plan, 126, 135–136, 139, 153
Cuba, 1–2
    US occupation of and fight against disease in, 17–20, 62, 63, 87
Cumming, Hugh
    Children's Bureau and, 78, 121–122, 143–144
    Lumsden and, 76, 86, 92–93
    Parran as replacement for, 104 (see also Parran, Thomas)
    pellagra and, 77
    Social Security Act and, 121–122
    as surgeon general, 76
Cushing, Harvey, 109, 118, 120
CWA (Civil Works Administration), 96–97
    antimalaria effort, 108
    drainage project, 130
    PHS and, 104–105
    privy building, 135

Davis, Michael M.
    on CCMC, 99
    CES and, 108, 109
    on labor and PHS, 154–155
    Roosevelt and, 171
    Rosenwald Fund and, 99, 103
DDT, 169, 174
DeKruif, Paul, 88, 89, 132–134
dirt eaters
    hookworm symptoms and, 24–25, 30, 126
    See also hookworm
disability insurance
    AALL and, 47
    in Great Britain, 46
    in the United States, 145, 151, 153, 171, 187

drainage, as antimalaria measure, 62–64, 97, 104–105, 127–130
Draper, Warren
    rural sanitation program and, 80, 91–94
    United Mine Workers health fund and, 177
drought of 1930–1931, 7, 76, 92–95, 104

Ebola, 202
EIS (Epidemiological Intelligence Service), 185
Eisenhower, Dwight, 185–187
Emergency Maternity and Infant Care Program, 169
Epidemiological Intelligence Service. See EIS (Epidemiological Intelligence Service)
Evans, Walker, 126–127
Ewing, Oscar
    hospital insurance plan and, 186
    Parran and, 179–180
    Southern Democrats and, 183–184, 185
exclusion of farm workers and domestics from SSA old-age pensions, 115, 148, 162, 171
extracantonment zones, 59–61
    domestic health work during World War II, in comparison to, 159–160, 167
    malaria control in, 61–64
    Mountin and, 144, 158
    Parran and, 97
    post–World War I PHS plans and, 66, 70, 73, 75

Falk, Isidore
    on AMA endorsements of federal public health work, 111, 174–175
    CCMC and, 99, 101–102
    CES and, 106–107, 110, 111–115, 119
    hospital insurance for the elderly and, 186